Speech Development Guide for Children with Hearing Loss

Speech Development Guide for Children with Hearing Loss

Frederick S. Berg, Ph.D.

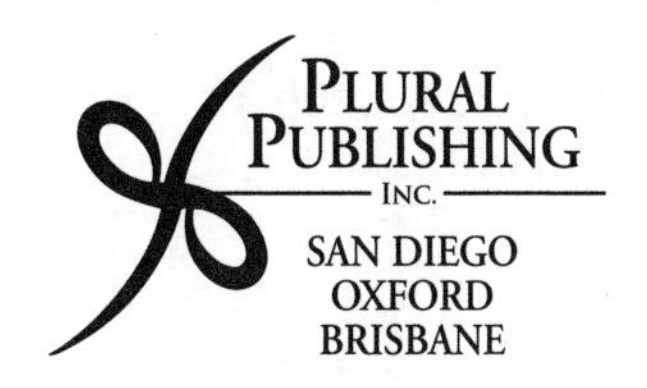

9769

KH

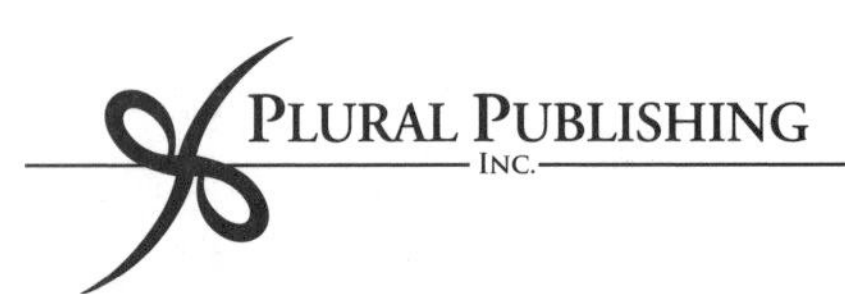

5521 Ruffin Road
San Diego, CA 92123

e-mail: info@pluralpublishing.com
Web site: http://www.pluralpublishing.com

49 Bath Street
Abingdon, Oxfordshire OX14 1EA
United Kingdom

Typeset in 11/13 Garamond by Flanagan's Publishing Services, Inc.
Printed in the United States of America by McNaughton and Gunn

Library of Congress Cataloging-in-Publication Data

Berg, Frederick S.
Speech development guide for children with hearing loss / Frederick Berg.
p. ; cm.
Includes bibliographical references and index.
ISBN-13: 978-1-59756-248-5 (alk. paper)
ISBN-10: 1-59756-248-3 (alk. paper)
1. Hearing impaired children—Language. 2. Hearing impaired children—Rehabilitation.
3. Speech therapy for children.
[DNLM: 1. Rehabilitation of Hearing Impaired. 2. Speech Therapy—methods.
3. Child. 4. Speech. WV 271 B493s 2007] I. Title.
RF291.5.C45B466 2007
617.80083–dc22

2007050048

4/3/23

Contents

Preface

I was introduced to the speech of deaf children while enrolled in a teacher training program at the Central Institute for the Deaf (CID), a private oral school, in 1950. Their speech had many errors but was somewhat intelligible because of extraordinary efforts of highly committed teachers and a speaking environment in and out of school. After graduating from the eighth grade at CID, the majority of these children graduated from regular high schools and then hearing colleges. Few elected to go to Gallaudet College, where speech is seldom used by the majority of the student body.

In 1960, I began preparing college students to teach speech to children at the Oregon School for the Deaf (OSD), a public residential facility through the 12th grade. However, most of their teachers provided little speech training, and the deaf children communicated through signs outside of classes. The speech of those children was not as intelligible as that of the deaf children at CID. When they completed school at OSD, they seldom attended regular high schools or colleges. Some attended Gallaudet College.

Since 1965, the teaching of speech in public schools for the deaf has received even less emphasis, although it has continued to be emphasized in private oral schools for the deaf. The great majority of teacher training programs for the deaf have become sign-based. Recently, however, new technologies, including cochlear implants, have overtaken deaf education. Nearly all children with permanent hearing loss are being discovered soon after birth, and the great majority of their parents are electing cochlear implants and speech training for them rather than sign language. Cochlear implant surgery restores much a deaf child's hearing. When performed on babies, whose brains are still developing, who afterwards are given listening and speech training, these children can acquire almost normal speech. Listening and speech training methodology for children with hearing loss has become more widely used in private schools and early childhood programs for the deaf since the 1970s.

During 1976 my book, *Educational Audiology: Hearing and Speech Management*, detailed new listening and speech technologies. Two years later, I also wrote the *Listening and Speech Package*, which included hundreds of data-based programs. I also developed speech technology for the Vocal Scope and a Speech Shaping Target, which greatly help in teaching and learning speech sounds.

During 1998 and 1999, my wife and I created an illustrated speech package for children with hearing loss entitled *Targeting Speech Articulation: English Version*. Copies were printed in India, where I taught speech to young children with hearing loss and assisted in the training of speech-language pathologists, audiologists, and educators of the hearing impaired for the Southern Regional Branch of the Ali Yavar Jung National Institute for the Hearing Handicapped.

During the past two years I have reorganized my previous work and added procedures and materials for this book entitled *Speech Development Guide for Children with Hearing Loss*. It includes chapters on the basics of speech acquisition, the learning of speech skills, as well as a chapter with an extensive number of speech lessons. The testing and training materials contained therein are developmentally arranged. Also, a recording system tracks incrementally accuracy and improvement in speech sound production.

This book describes and illustrates (1) speech sounds and blends and how to shape them; (2) sensory clues and aids; (3) the Speech Shaping Target; (4) a recording form for further speech development; (5) breath control, syllable, and prosodic drills; (6) additional words for speech transfer; (7) a sample lesson plan; (8) a sample progress and final report; and (9) guidelines for parents. An appendix describes the incidental learning of speech and the use of the Vocal Scope and an analog sound level meter in speech instruction.

The technologies and materials of this book should make a significant contribution to the teaching speech skills to children with hearing loss, particularly if applied early, with care, and in conjunction with incidental learning of speech and use of hand cues for acquisition of spoken language.

Many individuals have contributed to and made possible the development and publishing of this book. My wife Edna has drawn illustrations and taken photos. My daughter Karen Roylance, her husband Mark, and David Sorenson, Chris Olsen, and John Pratt have helped with digital images. Sadanand and Angie Singh and other staff of Plural Publishing have given consistent support. Other persons and organizations have contributed several figures and tables. References and a glossary are included.

1

Basics of Speech

Speech Phenomena

Speech is a highly desirable human asset. It is our main vehicle for expressing our thoughts and feelings to other people. It is a multifaceted and yet learnable system, even for children who are deaf.

The control centers of speech are in the brain. The speech act is powered by air in the lungs. The larynx (voice box) transforms the steady flow of air from the lungs into a series of puffs, which provide the source for the voiced sounds. Constrictions of the throat and mouth are sources of voiceless sounds. The closing or opening of a valve (velopharyngeal port) in the back of the mouth determines whether a sound is produced through the mouth or the nose. Each vowel and consonant of speech is a unique combination of tongue, lip, and lower jaw positioning. The pitch of the voice is determined by the tension of vocal folds in the larynx. The loudness of the voice depends on the air pressure from the lungs. The duration of each syllable of speech is determined by chest muscles (Berg, 1987).

Seven features of the speech mechanism are detailed below, some of which can be seen in Figure 1-1.

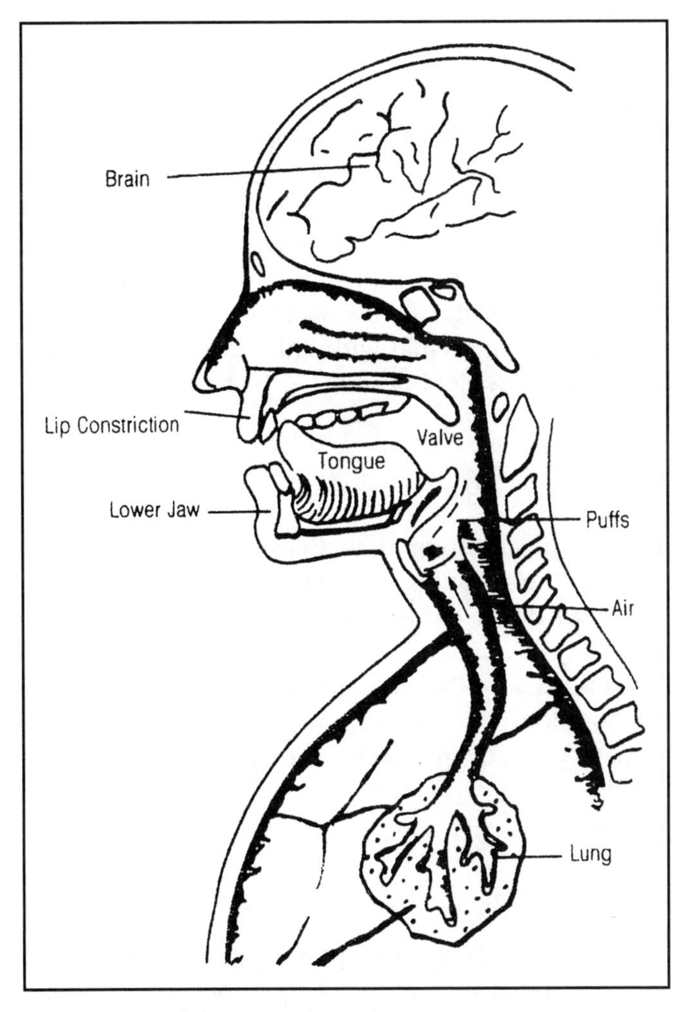

Figure 1–1. Parts and processes of the mechanism for producing speech sounds. From *Visible Speech* (p. 32), by R. Potter, G. Kopp, and H. Green, 1966, New York: Dover. Copyright 1966 by Dover. Adapted by permission.

Breath

A breath stream from the lungs powers the speech act. It sets the vocal folds into vibration for voiced sounds. It also moves through the throat and mouth, making possible the production of voiceless sounds. To speak, a person must be able to produce a steady and a pulsed (voiced) breath stream that coordinates with and supports production of other features of speech. This skill is lacking in the speech of many deaf children.

Stress

The syllables of speech are produced with varying degrees of stress. The word *Mississippi* (mɪ sɪ sɪ pɪ), for example, has most stress on the third syllable, next most on the first syllable, least on the second syllable, and next least on the last syllable. If stress patterns are not a part of speech, communication is adversely affected. A child with little or no hearing often has a problem in appropriately stressing syllables and words.

Voice

Most sounds of speech are voiced. This requires that the vocal folds of the larynx vibrate. The voice is pleasant when the vocal folds vibrate precisely. Vocal disorders occur when they are not coming together or separating on target. The quality of voice is largely determined by the precision of vocal fold vibration during speech. A child with little or no hearing often has a voice problem.

Pitch

When a speech sound is vocalized it has a pitch. The pitch of the voice is determined by the rate at which the vocal folds vibrate. While saying a sentence, a person uses a range of pitches. People have different pitches because their vocal folds vary in length. Pitch, or vibration rate, also depends upon vocal fold tension. It must be precisely adjusted or pitch will be inappropriate.

Intonation

When a polysyllabic word, phrase, or sentence is being said, the pitch of a person's voice normally changes continuously. This melody of speech is referred to as intonation. A sequence of pitch changes, called an intonation contour, extends from each fully stressed syllable, for example, the third syllable of the word *Mississippi*. Meanings are affected by changing intonation contours in sentences. Intonation is normally present in the vocalizations and speech of very young children. A child must be able to sense precise pitch differences to use normal intonation while speaking. A child with little or no hearing often has monotonous or uncontrolled intonation.

Nasality

Speech sounds naturally exit the mouth, except for the three nasal consonants /m/, /n/, and /ŋ/, which exit the nose. The positioning of the velum in the back of the mouth determines whether a speech sound is orally or nasally emitted. If the velopharyngeal port is closed, the sound comes through the mouth; if open, the sound comes through the nose. When the velum is down when it should be up, sound that should be orally emitted spills into the nose and severely disturbs speech output. The vowels tend to be blurred, and the consonants lose their precision and crispness. Knowing whether the velopharyngeal port is shut or open during speech ordinarily requires hearing. A child with a hearing loss often has speech that is too nasal.

Articulation

Speech is also characterized by the forming and joining of the tongue, lips, and lower jaw to produce vowels and consonants in syllables, words, and sentences. This articulation process is normally the last of the speech phenomena to fully mature. Many subskills have to be reached before this achievement occurs. Each vowel or consonant is a unique combination of the activity of the vocal folds, the valve in the back of the mouth, the constriction of the air stream in the mouth, and the place where articulation is occurring. Bilateral hearing loss complicates the mastery of speech sound articulation.

How We Speak

Speech planning takes place in the brain before speech production occurs in the vocal tract. In the brain, meanings or ideas are coded into language and motor correlates before motor commands can be sent to the vocal tract to cause speech movements (MacNeilage,

Studdert-Kennedy, & Lindblom, 1985). The language forms include semantic, syntactic, morphologic, and phonemic subforms. Semantic refers to the meaning of words, syntactic to sentence structure, morphologic to word structure, and phonemic to speech sound classes. We speak in a "hierarchy from phonemic feature, to phoneme, to syllable, to word, and to phrase and sentence" (Hirsh, 1985). Each phoneme produced includes several phonemic features. A feature of each vowel phoneme, for example, is absence of pressure buildup in the vocal tract, in distinction to each consonant phoneme, which has pressure buildup (Stevens, 1985). Stress and intonation features are also inherent in the syllables, words, phrases, and sentences of the speech act.

Speech can be meaningful or nonmeaningful. If meaningful, it is spoken language. If not, it is just a motor activity. In early speech development, the child babbles in nonmeaningful syllables. Later, the child speaks in words and sentences. As the child moves up the hierarchical ladder of speech from phonemes to long and complex sentences, speaking becomes more difficult. This difficulty is offset in part by hierarchical organization of speech units. Vowels, consonants, and syllables, for example, are incorporated into intonation and rhythmic patterns. Children use a self-organizing process to master the complicated interactive systems used to produce speech (Kent, 1985; Lauter, 1985).

Speech takes place over time. We speak at a rate of about 14 segments per second (MacNeilage et al., 1985). To say all possible sounds, syllables, words, and sentences intelligibly and fluently requires either preplanning (speech targets selected well in advance of speech movements), rapid sensory feedback with servo control, a cognitive schema that is highly responsive to various situational demands, or some combination of these (Bowe, 1985). There is evidence that the nerves cannot carry impulses fast enough to enable feedback to exercise moment-to-moment control over speech production. Ling (1976) has stated that feedback can only allow us to determine whether production has satisfied intention. Speech is functional when it is automatically or fluently produced. This occurs when we can concentrate on what we are saying rather than have to be concerned with how to produce speech (Stelmach & Hughes, 1985).

When people speak, they hear what they say through air conducted and bone conducted sound. They also receive tactile feedback as their articulators (lips and tongue) lightly touch other surfaces, and proprioceptive feedback as their joints, tendons, and muscles of respiration, phonation, and articulation are stimulated (Warren, 1976). Feedback loops within the brain or central nervous system also exist (Borden & Harris, 1984). Children depend on various sensory loops to learn speech, and when they cannot hear well, they can depend on a visual loop if one is made available to them (Berg, 1976).

The speaker has to breathe in a unique way while speaking. In comparison with quiet breathing, more air is inspired, and more quickly, and expiration is much longer (Lauter, 1985). A word or sentence may be produced during the expiration of one breath. The brain's control of speech respiration must be closely orchestrated with its control of speech articulation. The air pressure from the lungs must continuously change in step with each successive phoneme produced.

Air pressure from the lungs must also be sufficient to assist with phonation or voice. During each cycle of phonation (vibration), pressure forces the vocal folds in the larynx to open and move outward. The outward movement continues because of momentum but is stopped and reversed by the elastic tension of the vocal folds. As the folds move inward and approach a closed position, the Bernoulli effect (sudden pressure drop due to narrow opening between folds) causes them to close abruptly. Air pressure from the lungs and the elasticity of the closed folds cause this cycle to repeat itself (Pickett, 1980). The elasticity, tension, and mass of the folds determine the number of times this outward-inward cycle occurs per second. Adult men have the greatest vocal fold mass and therefore the lowest frequency (cycles per second) of vocal fold vibration. Adult women have less vocal fold mass, but they still have more than children, who have the highest vocal pitch. If air pressure from the lungs is increased, the folds will open wider during each vibration cycle, producing a more intense voice (Borden & Harris, 1984).

"When we generate an utterance, we attempt to control the positions and movements of the articulatory structures and the respiratory system so as to achieve certain patterns of acoustic goals or targets" (Stevens, 1985, p. 38). For an utterance to be understood by a listener, some aspects of these goals must be achieved with precision while others can be approximated. Within a speaker-listener's brain is an inventory of more acoustic features than needed to produce or perceive the sounds and words of a language. To produce or perceive "bead" and "beet," for example, the /d/ is different from the /t/ on the basis of (a) presence or absence of voicing, (b) duration of the preceding vowel, and (c) intensity or duration of the burst of noise as these words are released or terminated. Speech is also more understandable when it is slowed down, allowing the listener additional time to decode the parts of an utterance (Stevens, 1985).

Speech Perception

Children ordinarily perceive prosodic and phonetic features of the vocal tract primarily through hearing. Figure 1–2 illustrates six of these phenomena: stress, intonation, voicing, oral-nasal distinction, locality of

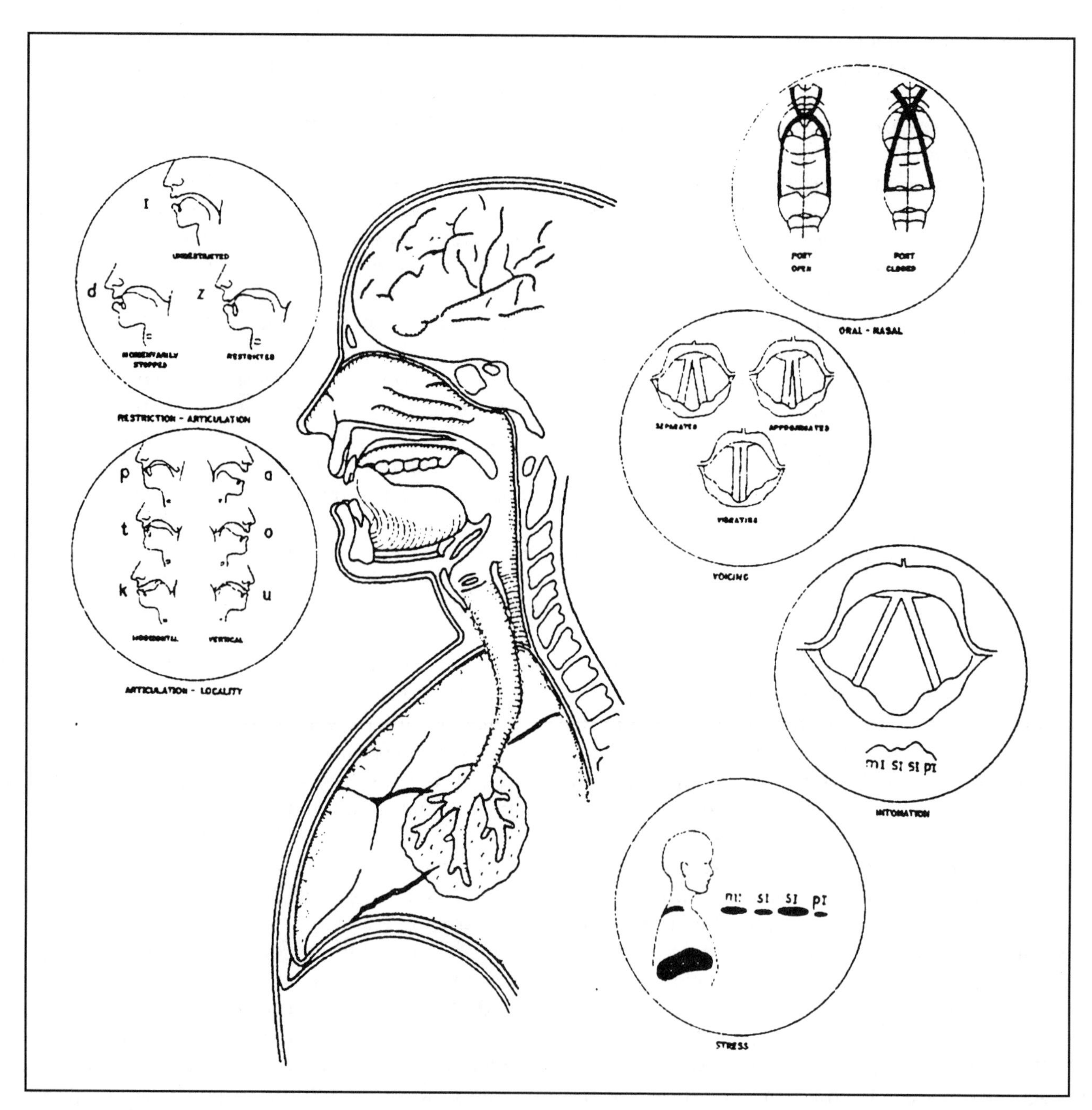

Figure 1–2. Vocal, prosodic, and articulatory features of speech within the vocal tract. From *Visible Speech* (p. 32), by R. Potter, G. Kopp, and H. Green, 1966, New York: Dover. Copyright 1966 by Dover. Adapted by permission.

articulation, and restriction of articulation. Table 1-1 compares the perception of these features by a near-deaf client through vision (lipreading or speechreading) and audition. For example, whereas two to three of four levels of stress may be perceived through audition, none of them are perceived through speechreading. This assumes that a powerful hearing aid or a cochlear implant is used by the client (Berg, 1987).

However, if the clinician uses a speech aid to display visual correlates of acoustic features of speech, the client can learn to perceive these features. Figure 1-3, for example, displays Lissajous patterns from the Vocal Scope for the author saying 36 vowels, diphthongs, and consonants into its microphone. The author trained a near-deaf college student to identify with phonetic symbols each of these visual patterns without error (Berg, 1976).

KayPENTAX manufactures a wide range of speech aids for visually displaying acoustic as well as motor features of speech production. They include real-time spectrographic, nasal, pitch, and articulation displays with hand-held microphone inputs. The Sona-Speech II unit for speech articulation is the least expensive, and incorporates a laptop computer and screen. A palatometer shows linguapalatal (tongue to palate) contact, with visual screens for therapist and child (Speech Analysis and Feedback Products, 2006).

Speechreading and Tactile Clues

Noninstrumental speech training relies on use of speechreading and tactile clues. While the therapist provides a speech model for imitation, the child looks at him or her. The child may also have his or her fingertips on the throat or nose of the therapist, or at times in front of the mouth of the therapist. The speechreading and tactile clues contribute to the perceptual pool which guides the child to a correct response.

The clues from speechreading include features of lip positioning, mouth opening, mandibular depression, and tongue positioning and contact. A different combination of these features characterizes the visual aspect of each phoneme. However, the visual differences among consonant cognates are subtle. For example, the /f/ and the /v/ look alike, except that the point of articulation of the teeth on the lower lip may be located at a slightly different spot.

The articulation information is only partially visible through speechreading. For example, the voiced-voiceless, and the oral-nasal distinctions are hidden from view. In addition, closing the teeth hides the tongue positioning information that is related to the production of many phonemes. Furthermore, it is impossible to note the glottal approximation for /h/ and difficult to see the linguavelar articulation of the /k/, /g/, and /ŋ/.

During speech modeling it is helpful to use a mirror and to employ a flashlight. Thus the child can compare his articulation of a given phoneme with that of the therapist more clearly.

As the child imitates speech, the therapist slows down the stimulus presentation. This helps the child to study the visible clues from formations and locations of articulation and to couple this information with the auditory speech clues that he or she may perceive. Furthermore, tactile speech clues provide the child with still additional perceptual information for shaping speech sounds.

Table 1–1. Possible Perception of Speech Features by a Child with a 100 dB Bilateral Loss

Speech Feature	Hearing	Lipreading
1. Stress patterns	Mainly perceived	Not perceived
2. Pitch patterns	Broad changes perceived	Not perceived
3. Voiced-voiceless	Perceived if syllable stressed	Not perceived
4. Oral-nasal	Perceived if syllable stressed	Not perceived
5. Unrestricted, restricted, or momentarily stopped	Perceived if syllable stressed	Perceived if syllable stressed
6. Tongue position primarily; lip and jaw position and other points of articulation	Mainly perceived if syllable stressed	Partially perceived if syllable stressed

Note. From *Facilitating Classroom Listening* (p. 58) by F. Berg, 1987, Boston: College-Hill Press. Copyright 1991 by PRO-ED. Reproduced by permission.

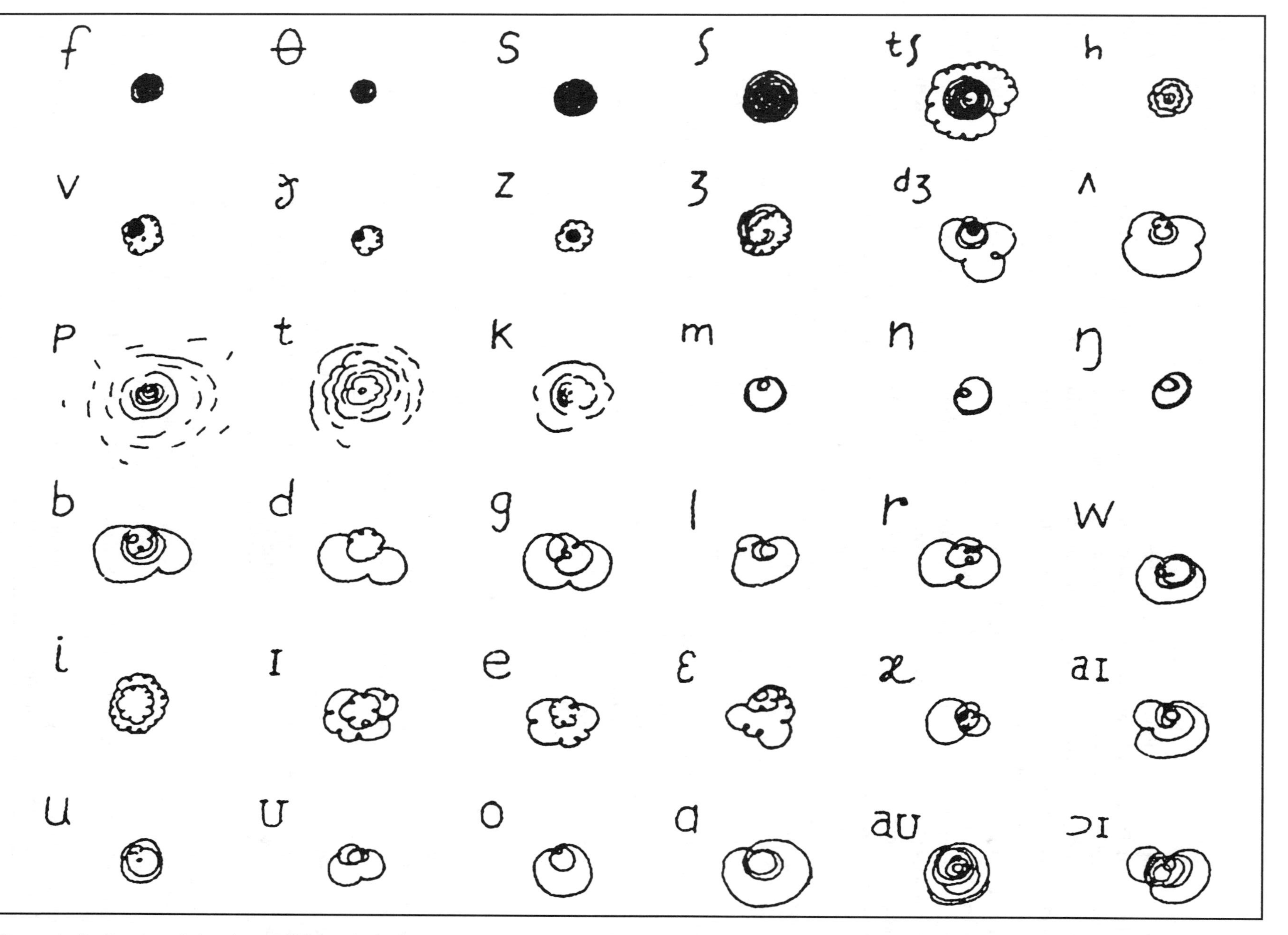

Figure 1–3. Freehand drawings of Video Articulator patterns for 36 isolated phonemes articulated by the author. From *Educational Audiology: Hearing and Speech Management* (p. 198), by F. Berg, 1976, New York and London: Grune & Stratton. Copyright 1976 by Grune & Stratton. Reproduced by permission.

The tactile speech clues include vibration from the throat to indicate voicing and vibration from the nose to indicate nasal production. Air flow or expulsion from the mouth indicates a voiceless sound, and its amount and location even reveal production of a specific phoneme. Mandibular position, movement, and tension reveal information relevant to the production of specific phonemes, for example, /i/ versus /e/.

Although tactile clues assist the child in imitating the therapist, their use is largely restricted to the initial shaping of phonemes and core words. Thereafter, taction is phased out because it is cumbersome and tiring for the child to place his or her hand on the throat or nose of the therapist. Also tactile information is often less refined than other sensory input. A child may tend to develop laryngeal tension with resultant voice disorder if the therapist is not cautious and conservative in utilizing tactile speech clues.

In short, tactile speech clues are valuable in the initial shaping of phonemes and core words, when the child needs as much information as possible about the vocal tract phenomena of voicing, velopharyngeal (valve) posture, restriction, and locality of articulation. However, they need not be used when sufficient perceptual information is available from audition and speechreading, and when articulations are shaped so that habit patterns are established. By this time the clinician can utilize notations or can even point to specific anatomic locations to signal that a particular vocal tract phenomenon is being omitted or should be included (Berg, 1976; Berg, 1987).

Electro-Visual Speech Clues

The author has made extensive use of Lissajous patterns from a Vocal Scope to supplement speechreading and tactile speech clues for shaping phonemes that cannot be fully heard. As speech is said precisely within 2 inches of its microphone, the visual display is shown as a different unique pattern for each phoneme. For a voiceless sound, for example the /s/ in Figure 1–4, each person saying it will produce the same Lissajous pattern for that sound. For a voiced sound, each person saying it will produce a similar Lissajous pattern.

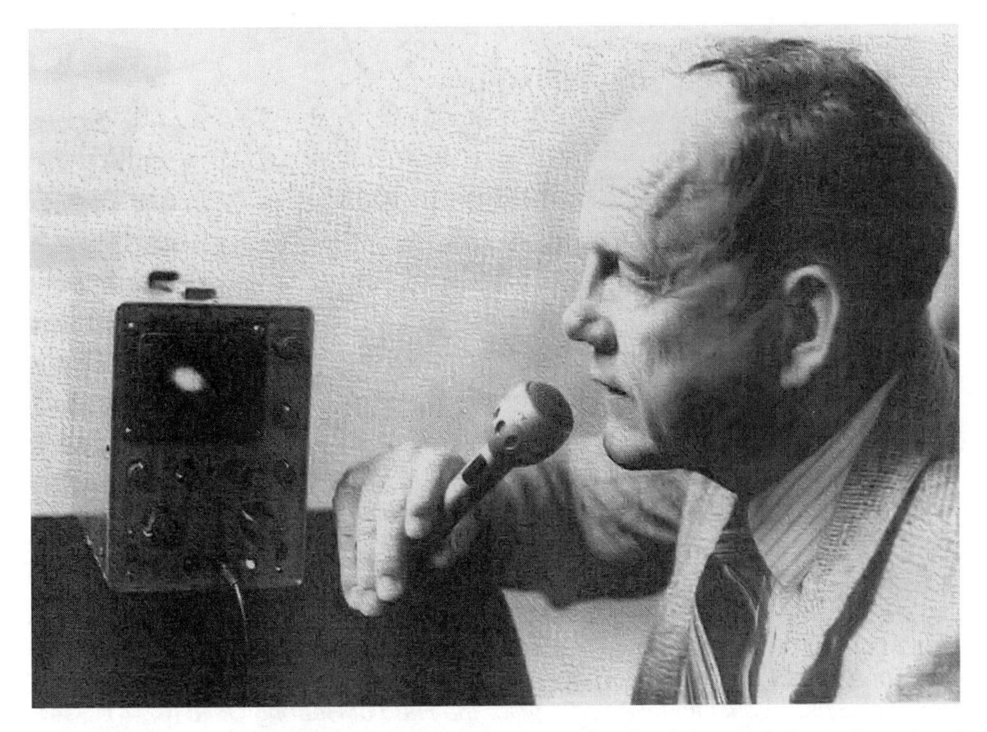

Figure 1–4. Vocal Scope with Lissajous pattern for the /s/ sound. Compliments of Amera Incorporated, Logan, Utah.

When a child produces a response that is desirable, the corresponding Lissajous pattern becomes the model to duplicate (Berg, 1976).

The author used these electro-visual clues in combination with speechreading and tactile clues to shape the articulation of a 10-year-old boy who could not hear. After 10 training sessions, the child greatly improved accuracy of articulation of 36 vowel, diphthong, and consonant targets in error. Figure 1-5 shows baseline versus final measurements of accuracy (Berg, 1976).

The author also found Lissajous clues very helpful in shaping vowel, diphthong, and consonants sounds of deaf and severely hard of hearing preschoolers he taught (Berg, 2000). He also recommends their use in articulation training provided for children with nor-

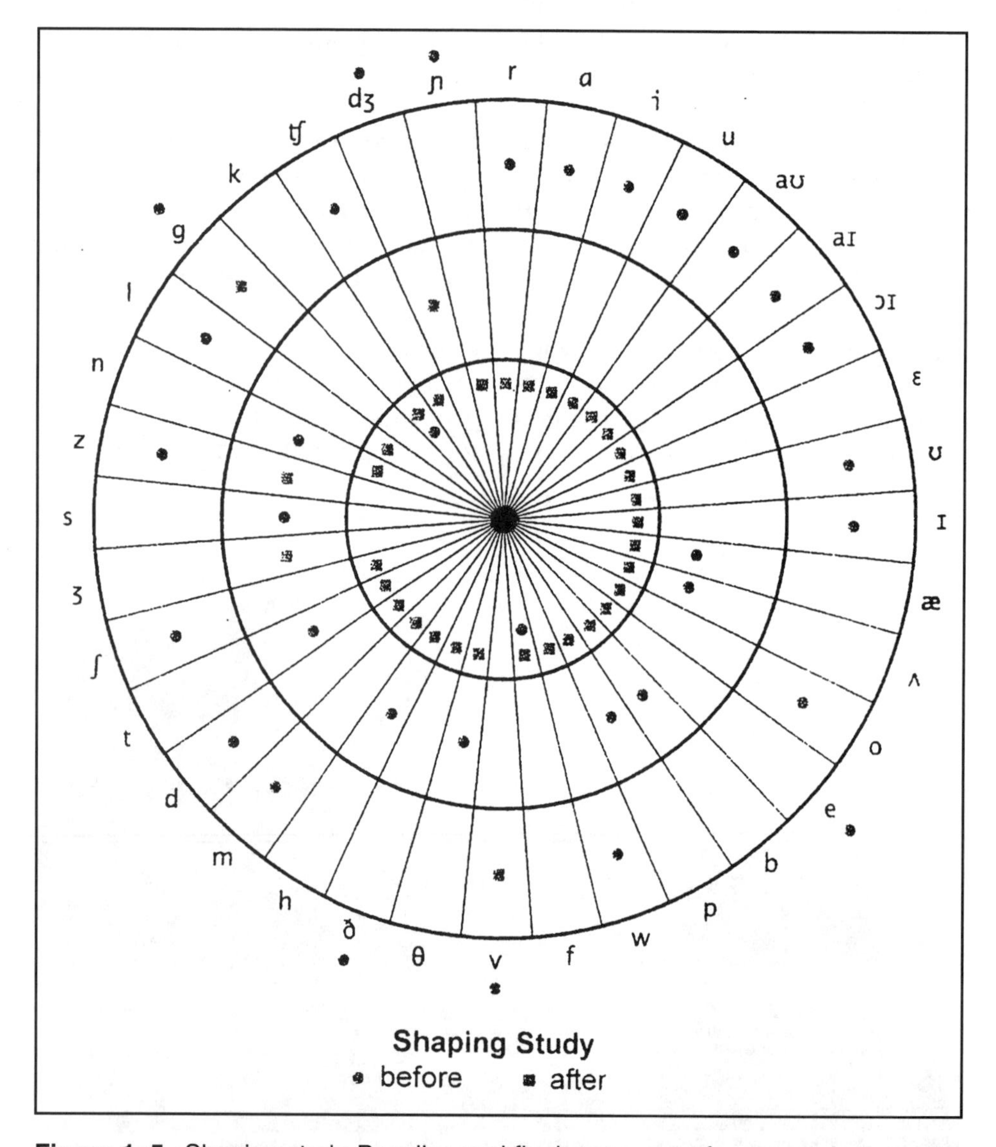

Figure 1–5. Shaping study. Baseline and final measures of accuracy in the articulation of 36 vowels, diphthongs, and consonants by a deaf child. From "Listening and Speech Skills," by F. Berg, 1986. In F. Berg, J. Blair, S. Viehweg, and A. Wilson-Vlotman (Eds.), *Educational Audiology for the Hard of Hearing Child* (p. 147). New York and London: Grune & Stratton. Copyright 1978 by Grune & Stratton. Reproduced by permission.

mal hearing. The Lissajous patterns motivate a child to attend to a speech stimulus and clarify the child's perception of it.

A predecessor of the Vocal Scope was a Lissajous device described by Pronovost,Yenkin, Anderson, & Lerner (1968) called the Voice Visualizer. As seen in Figure 1-6, it clearly showed the articulatory distinction between the sibilant voiceless and voiced cognates /s/ and /z/. The /s/ pattern includes many juxtaposed circles. The /z/ pattern has a similar circular display but also evidence of vocal fold vibration.

The Lissajous display provides electro-visual feedback on all acoustic features of speech. The basic Lissajous pattern is a single circle for a pure tone. The Lissajous patterns for speech sounds, each of which includes a different combination of many pure tones, result in various combinations of many circles.

Auditory, Speechreading, and Hand Clues

Auditory clues, even when combined with speechreading clues, do not ordinarily enable deaf children to learn to fully perceive the phonemes of speech with the use of hearing aids or cochlear implants. For example, in a sensory aids study conducted at the Central Institute for the Deaf, only 5 of 52 deaf children were able to identify words in open sets after 3 years of intense auditory and speech training. Four of the 5 were among 13 children who used cochlear implants (Geers & Moog, 1994).

If a deaf child cannot recognize each phoneme when using a hearing aid or a cochlear implant, he or she can learn to recognize them visually from hand clues in addition to speechreading clues. The 8 hand shapes and 4 hand placements, combined with speechreading clues, called cued Speech (CS), open the door to early spoken language development, in contrast to much slower spoken language development achieved through auditory, or combined auditory-speechreading, training for deaf children (Berg, 2001).

Hand shapes and locations for all phonemes are shown in Figure 1-7. The consonants are indicated by the shapes, and the vowels and diphthongs by the locations. Either the right hand or the left hand or both can be used. The back of the hand faces the child. The arm is held upright with the elbow at the side. Once a parent or other family member learns to add all these hand cues to speechreading cues (clues), the child can

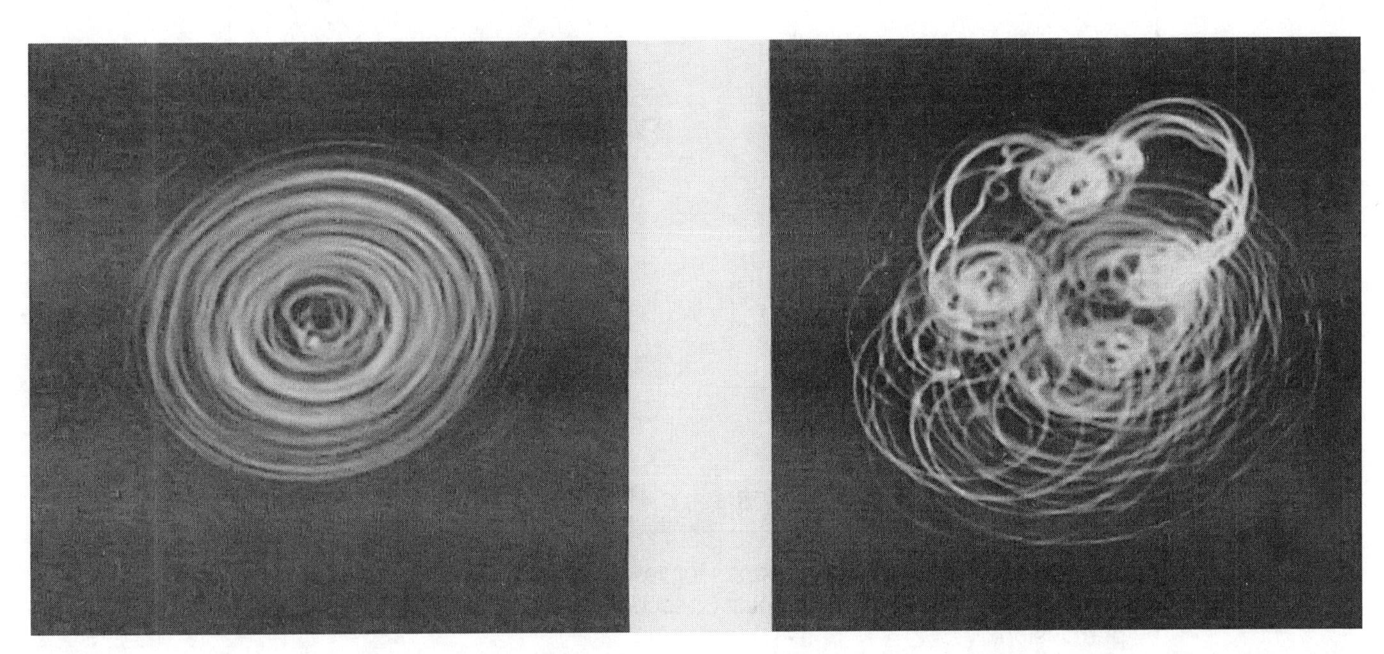

Figure 1–6. Lissajous patterns for the cognates /z/ (right) and /s/ left. From "The Voice Visualizer," by W. Pronovost, L. Yenkin, D. Anderson, and R. Lerner, 1968, *American Annals of the Deaf, 113*(2), pp. 230–238. Reproduced by permission.

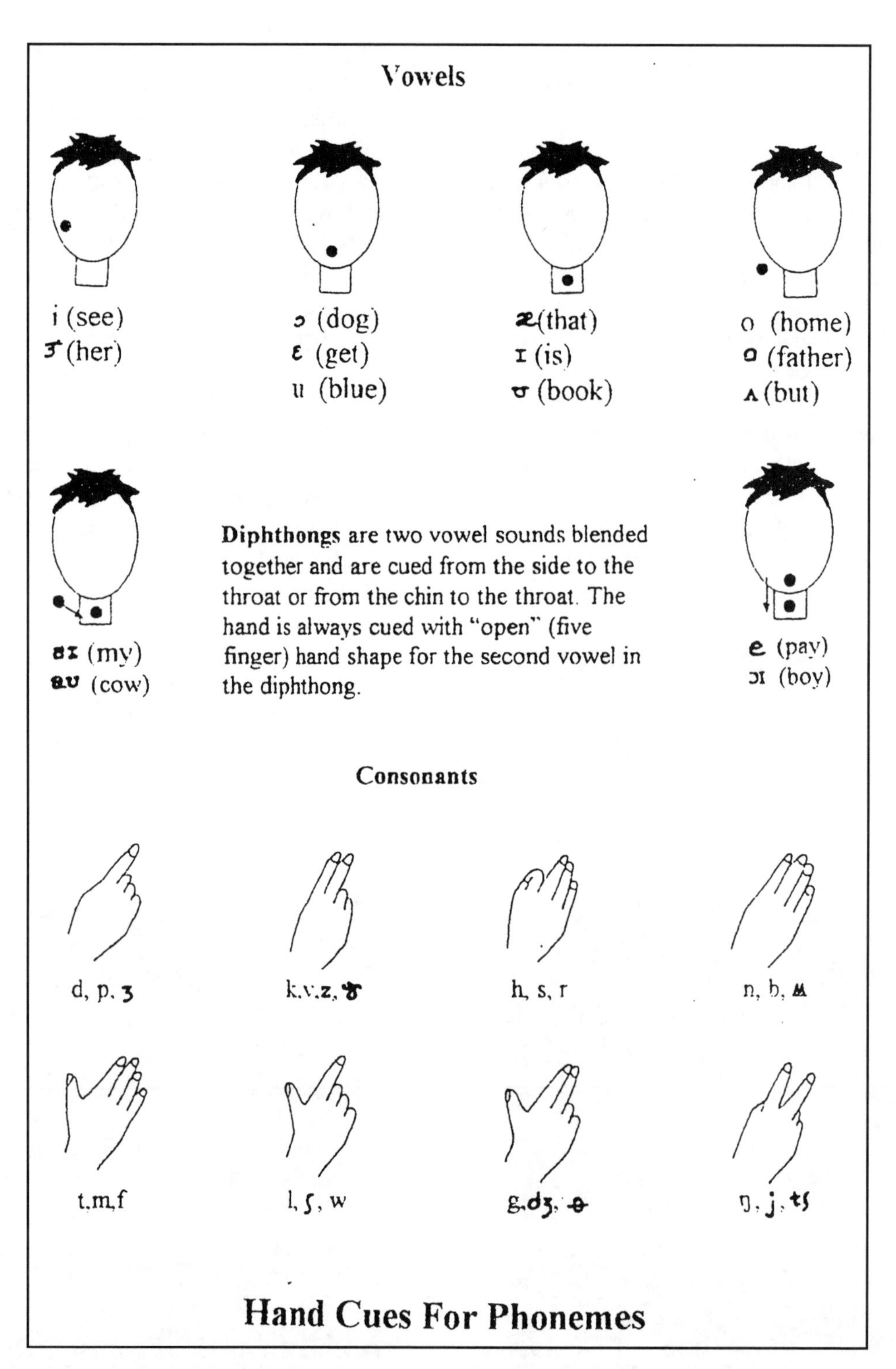

Figure 1–7. Hand positions and shapes for vowels, diphthongs, and consonants of cued Speech. Modified from West Coast Speech Programs by J. Rupert. Reproduced by permission.

begin learning to perceive the vocabulary of spoken language. With repeated exposure, the child will learn to perceive the thousands of words and multitude of sentences of spoken English.

Mastering the basics of CS requires up to a week of training provided through a CS workshop or videocassette. Three preliminary goals are to learn: (a) phonemes of words, (b) speechreading clues (cues), and (c) hand cues (clues) and (d) how to combine them in the syllables of speech.

To say the syllable /pi/, for example, the speaker includes the lip shut and forefinger cues for the /p/, and the lip spread and mouth corner cues for the /i/. This is done easily by placing the tip of the forefinger next to the corner of the mouth at the same time the /pi/ is said. Refer to Figure 1-7.

In 1966 Orin Cornett invented CS. Soon afterwards he taught it to a mother of a young deaf child. The mother's name was Marie Elsie Henegar (now Daisey). The child's name was Leah. She was 2½ years old and had no spoken language vocabulary. Marie quickly learned the additional cues and began using them as she spoke to Leah. A year later Leah could recognize 450 words spoken by her mother. She also learned to speak. At age 6 she started the first grade with normal hearing children. She is now a highly literate and educated adult (Cornett & Daisey, 1992).

Children taught CS also have a head start in learning to speak. The spoken language they have already learned helps them follow speech training directions. They also already recognize phonemes and know the meaning of many words and sentences. They also perceive the order and number of phonemes in words, and several prosodic features of speech (Berg, 2000; Berlin, 1995).

A child with a hearing loss can learn spoken language and speech more rapidly if the child's family will begin cueing to the child during the time the child's speech normally develops. A case in point is Courtney Branscombe. By age 2 this deaf girl could not only understand language through CS but also express it. A speech therapist learned CS to help her do this. Courtney could cue the names of the Sesame Street characters on TV. Also, she could articulate sounds well enough for her mother to understand her. For example, her mother picked her up at a friend's house and Courtney pointed out their TV set and said, "No pooh bear." She then smiled and said, "Pooh Bear at home" (Cornett & Daisey, 1992).

Literacy and Speech

A deaf or hard of hearing child can learn speech and spoken language best during the preschool years. This can be done through a combination of Cued Speech and speech instruction that enables the child to perceive the acoustic features of vowels, consonants, words, phrases, and sentences, or their visual correlates.

The normal child knows the spoken language well before he or she starts to learn to read. Not only is it the language on which reading is based, it is the language in which everything is taught at school. Without a solid prior knowledge of this language, the typical prelingual deaf child is doomed to slow, laborious learning (Cornett & Daisey, 1992).

The normal child also develops speech at the same time he or she acquires a native language. During the 1950s Mildred Templin of the University of Minnesota studied the development of speech sounds among 480 children from 3 to 8 years of age. She published her findings (see Table 1-2) and then collaborated with Fred Darley of the University of Iowa to develop a standardized speech articulation test based upon these data (Berg, 1970; Berg, 1976; Templin, 1957; Templin & Darley, 1960).

Afterwards, Berg (1970, 1976) recorded the speech and language development of his son Sven during the first 5 years of his life. Table 1-3 includes a sample of words uttered by Sven that reveals he had learned to articulate most phonemes during the first 3 years of life (Berg, 1970, 1976).

By 12 months of age a child normally vocalizes, repeats syllables, and says a few words. At age 3 years, the child normally understands and says a great many words and sentences, including all the vowels and diphthongs and most of the consonants. During the remainder of the preschool years, the child masters additional consonants and many word-initial and word-final blends. These are incorporated in an expanding vocabulary and sentence structure, such as Sven's further language growth shown in Table 1-4. This provides the child with sufficient speech and spoken language for learning the basics of reading and writing.

The relationship between early language development and school success for a deaf child is illustrated by the life of Dorothy Jane Crosby. Her parents learned

Table 1–2. Earliest Age at Which 75 Percent of All Subjects Produced Each of 176 Test Sound Elements Correctly

CA	Sound Elements
3	Vowels: e, i, e, a, o, u, o, o͝o, o͞o, ō, ô, ȧ, ûr Dipthongs: u, a, i, ou, oi Consonants: m-, -m-, -m, n-, -n, -ng-, -ng, p-, -p-, -p, t-, -t, k-, -k-, b-, -b-, d-, -d-, g-, -g-, f-, -f-, -f, h-, -h-, w-, -w- Double-consonant blends: -ngk
3.5	Consonants: -s-, -z-, -r, y-, -y- Double-consonant blends: -rk, -ks, -mp, -pt, -rm, -mr, -nr, -pr, -kr, -br, -dr, -gr, -sm
4	Consonants: -k, -b, -d, -g, s-, sh-, -sh, -v-, j-, r-, -r-, l-, -l- Double-consonant blends: pl-, -pr, tr-, tw-, kl-, kr-, kw-, bl-, br-, dr-, gl-, sk-, sm-, sn-, sp-, st-, -lp, -rt, -ft, -lt, -fr Triple-consonant blends: -mpt, -mps
4.5	Consonants: -s, -sh-, ch-, -ch-, -ch Double-consonant blends: gr-, fr-, -lf
5	Consonants: -j- Double-consonant blends: fl-, -rp, -lb, -rd, -rf, -rn, -shr Triple-consonant blends: str-, -mbr
6	Consonants: -t-, th-, -th-, -th, v-, -v, th-, -l Double-consonant blends: -lk, -rb, -rg, -rth, -nt, -nd, -pl, -kl, -bl, -gl, -fl, -sl Triple-consonant blends: skw-, -str, -rst, -ngkl, -nggl, -rj, -ntth, -rch
7	Consonants: -th-, z-, -z, -th, -zh-, -zh, -j Double-consonant blends: thr-, shr-, sl-, sw-, -lz, -zm, -lth, -sk, -st Triple-consonant blends: skr-, spl-, spr-, -skr, -kst, -jd
8	Double-consonant blends: -kt, -tr, -sp

*hw-, -hw-, -lfth, and -tl are not produced correctly by 75% of the subjects by eight years of age. Templin, 1957, p. 51.

Note. From "Certain Language Skills in Children," by M. Templin, 1957, *Institute of Child Welfare Monograph No. 26* (p. 51), Minneapolis: University of Minnesota Press. Reproduced by permission.

she was deaf when she was 2 years of age. They learned signs with her, and then CS, which enabled her to begin learning spoken language. First came receptive language, and when she started learning expressive language, it came so fast her father called it a rocket ride. At age 10.75 Dorothy Jane read better than 95% of the children her age (Cornett & Daisey, 1992).

Beck (1999) has summarized group research studies supporting CS. One study showed that 30 deaf children who used CS scored as well in reading as a matched group of 30 hearing students. Another study showed that deaf children exposed to CS scored higher on language structure than 92% of hearing-impaired children generally. Still another study showed that using CS improved speechreading.

In the early 1970s, a National Cued Speech Center was established at Gallaudet College, providing CS workshops for families of deaf children. Edward C.

Table 1–3. Speech Responses and Emerging Phonemes of Sven during the 1st, 2nd, and 3rd Years of Life.

Year	Response	New Phoneme
1	dædæ, mamə, baʊwʊu, haɪ, helo, kʊkɪ	/d/, /æ/, /m/, /a/, /ə/, /b/, /w/, /aʊ/, /h/, /aʊ/, /ɛ/, /o/, /k/, /ʊ/
2	go, no, ɪə (ear), mgoaʊt foə (for), bip	/g/, /n/, /ɪ/, /ə/, /t/, /f/, /i/, /p/
3	jɛwo (yellow), wet (late), tu, bæŋ, ju fid, bɔɪ	/j/, /e/, /u/, /ŋ/, /ju/, /aɪ/

Note. From *The Hard of Hearing Child: Clinical and Educational Management*, by F. Berg, 1970, New York and London: Grune & Stratton. Copyright by Grune & Stratton. Reproduced by permission.

Table 1–4. Sentences Said by Sven While 36 to 54 Months of Age

Month	Remarks
36	I am not going home because I am going to New York City with Louis Nils Berg.
48	I looked in the microscope and Glenn has chicken pox all over him.
54	My tummy hurts so much it's going to cry its heart out.
56	He's a house hopper. If he was on the pavement, he'd be called a pavement hopper. If he was on the grass, he'd be called a grasshopper like he usually is.
56	I'm so irritated, I'm just frustrated. It astonishes me.
57	I'd like to have an electric motor to widen my shoe when I put my foot into it.
60	When I push the button, I'll go up to the top of the house, or to outer space, or to the top of outer space.
61	I made a rule for myself. When I'm watching TV, do not leave until the program is over. This is the first rule I've made.
62	I lost my mind on projects. I'm not wanting any more projects. My mind is off from the projects. Maybe I'll have some after I see the World's Fair.
64	Well, breakfast is when you wake up, and dinner is before you go to bed, and lunch is in the middle of the afternoon. Lunch is between morning and afternoon.

Note. From *The Hard of Hearing Child: Clinical and Educational Management*, by F. Berg, 1970, New York and London: Grune & Stratton. Copyright 1970 by Grune & Stratton. Reproduced by permission.

Merrill was then the president of Gallaudet and gave the center strong support. In 1995, T. King Jordan, who had become president of Gallaudet College, closed the center (Beck, 1999).

In retirement, Merrill stated that after 20 years, substantial data on cued Speech showed that through it deaf children attained competency in English at the level of hearing students, grade by grade, and that no other system had enabled this to happen (Merrill, 1992). Recently CS has come to be used by families of deaf children in more than 60 languages and spread to every continent in the world.

CS continues to grow in numbers of users and numbers of influential advocates. Among these is

Charles Berlin, a widely known audiologist, who has stated that CS prepares a child for English language comprehension and reading in a most efficient and useful way, independent of amplification success or failure (Berlin, 1995).

During 2006 the National Cued Speech Association (NCSA) held a 40th anniversary conference. Attendees from countries outside the United States met with local representatives to establish a World Cueing Alliance (World Cueing Alliance, 2007).

2

Learning Speech Skills

The learning of speech skills by a young child with hearing loss may be classified into three overlapping tasks:

1. Articulation—learning to say each speech sound and each word-initial and word-final blend.
2. Voice control—learning to sustain breath during speech.
3. Prosody—learning to incorporate stress and intonation patterns in speech.

Learning speech skills occurs naturally as a part of spoken language development. It begins to take place after a young child is fit with a hearing aid or cochlear implant. This incidental learning of speech is described in Appendix A.

Speech Shaping Target

Speech skills are further learned through structured speech training described in this guidebook. An initial training tool the author has developed is the Speech Shaping Target and Recording Form of Figure 2-1 (Berg, 1976; Berg & Berg, 1999). It documents improvement in the child's ability to shape the vowels, diphthongs, and consonants of the English language. These speech sounds and related acoustic and physiologic features are summarized in Table 2-1. L, M, and H = low, mid, and high speech frequencies, Rnd = round lips, Squ = square lips, Ns = noiselike, Bz = buzz or vibration of the lower lip or tongue, Stp = stop, Hgh = high tongue, Fnt = front of mouth, + = present, and – = absent.

Voiced sounds are indicated by pluses. Their vocal fold vibration may be felt by placing the tips of the thumb and forefinger on the throat in the vicinity of the thyroid cartilage. Voiceless sounds are indicated by minuses. Nasal sounds are indicated by pluses. Their nasal production may be felt by placing the tips of the thumb and forefinger on the sides of the bridge of the nose near the corners of the eyes. The other sounds are oral as indicated by minuses.

The child's audiograms for the two ears indicate the extent to which he or she may hear low, mid, and high speech frequencies when wearing a hearing aid. Many children with hearing loss use cochlear implants, permitting them to hear within low, mid, and high frequency ranges. However, this does not ensure they can discriminate completely between speech sounds with similar frequencies within these ranges. A cochlear implant provides frequency discrimination in that it has 22 or 24 frequency channels, whereas a normal cochlea has thousands of hair cells, allowing more refined speech frequency discrimination.

A deaf child can learn, however, to differentiate all speech sounds. One way is through their Lissajous patterns, which are visual correlates of sounds. The other way is through combinations of hand and speech-reading clues. Speechreading clues alone cannot help the child do this because (a) speech articulation is largely hidden from view and (b) most speech sound articulations look almost exactly like other speech sound articulations to the speechreader.

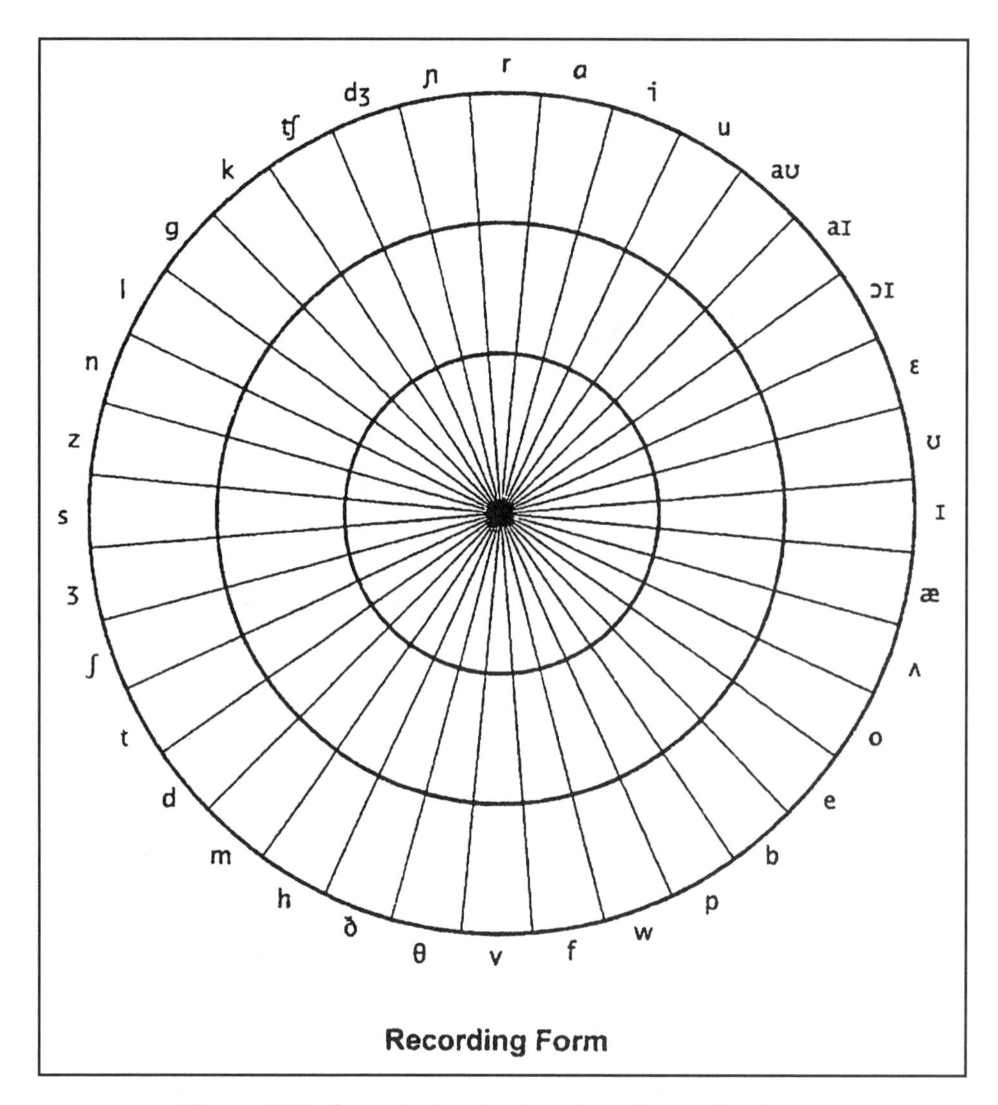

Figure 2–1. Speech shaping target and recording form.

The International Phonetic Alphabet (IPA) symbols for all these sounds encircle the Speech Shaping Target and Recording Form. They are placed clockwise, beginning with /ɑ/ at the top of the target. The symbol for next sound is /i/ as in the word *bee*, and for the last sound is /r/ as in the word *rate*. The symbols encircle the target in the general order in which speech sounds develop in normal speech.

The target is divided into 36 sectors, one for each vowel, diphthong, or consonant. During a lesson, go through all of these sounds with the child in about 5 minutes. Start with the /ɑ/. Instruct the child to say it after you. Say it, and then look at and listen to the child as he or she says it.

Mark a dot in the sector of the circle for the /ɑ/. For a precise articulation mark the dot in the center of the center circle (bull's-eye). For a mild distortion, mark the dot in the inner ring. For a severe distortion, mark the dot in the outer ring. For a gross distortion, or a substitution with another sound, mark a dot outside the target. Follow the same procedure for /i/ and each succeeding sound. During this process, provide the child with all helpful sensory clues: auditory, tactile, and visual.

A speech therapist will find that his or her speech sound articulations and associated speechreading and tactile clues can be useful models for most phonemes when the goal is to move a production onto target.

Table 2–1. Speech Features for Each of 36 Vowels, Diphthongs, and Consonants

Sound	Word	Voiced	Nasal	Freq	Rnd	Squ	Ns	Bz	Stp	Hgh	Fnt
1. ɑ	arch	+	–	L-M	–					–	–
2. i	bee	+	–	L-H	–					+	+
3. u	moon	+	–	L	+					+	–
4. aʊ	house	+	–	L-M	–+					–+	–
5. aɪ	bike	+	–	L-H	–					–+	–+
6. ɔɪ	boy	+	–	L-H	+–					–+	–+
7. ɛ	jet	+	–	L-H	–					+	+
8. ʊ	hook	+	–	L-M	+					+	–
9. ɪ	fish	+	–	L-H	–					+	+
10. æ	man	+	–	L-M	–					–	+
11. ʌ	bus	+	–	L-M	–					–	
12. o	bow	+	–	L-M	+					+	–
13. e	baby	+	–	L-H	–					+	+
14. b	bat	+	–	L-M	–				+		
15. p	push	–	–	L	–				+		
16. w	walk	+	–	L	+					+	–
17. f	foot	–	–	H	–		+				
18. v	van	+	–	L-H	–		+	+			
19. θ	thumb	–	–	H	–		+				
20. ð	these	+	–	L-H	–		+	+			
21. h	hike	–	–				+				
22. m	moth	+	+	L	–						
23. d	dive	+	–	L-M	–				+	+	+
24. t	top	–	–	L-M	–				+	+	+
25. ʃ	shine	–	–	M-H		+	+			+	+
26. ʒ	mirage	+	–	M-H		+	+	+		+	+
27. s	soap	–	–	H	–		+			+	+
28. z	zipper	+	–	L-H	–		+	+		+	+
29. n	nose	+	+	L	–					+	+
30. l	leg	+	–	L-H	–					+	+
31. g	gun	+	–	L-H	–				+	+	–
32. k	cow	–	–	L-H	–				+	+	–
33. tʃ	chick	–	–	L-H		+	+		+	+	+
34. dʒ	jar	+	–	L-H		+	+		+	+	+
35. ŋ	king	+	+	L	–					+	–
36. r	rate	+	–	L-M		+				+	+

The auditory speech clues may assist in refining speech into the outer ring of the target, and even the inner ring. Lissajous clues will help the child produce bull's-eye speech responses.

When Lissajous patterns are unavailable, use an analog sound level meter with a needle indicator and fast response setting to indicate a fewer number of electrovisual clues (see Figure 2–2A and Figure 2–2B). Also, use a paper strip held in front of the mouth to provide breath clues of consonants, especially voiceless ones (see Figure 2–2C). In addition, use a flashlight to highlight mouth openings and shapes and visible tongue elevations.

Syllable Practice

Once a deaf child can say a vowel, diphthong, or consonant in isolation, teach him or her to say it in syllables, using voice control and correct stress and intonation. Each lesson of the next chapter includes syllable drill or prosodic drill that incorporates these tasks. They prepare the child to fluently and automatically say the syllables of thousands of words and sentences.

There are vowel (V), vowel-consonant (VC), CV, CVC, CCV, CCCV, VC, VCC, and VCCC syllables. For example, the words *moon* and *ball* are CVC syllables, and the words *tree* and *ask* are CCV and VCC syllables, respectively.

Use three types of syllable drills: (a) sustaining a syllable, e.g., /bɑ-----/; (b) repeating a syllable, e.g., /bɑbɑbɑ/, and (c) alternating between two or more syllables, e.g., the four syllables of the word *Mississippi* (mɪ sɪ sɪ pɪ).

Teach the child to repeat syllables at different rates: e.g., five times a second, four times a second, and three times a second, each on a breath or all on one breath separated by pauses. These rates are clarified below.

fi fi fi fi fi (5/second) fi fi fi fi (4/ second)
fi fi fi (3/second)

Teach the child to (a) repeat sequences of syllables, e.g., fa fa fa, fi fi fi, fu fu fu, fe fe fe, fo fo fo, and to (b) alternate these syllables with other syllables, e.g., fali falo falu fale fami famo famu fame, fili filo file fimi fimo fimu fime, lifa lofa lufa lefa, mifa mofa mufa mefa—which lead to such words as *fall*, *flow*, *feel*, *leaf*, and *loaf*.

Teach the child to use correct stress patterns when saying syllables of a word or a sentence. For example, if saying the word *Mississippi*, give primary accent to the third syllable and secondary accent to the first syllable. The second and fourth syllables are unaccented.

When a syllable is stressed, which is primarily lengthening its duration and secondarily increasing its intensity, the pitch of the syllable rises. Thus, the intonation contour naturally follows the stress pattern, and need not be taught separately.

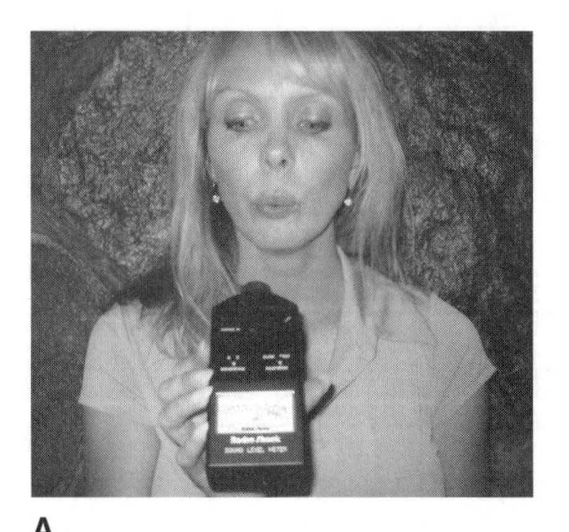
A

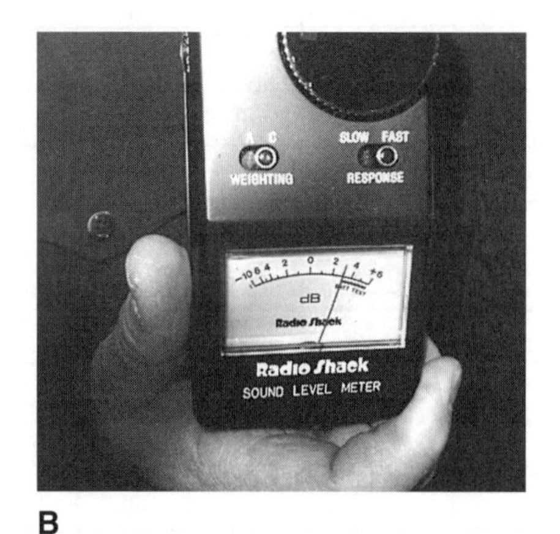

B

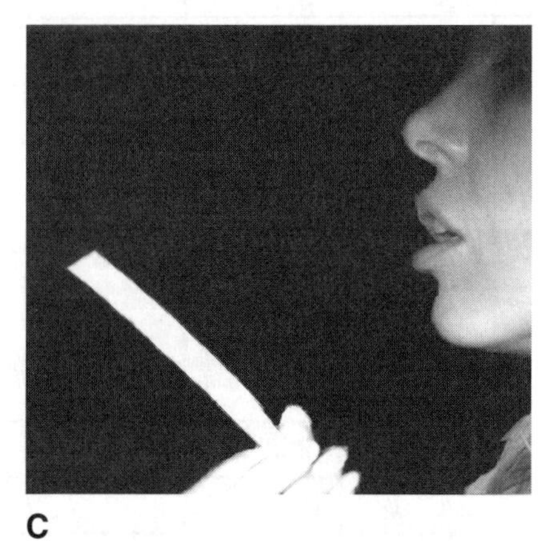
C

Figure 2–2. Speech shaping aids. **A.** Radio Shack sound level meter used in conjunction with the articulation of the /u/ sound. **B.** Close-up of sound level meter reading. **C.** Paper strip movement in conjunction with the articulation of the /ʃ/sound.

Word and Sentence Transfer

Once a deaf child can say a vowel, diphthong, or consonant in isolation, and incorporate it into syllables, teach him or her to transfer this speech skill into words and sentences. Also teach the child to transfer his or her skill in saying simple consonants to saying consonant blends and syllables, words, and sentences incorporating them.

In each lesson a picture, a printed word, and an incomplete sentence serve as stimuli for transferring a speech skill. In each lesson additional printed words serve as stimuli for further transfer of that speech skill as well as for testing for generalization of it.

A Word Test Form (see Table 2-2) is used to keep track of progress in speech development. It includes (a) IPA symbols for each of 117 speech sounds and blends, (b) a printed word for each of these, and (c) a space for recording a child's accuracy in saying each speech sound and blend. The marking key is: 1 = precise articulation, 2 = mild distortion, 3 = severe distortion, and 4 = gross distortion or substitution of another sound. This applies only to the target sound or consonant blend of each word. It should not be affected by how well the child articulates other sounds in the word.

Chapter 3 of this guidebook includes lessons for assisting a deaf or hard of hearing child to learn to articulate, and use in everyday speech, each of 117 speech sounds and word-initial and word-final consonant blends. Each lesson includes the following:

1. The IPA symbol(s) for the speech sound or consonant blend to be taught.
2. One or more side view drawings of how the sound or blend is made.
3. One or more front view photographs of a speaker saying the sound or blend.
4. A printed description of the sound or blend, and how to teach it.
5. A breath control and syllable drill or prosodic drill for the sound or blend.
6. A picture of a word that includes the sound or blend.
7. The printed form of that word.
8. A sentence to repeat and complete with the word.
9. Additional words that include the sound or blend.

Lesson Planning

Speech training will be more effective if planned. Goals should be set, materials compiled, procedures outlined, and results recorded. A lesson plan should not be set in concrete. A child should be encouraged to progress as rapidly as possible. No limit should be placed on him or her. A sample lesson plan is outlined below.

Lesson Plan

Child: Michael Johnson *Date:* April 30, 2007

Goals:
1. Say each speech sound in isolation.
2. Say /f-/ in prosodic drills.
3. Transfer /f/ in the word *fish* to additional words and sentences.

Materials: 1. Copy of Speech Shaping Target and Recording Form, 2. Lesson #21, 3. Colored pencils

Procedure	***Result***
1. Help Michael say 36 speech sounds in isolation. Compare dots to yesterday's (different colored) dots.	Slight improvement—3 minutes
2. Combine /f/ with /ɪ/ in prosodic drills, with stress on various /fɪ/ syllables. Compare with yesterday.	Learned to do—3 minutes
3. Say /f/ in picture word and complete sentence.	Learned to do—2 minutes
4. Say /f/ with other vowels in 11 additional words.	Learned to do—2 minutes
5. Say /f/ in three original words and sentences. *Tiffany* (sister), *fun*, *funny*. *Tiffany is fun. Tiffany is funny.*	Rewarding to him!—2 minutes

Progress Reports

Progress reports on the child's training should be kept. A progress report includes what has been accomplished since the beginning of training or since the last progress

Table 2–2. Recording Form for Speech Development

1. ɑ ___ car
2. i ___ key
3. u ___ shoe
4. aʊ ___ house
5. aɪ ___ bike
6. ɔ ___ ball
7. ɔɪ ___ boy
8. ɛ ___ egg
9. ʊ ___ foot
10. ɪ ___ fish
11. æ ___ cap
12. ʌ ___ cup
13. o ___ rope
14. e ___ gate
15. b- ___ bat
16. –b ___ rib
17. p- ___ pen
18. –p ___ rope
19. w- ___ wire
20. ʍ- ___ wheel
21. f- ___ fish
22. –f ___ knife
23. v- ___ vase
24. –v ___ glove
25. θ- ___ thumb
26. –θ ___ teeth
27. ð- ___ there
28. –ð ___ bathe
29. h- ___ hook
30. m- ___ match
31. –m ___ thumb
32. d- ___ door
33. –d ___ bed
34. t- ___ table
35. –t ___ mitt
36. ʃ- ___ shoe
37. –ʃ ___ dish
38. –ʒ ___ television
39. s- ___ soap
40. –s ___ bus
41. z- ___ zipper
42. –z ___ eyes
43. n- ___ knife
44. –n ___ pan
45. l- ___ log
46. –l ___ mail
47. g- ___ gal
48. –g ___ bag
49. k- ___ coat
50. –k ___ book
51. tʃ- ___ chair
52. –tʃ ___ match
53. dʒ- ___ jam
54. –dʒ ___ badge
55. –ŋ ___ ring
56. r- ___ rock
57. –r ___ door
58. sm- ___ smell
59. sp- ___ spill
60. sw- ___ sweet
61. sk- ___ school
62. sl- ___ sled
63. sn- ___ snake
64. st- ___ star
65. θr- ___ thread
66. bl- ___ block
67. br- ___ broom
68. fl- ___ floor
69. fr- ___ frame
70. kw- ___ quail
71. pl- ___ plug
72. pr- ___ prayer
73. dr- ___ dress
74. gl- ___ glass
75. gr- ___ grape
76. kl- ___ cloth
77. kr- ___ crack
78. tr- ___ tree
79. spl- ___ splash
80. spr- ___ spray
81. str- ___ stream
82. –fs ___ muffs
83. –lz ___ balls
84. –mz ___ thumbs
85. –nz ___ coins
86. –sn ___ listen
87. –vz ___ knives
88. –rn ___ yarn
89. –ft ___ lift
90. –ld ___ filled
91. –lp ___ whelp
92. –mp ___ lamp
93. –nd ___ hand
94. –nt ___ paint
95. –ntʃ ___ bench
96. –ŋk ___ sink
97. –sp ___ clasp
98. –st ___ fist
99. –sk ___ desk
100. –vd ___ curved
101. –rk ___ fork
102. –bl ___ table
103. –dl ___ needle
104. –dz ___ beads
105. –ps ___ ropes
106. –tl ___ bottle
107. –tn ___ mitten
108. –ts ___ coats
109. –kt ___ packed
110. –pt ___ taped
111. –nts ___ points
112. –tnz ___ mittens
113. –kl ___ pickle
114. –ks ___ socks
115. –pl ___ apple
116. –fts ___ lifts
117. –plz ___ apples

report and recommendations for the next period of training. These reports should be made at least once a month, and can be made more often, particularly if a major problem or improvement has taken place.

Progress reports should be kept in a file along with test and other information on the child. Each report should include the child's name, the date, and the name of the person preparing the report. These reports should be placed chronologically in the file. When the training is completed or discontinued, a full progress report should be written and filed. It should describe the training given, the accomplishment made, and recommendations for further training. Sample reports are described below.

Progress Report for April 2007

Child: Michael Johnson May 2, 2007
Prepared by Karen Smith

Accomplishments: Michael has learned to:

1. Precisely articulate /f-/, /-f/, /v-/, and /-v/ in isolation, prosodic drills, words, and sentences, with breath control and correct stress and intonation.
2. Precisely articulate the consonants /θ/, /ð/, /s/, and /z/ in isolation.

Recommendations: During the next month Michael should learn to:

1. Precisely articulate /θ/, /ð/, /s/, and /z/ in syllable drills, words, and sentences, with breath control and correct stress and intonation.
2. Precisely articulate at least two additional consonants in isolation.

Final Report

Child: Michael Johnson December 1, 2007
Prepared by Karen Smith

Training Program: Speech Development Guidebook for Children with Hearing Loss

Accomplishments: Michael has learned to:

1. Precisely articulate all vowels, diphthongs, and single consonants in isolation, prosodic drills, words, and sentences, with breath control and correct stress and intonation.
2. Precisely articulate many consonant blends in isolation.

Recommendations: Michael should receive additional training so as to learn to:

1. Precisely articulate all the consonant blends in isolation, prosodic drills, words, and sentences, with breath control and correct stress and intonation.
2. Transfer the above skills into his everyday spoken language.

Guidelines for Parents

Parents can be of great help to speech pathologists or deaf educators. Guidelines for helping them participate in speech development are described below.

1. Encourage parents to study a copy of this guidebook and write down any questions they have.
2. Show parents how to correctly articulate each speech sound and each consonant blend. Instruct parents how to correctly repeat each sound and blend you say.
3. Share with parents the results of the speech evaluations you administer.
4. Explain the purpose and procedures of each speech lesson you give, and what they can do to reinforce the speech skills you are helping the child to produce.
5. Let parents observe the speech lessons unless it distracts the child from paying attention and learning.
6. Refer to the target form for phonetic symbols of all the sounds. Help the parents learn to associate them with the speech sounds.
7. Refer to the table that includes phonetic symbols and distinguishing features of speech sounds. Explain which speech frequencies (low, mid, and high) are contained in each sound. Relate this to the child's audiograms, which show his or her hearing losses in those frequency regions, with and without a hearing aid or cochlear implant.
8. Try to persuade parents to also do the following:
   - Show interest in what the child expresses.
   - Let the professionals take care of speech correction.

- Reward the child for what he or she says correctly. Don't punish the child for what he or she says incorrectly. Simply repeat what the child says, except say it correctly.
- Get down on the child's level as much as possible. Talk about what interests the child.
- Don't put pressure on the child to learn. Prompt the child but do not force him or her.
- Read to the child every day. As you read, slow down and pronounce words carefully. Select reading materials that interest the child. Encourage the child to look at pictures and words in books you read.
- Encourage the child to learn to print or write some words. Help him spell the words correctly.

3

Speech Lessons

Introduction

There are 117 speech lessons described in this chapter. Each incorporates the Speech Shaping Target and Recording Form, the Word Test Form, and the Vocal Scope or sound level meter and paper strip.

Initially teach the child to articulate each of the 36 vowels, diphthongs, and consonants in isolation, using copies of the Speech Shaping Target and Recording Form. Continue this procedure during each of the first 57 lessons.

Lessons 1–14 cover vowels and diphthongs. During each of these lessons teach the child breath control and syllable repetition. Lesson 1, for example, requires that the child (1) sustain /ɑ/, (2) sustain /bɑ/, and (3) repeat /bɑ/ in syllable groups of 2, 3, 4, and 5. Also, teach the child to repeat syllables at rates of 3, 4, and 5 per second.

Lessons 15–117 cover consonants and consonant blends. During each of these lessons spend some time on stress and intonation patterns. Teach the child to stress the first syllable of the three-syllable group, then the second syllable, and finally the third syllable. Follow a similar procedure with the four-syllable groups. Then make up syllable groups, each with syllables that alternate in composition.

Last, teach the child to say a word containing each target sound, e.g., /ɑ/, under three conditions: (a) repeating the word after the therapist, e.g., *car*, (b) saying it when looking at a picture of it, and (c) repeating and completing a sentence with the word: "This is a ______" (therapist says). "This is a car" (child responds).

At the completion of Lesson 1, record the accuracy with which the child repeats the /ɑ/ in the word *car* in the space preceding the word on the Word Test Form. Follow the same procedure with the speech sound or consonant blend for each lesson that follows.

As you move from lesson to lesson, review the target words of up to five previous lessons. For example, after recording the accuracy with which the child repeats the /i/ in the word *key* for Lesson 2 on the Word Test Form, again record the accuracy with which the child repeats the /ɑ/ in the word *car* for Lesson 1 on the Word Test Form, this time in the space following the word *car*. There is ample space after each word of the Word Test Form to follow this procedure.

Record other results directly on the lesson forms, for example, a check mark after successful completion of each part of a breath control and syllable drill of Lessons 1–14 or prosodic drill of Lessons 15–117. Also write numbers above additional words you ask the child to say at the bottom of each lesson to indicate the child's accuracy in transferring the speech skill of that lesson.

Lesson 1 /ɑ/

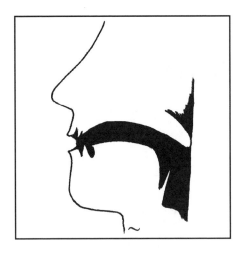

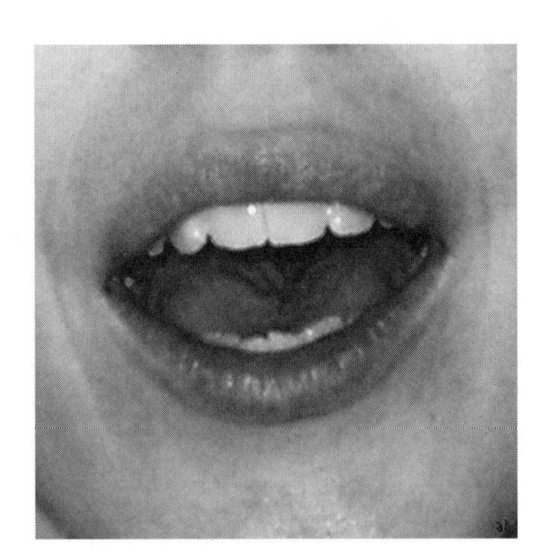

Tongue low in the mouth, mouth open, voice passes through. The articulation can be seen. Voicing may be felt on the throat. A low-mid frequency sound. A Lissajous pattern clarifies the acoustic clues.

Breath Control and Syllable Drill

ɑ ______________________________

bɑ ______________________________

bɑbɑ bɑbɑbɑ bɑbɑbɑbɑ bɑbɑbɑbɑbɑ

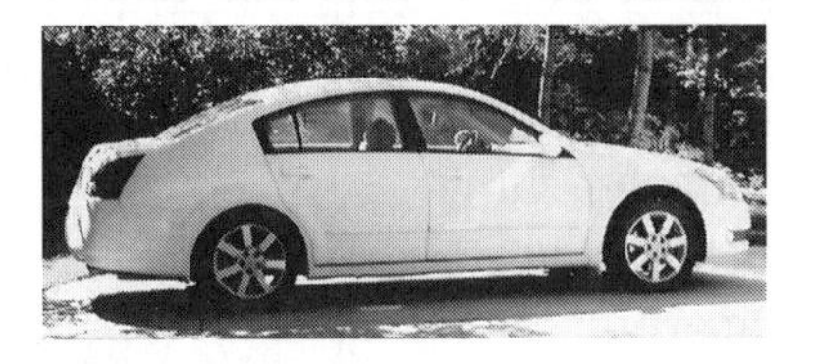

car

This is a ________.

arch bar bomb garage heart

large lock mop rock sock

Lesson 2 /i/

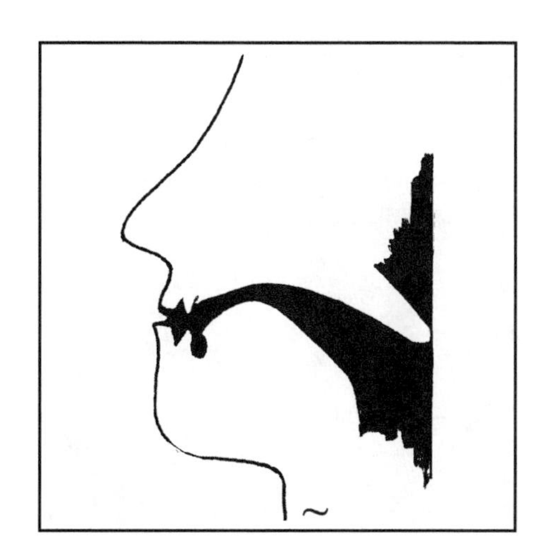

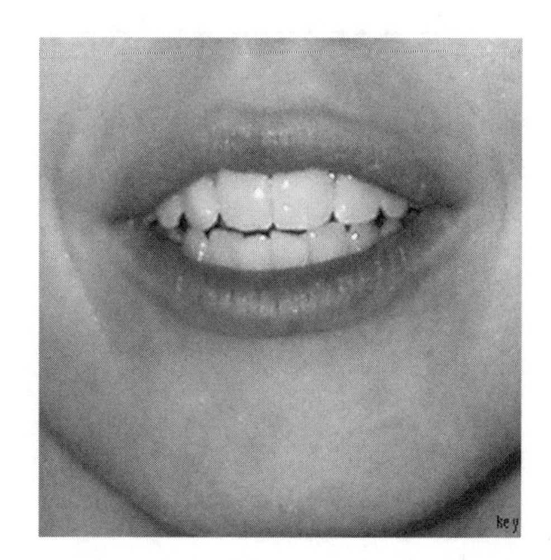

Front of tongue raised high, tongue tip behind lower front teeth, mandible dropped slightly, lips spread, voice passes through. Articulation can be seen when speaker opens mouth. Voicing may be felt on the throat. A low and high frequency sound. A Lissajous pattern clarifies the acoustic clues.

Breath Control and Syllable Drill

i ______________________________

bi _____________________________

bibi bibibi bibibibi bibibibibi

biba bibabi bibabiba bibabibabi

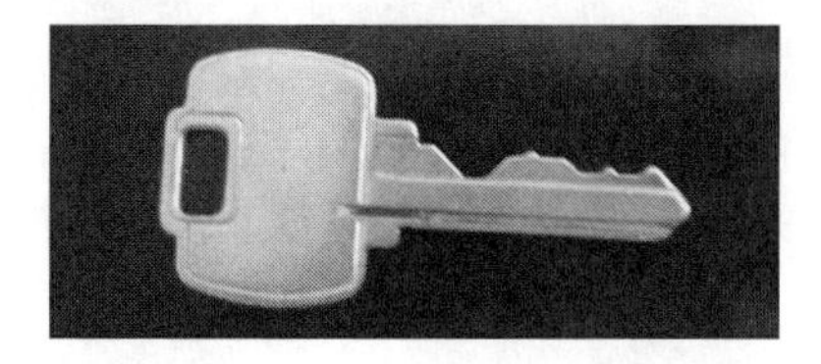

key

Turn the ________.

beam bean cheese deed feet

geese reel sheep teeth

Lesson 3 /u/

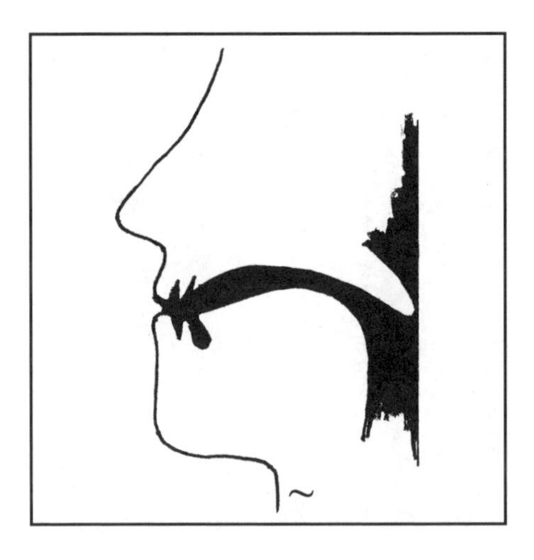

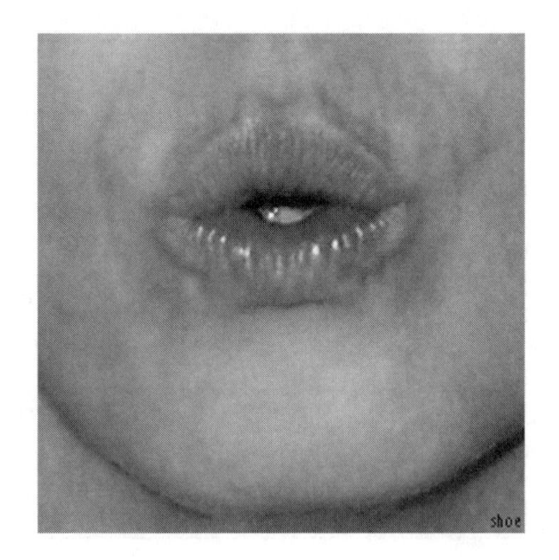

Back of tongue raised high, mandible dropped slightly, lips rounded and protruded with small opening, voice passes through. Articulation of tongue cannot be seen. Voicing may be felt on the throat. A low frequency sound. A Lissajous pattern clarifies the acoustic clues.

Breath Control and Syllable Drill

u ______________________________

bu ______________________________

bubu bububu bubububu bubububububu

bubi buba bubabi bubiba bubibabuba

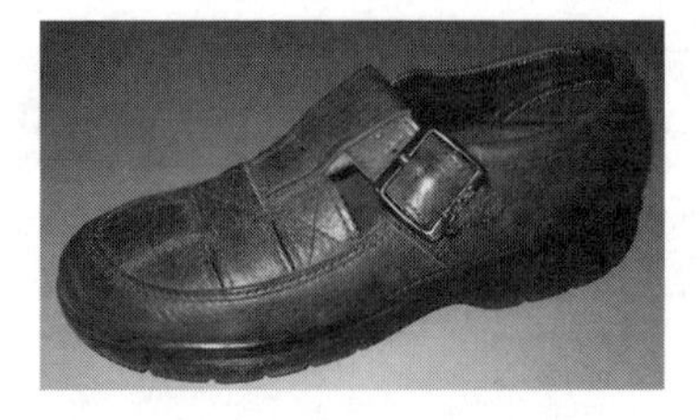

shoe

Shine the ________.

hoop moon noose room root

suit shoe tube zoo

Lesson 4 /aʊ/

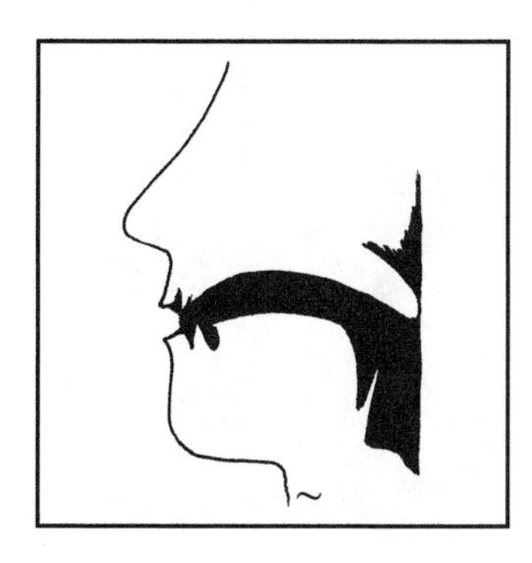
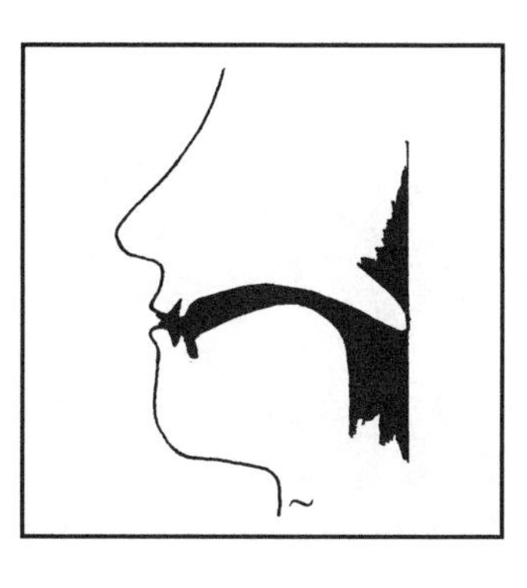
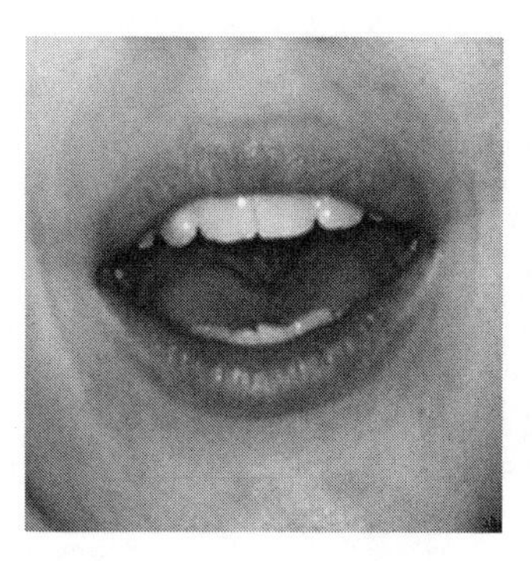
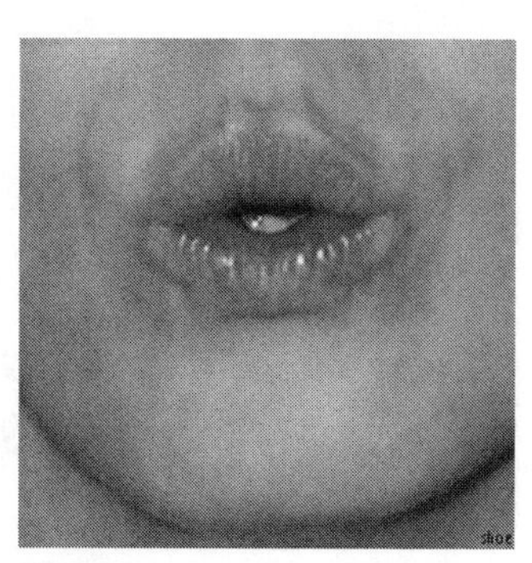

First part: Middle of tongue raised slightly, mandible down, lips relaxed. Second part: Back of tongue high, mandible up, lips rounded and protruded. Both parts: Voice passes through. Articulation of first part can be seen. Voicing may be felt on the throat. A low-mid to low frequency diphthong. A Lissajous pattern clarifies the acoustic clues.

Breath Control and Syllable Drill

aʊ ______________________________

baʊ ______________________________

baʊbaʊ baʊbaʊbaʊ baʊbaʊbaʊbaʊ

baʊbi baʊbo bobaʊ bibaʊ

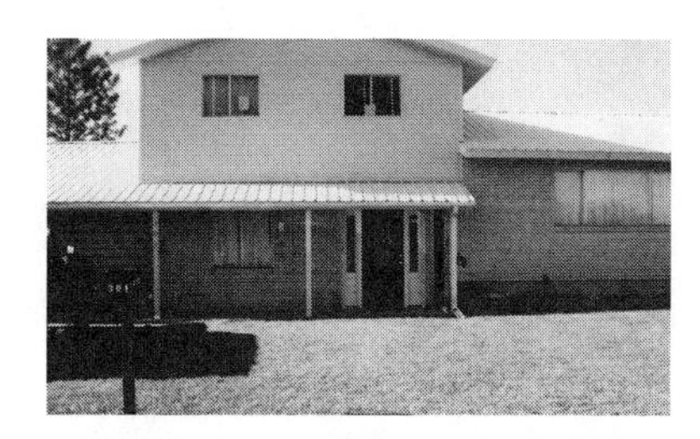

house

Live in the ________.

down mouse sow shout scout towel

Lesson 5 /aɪ/

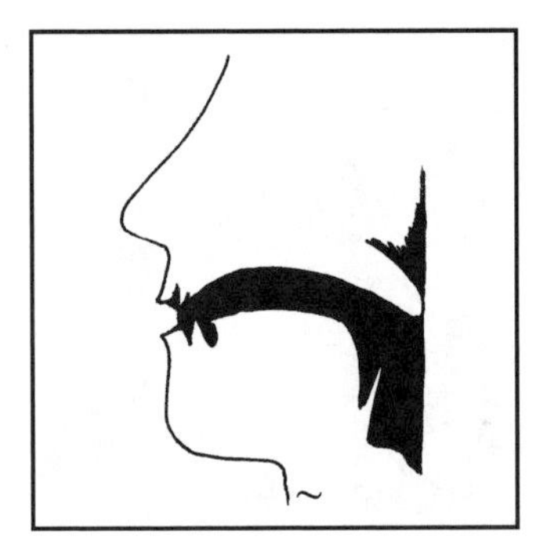
 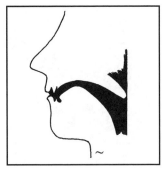
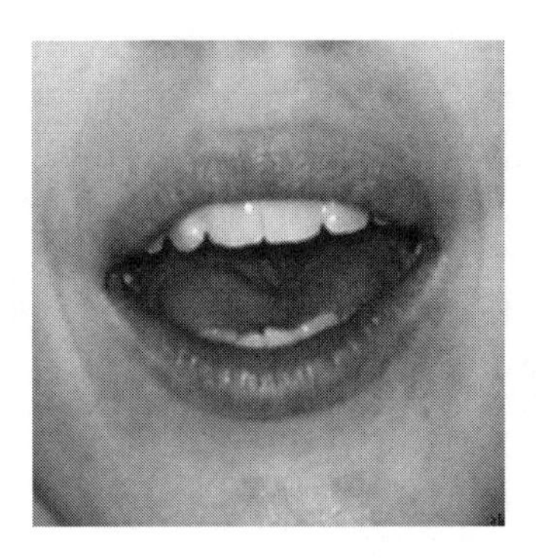
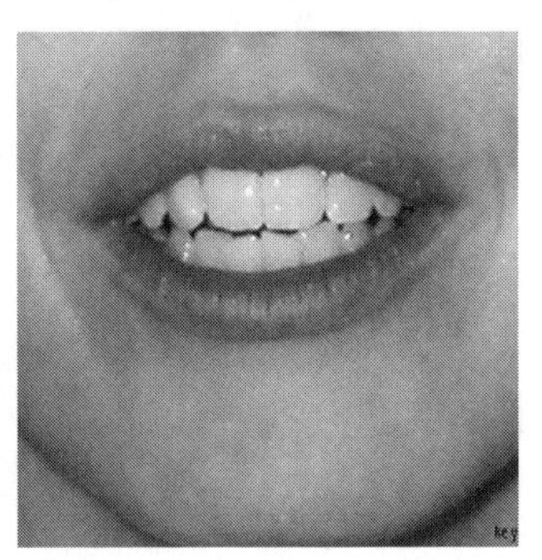

First part: Middle of tongue raised slightly, mandible down, lips relaxed. Second part: Front of tongue high, mandible up, lips relaxed. Both parts: Voice passes through. Articulation of first part can be seen. Voicing may be felt on the throat. A low-mid to low- high frequency diphthong. A Lissajous pattern clarifies the acoustic clues.

Breath Control and Syllable Drill

aɪ ______________________________

baɪ ______________________________

baɪbaɪ baɪbaɪbaɪ baɪbaɪbaɪbaɪ baɪbaɪbaɪbaɪbaɪ

baɪbaʊ baɪbɑ baɪbi baɪbu bubaɪ bɑbaɪ bibaɪ

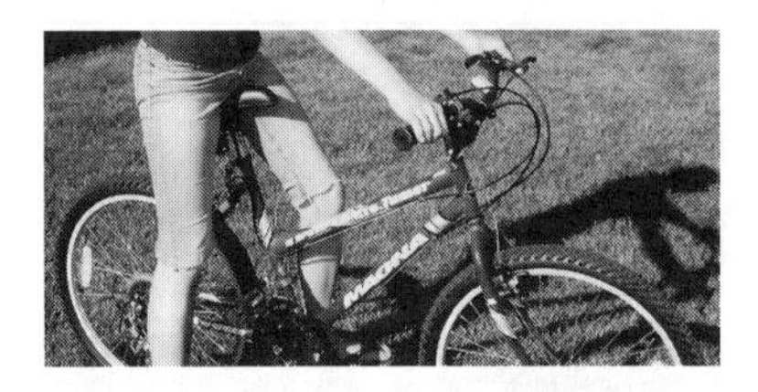

bike

Ride the ________.

fine five hive ice line

light pile thigh vine

Lesson 6 /ɔ/

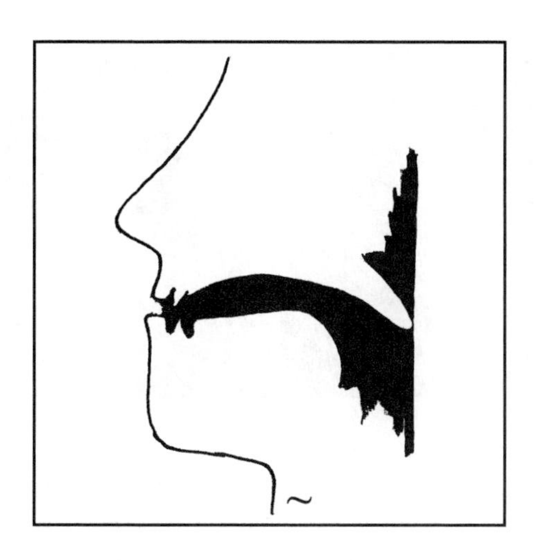

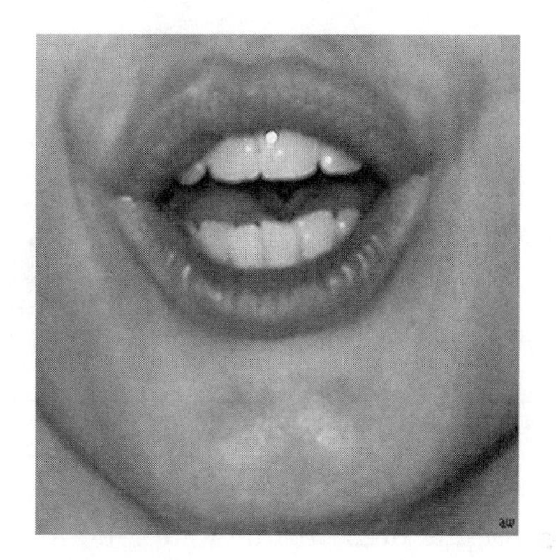

Back of tongue raised slightly, mandible down, mouth open, lips rounded, voice passes through. The articulation can be seen. Voicing may be felt on the throat. A low frequency sound. A Lissajous pattern clarifies the acoustic clues.

Breath Control and Syllable Drill

ɔ ________________________________

bɔ ________________________________

bɔ bɔ bɔ bɔ bɔ bɔ bɔ bɔ bɔ bɔ bɔ bɔ bɔ bɔ

bɔ bu bɔ bi bɔ bu bɔ bɑ bɔ bi

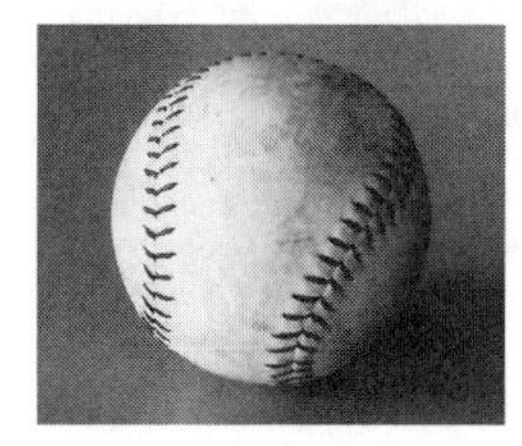

ball

Throw the ________.

bought hawk log moth

taut talk tong walk yawn

Lesson 7 /ɔɪ/

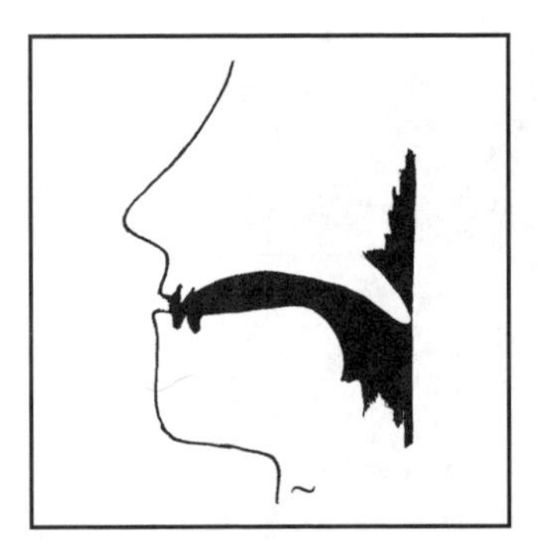
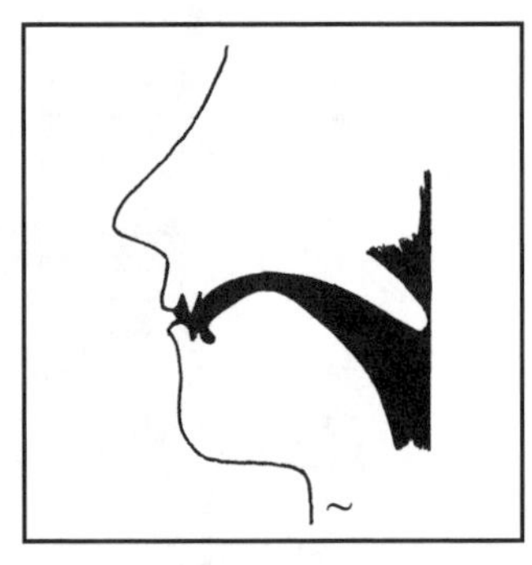
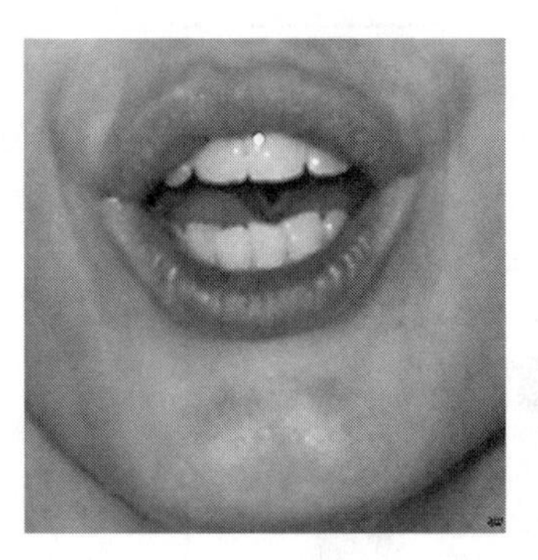
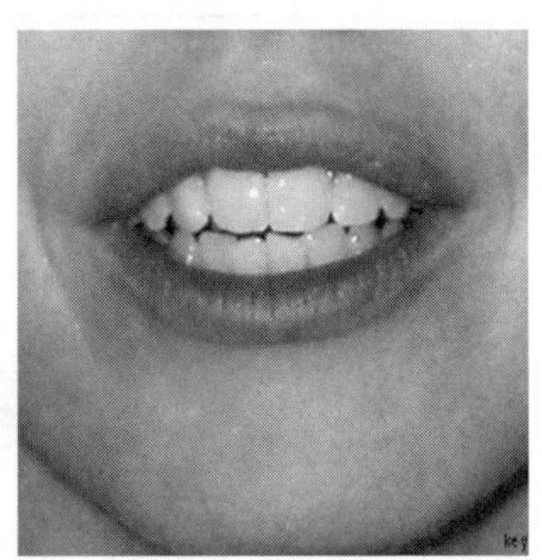

First part: Back of tongue raised slightly, mandible down, mouth open, lips rounded. Second part: Front of tongue high, mandible up, mouth closed, lips relaxed. Both parts: Voice passes through. Articulation of first part can be seen. Voicing may be felt on the throat. A low-mid to high frequency diphthong. A Lissajous pattern clarifies the acoustic clues.

Breath Control and Syllable Drill

ɔɪ ________________________________

bɔɪ ______________________________

bɔɪ bɔɪ   bɔɪ bɔɪ bɔɪ   bɔɪ bɔɪ bɔɪ bɔɪ   bɔɪ bɔɪ bɔɪ bɔɪ bɔi

bɔɪ bɑ   bɔɪ bi   bɔɪ bu   bɔɪ baʊ   bɔi baɪ

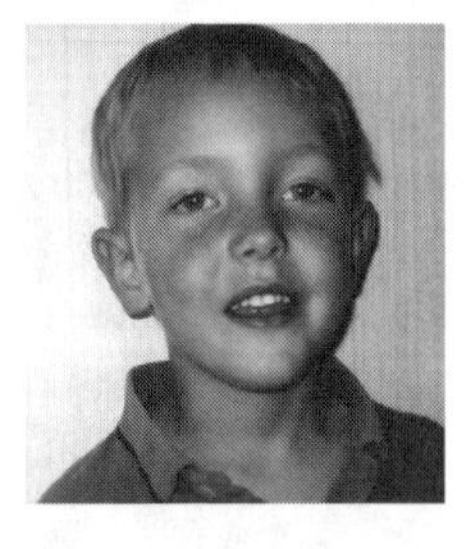

boy

He is a ________.

annoy   coil   foil   hoist   joy

poise   soil   toy   toil   voice   void

Lesson 8 /ɛ/

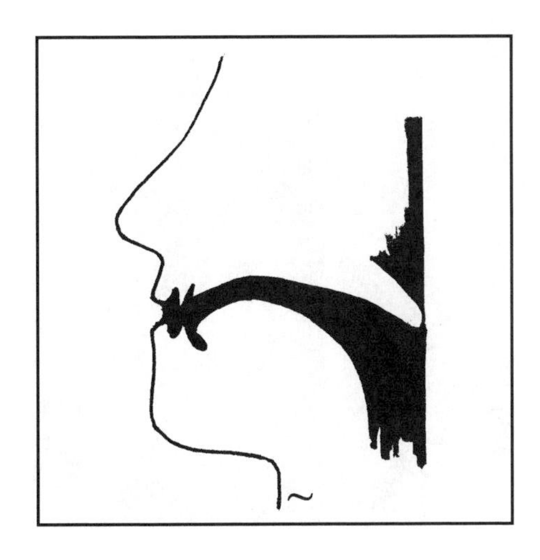

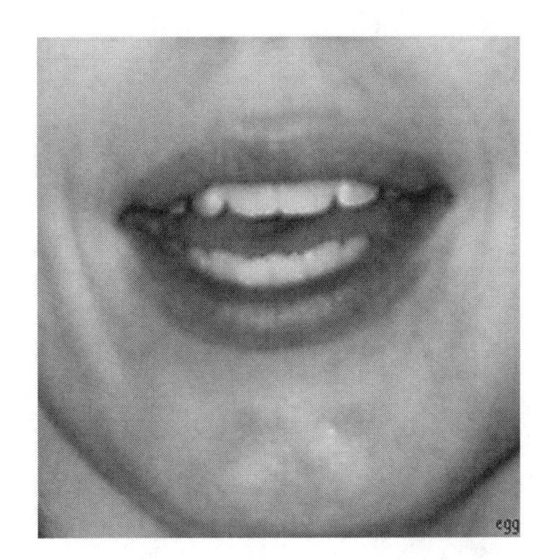

Front of tongue raised midway, tongue tip behind lower front teeth, mandible dropped midway, lips spread, voice passes through. The articulation can be seen. Voicing may be felt on the throat. A low-mid frequency sound. A Lissajous pattern clarifies the acoustic clues

Breath Control and Syllable Drill

ɛ ______________________________

bɛ ______________________________

bɛbɛ   bɛ bɛ bɛ bɛ   bɛ bɛ bɛ bɛ bɛ   bɛ bɛ bɛ

bɛbɑ   bɛbi   bɛbu   bɛbaʊ   bɛ baɪ   bɛ bɔɪ

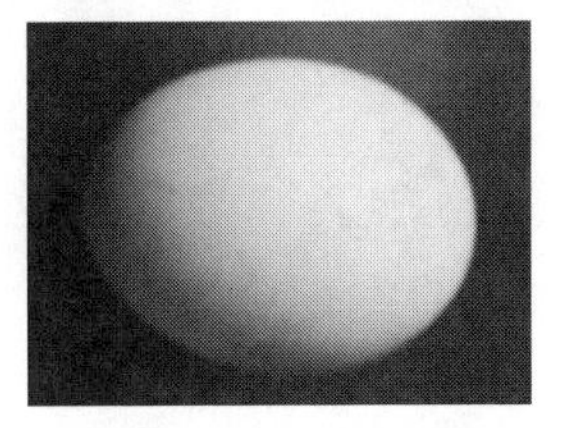

egg

Fry an ________.

bed   hedge   leg   ledge   men

net   pear   shell   ten

Lesson 9 /ʊ/

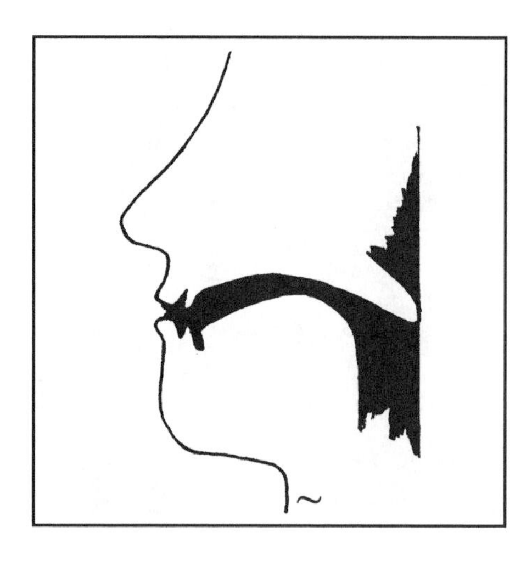

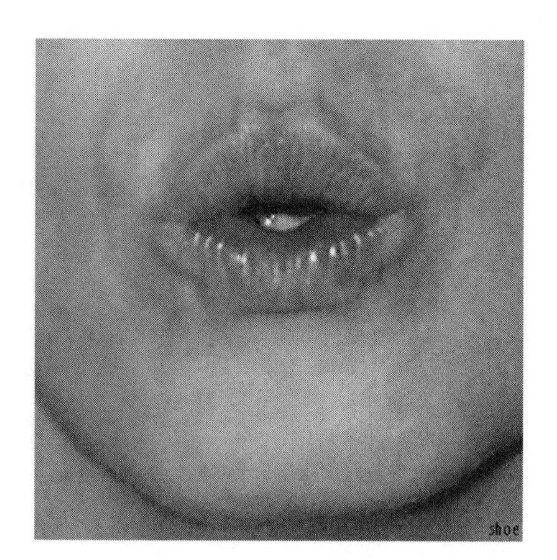

Back of tongue raised high, lips rounded and protruded some, mandible down some, mouth open some, voice passes through. The tongue cannot be seen. Voicing may be felt on the throat. A low frequency sound. Lissajous pattern clarifies acoustic clues.

Breath Control and Syllable Drill

ʊ ______________________________

bʊ ______________________________

bʊ bʊ   bʊ bʊ bʊ   bʊ bʊ bʊ bu   bʊ bʊ bʊ bu bʊ

bʊbu   bʊbi   bʊbɑ   bʊ bɔ   bʊ bɔɪ   bʊbaɪ

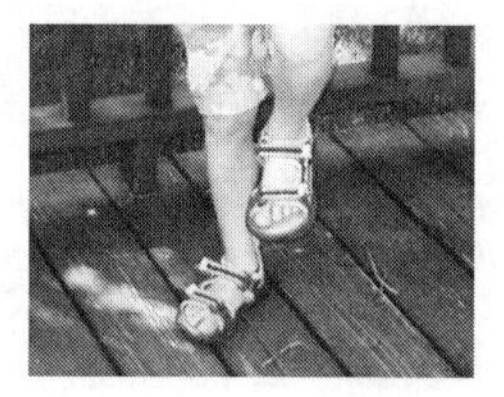

foot

Touch your ________.

bush   could   hood   push

pulled   roof   should   woods

Lesson 10 /ɪ/

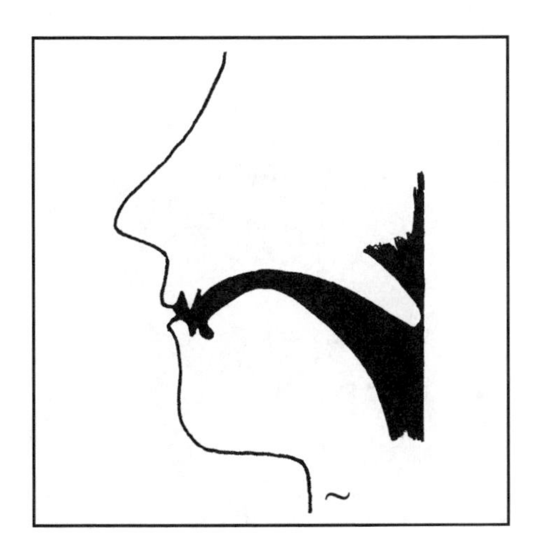

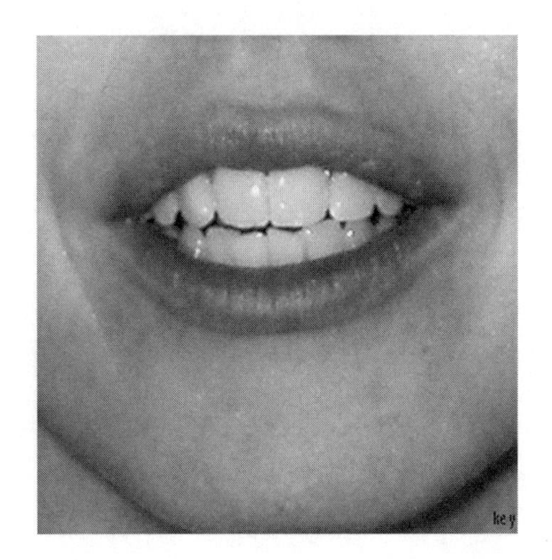

Front of tongue raised high, tongue tip behind lower front teeth, mandible dropped slightly, lips spread, voice passes through. Tongue articulation can be seen when speaker opens mouth. Voicing may be felt on the throat. A low and high frequency sound. A Lissajous pattern clarifies the acoustic clues.

Breath Control and Syllable Drill

ɪ ________________________________

bɪ ________________________________

bɪ bɪ   bɪ bɪ bɪ   bɪ bɪ bɪ bɪ   bɪ bɪ bɪ bɪ bɪ

bɪbi   bɪbɑ   bɪbu   bubɪ   bɪbɔ   bɪbɔɪ   bɪbʊ

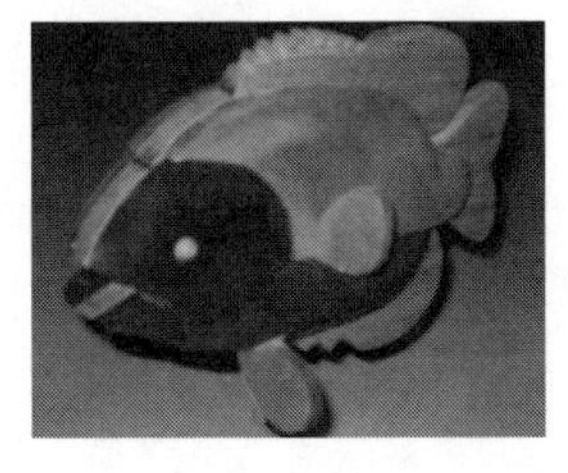

fish

Catch a ________.

bib   dig   fig   fin   hill   lid

mitt   knit   pit   sit   sing   ship   whip

Lesson 11 /æ/

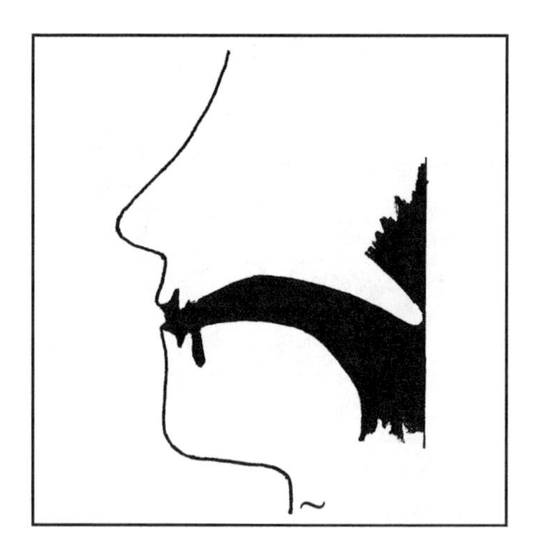

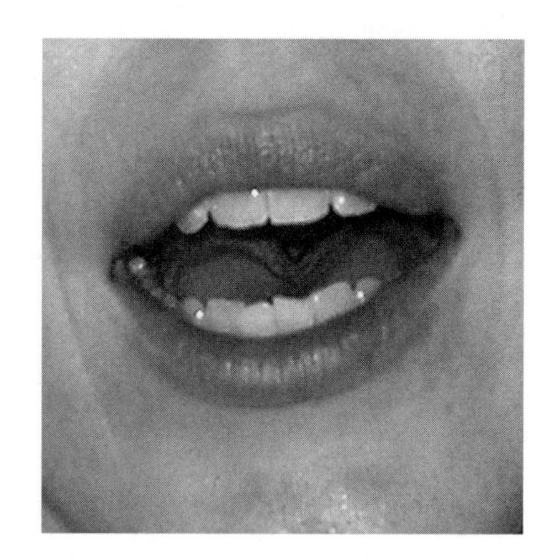

Front of tongue raised slightly, tongue tip behind lower front teeth, mandible dropped, lips spread, voice passes through. Tongue can be seen. Voicing may be felt on the throat. A low and mid frequency sound. A Lissajous pattern clarifies the acoustic clues.

Breath Control and Syllable Drill

æ ______________________________

bæ ______________________________

bæbæ bæbæ bæ bæ bæ bæ bæ bæ bæ bæ bæ bæ

bæbi bæbɑ bæbu bæbaɪ bæbɔɪ bæbɛ bæbʊ

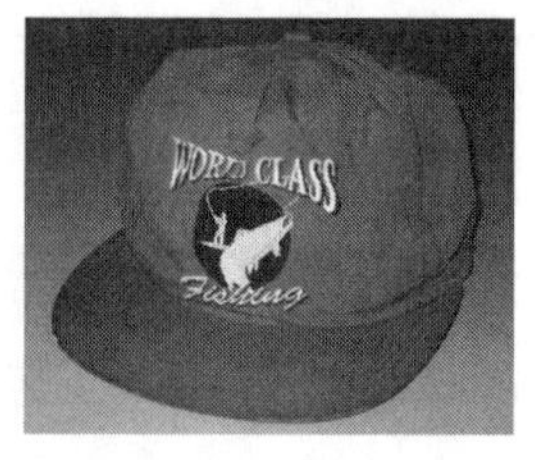

cap

Tip your ________.

bat badge cat catch fan happy jam

can lamb man mat patch sash vat

Lesson 12 /ʌ/

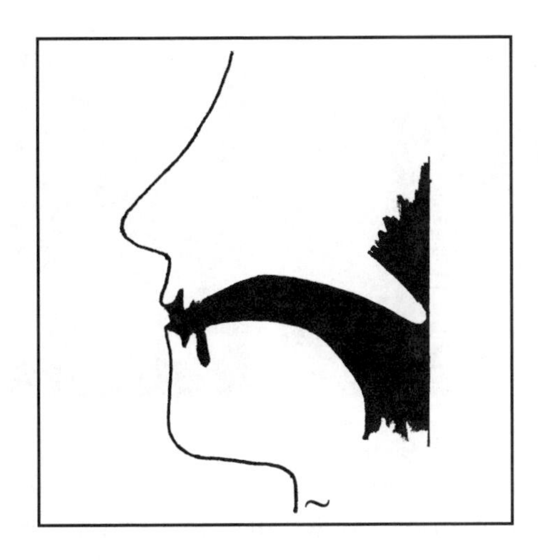

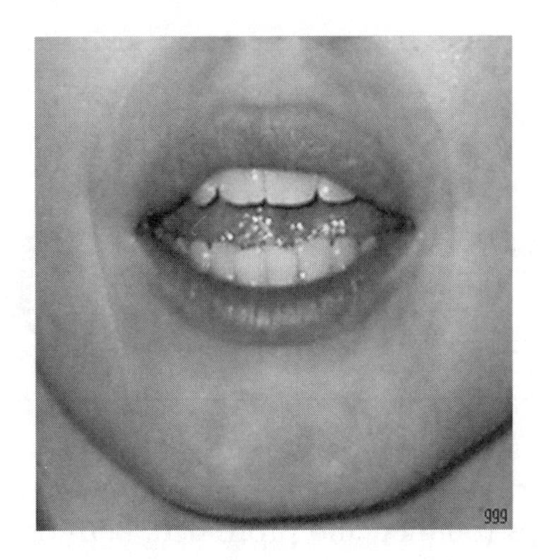

Tongue low in mouth, tongue tip behind lower front teeth, mandible dropped, voice passes through. Tongue position can be seen. Voicing may be felt on the throat. A low-mid frequency sound. A Lissajous pattern clarifies the acoustic clues.

Breath Control and Syllable Drill

ʌ ______________________________

bʌ _____________________________

bʌbʌ bʌbʌ bʌ bʌbʌ bʌ bʌ bʌ bʌ bʌ bʌ bʌ

bʌbo bʌbi bʌbɑ bʌ baʊ bʌbaɪ bʌ bɔ bʌbɔɪ

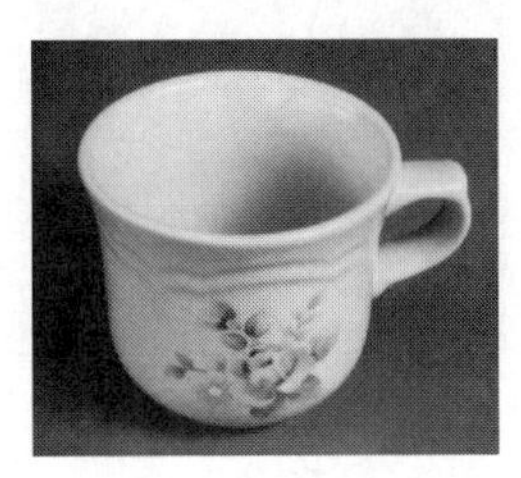

cup

Lift your ________.

bug bun cut dust fun gum hub

muss nut puck sun tub touch thumb

Lesson 13 /o/

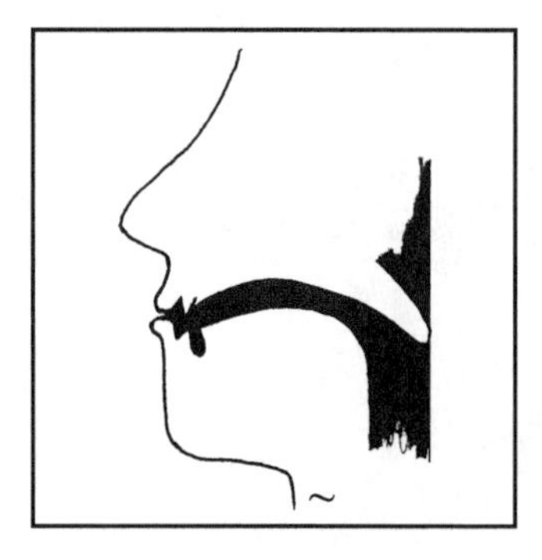
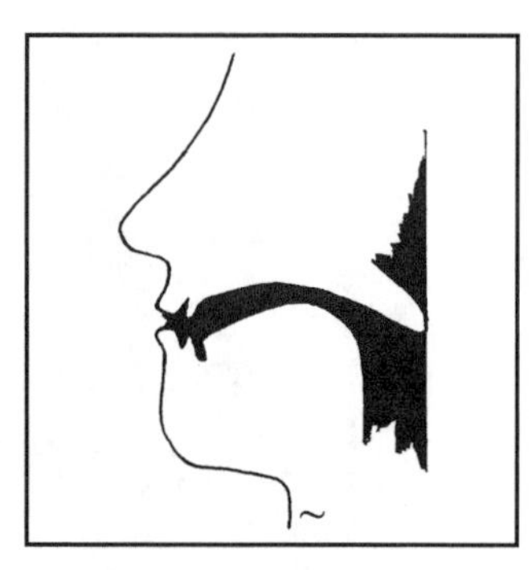
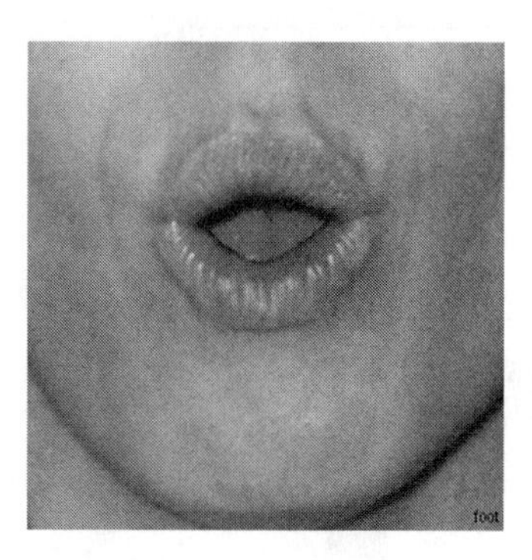
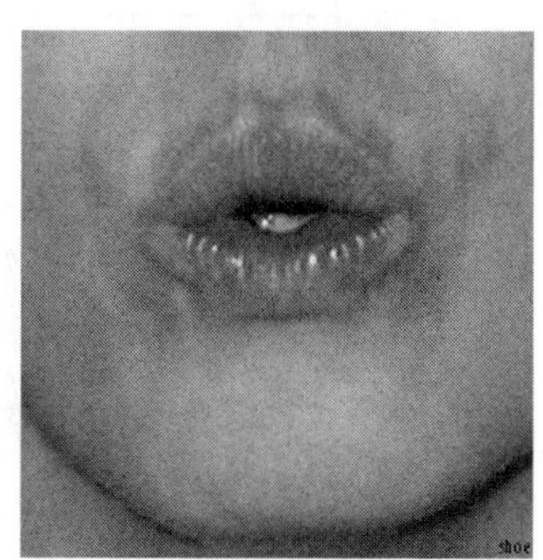

First part: Back of tongue raised, lips rounded, mandible down. Second part: Back of tongue raised high, lips rounded and protruded. Both parts: Voice passes through. Articulation of tongue hidden. Voicing may be felt on the throat. A low frequency diphthong. A Lissajous pattern clarifies the acoustic clues.

Breath Control and Syllable Drill

o ______________________________

bo ______________________________

bobo bobobo bobobobo bobobobobo

bobɑ bobi bobu bobaʊ bobaɪ

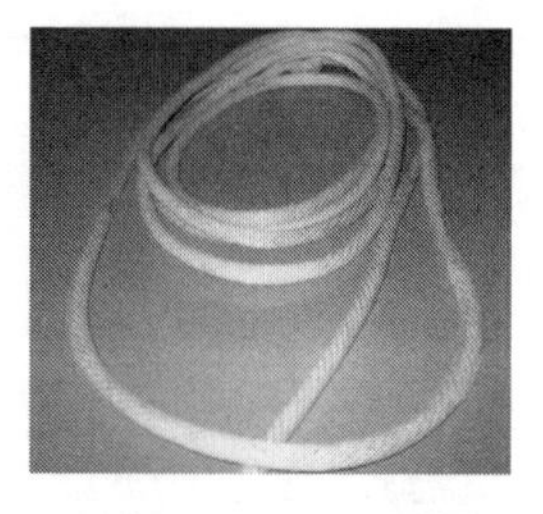

rope

Coil the ________.

boat cone coal fold goat goal hose

joke mole note phone roll sole told

Lesson 14 /e/

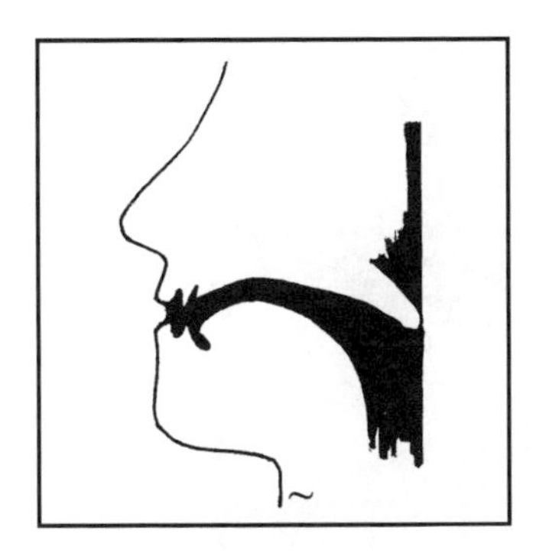
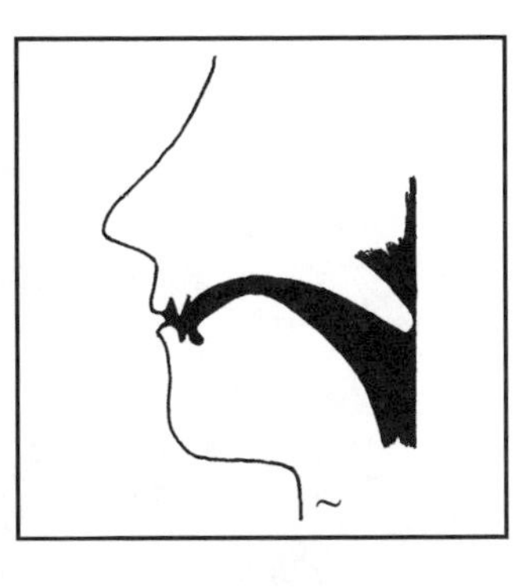
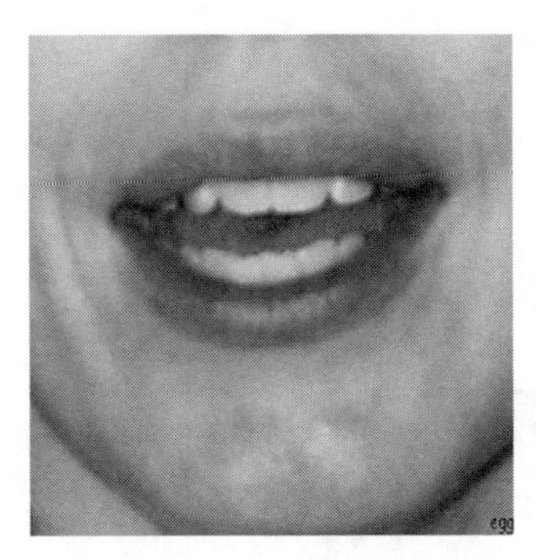
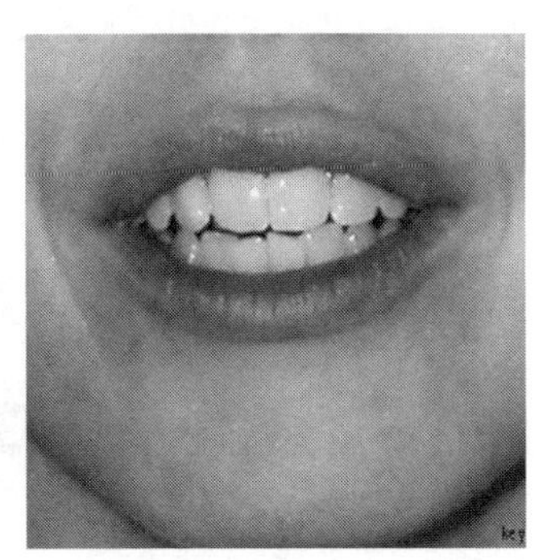

First part: Front of tongue raised, tongue tip behind lower front teeth, mandible dropped, lips spread. Second part: Front of tongue raised higher, tongue tip behind lower front teeth, lips spread. Both parts: Voice passes through. Articulation of tongue visible. Voicing may be felt on the throat. A low and high frequency diphthong. A Lissajous pattern clarifies the acoustic clues.

Breath Control and Syllable Drill

e ______________________________

be ____________________________

bebe bebebe bebebebe bebebebebe

bebɑ bebi bebu bebaɪ bebaʊ bebɔɪ

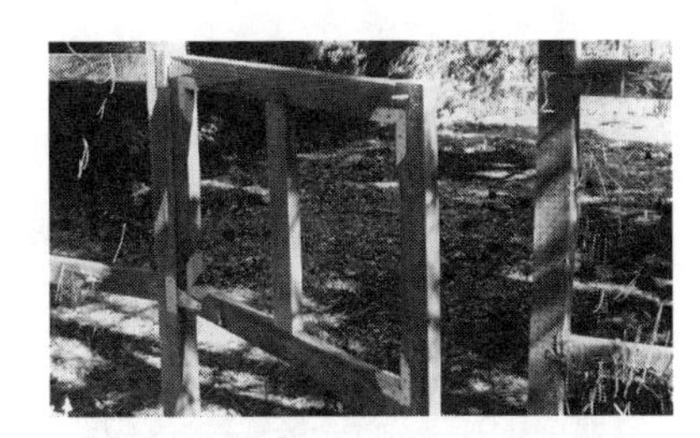

gate

Open the ________.

bait cake date face late

mail name pail rake sale whale

Lesson 15 /b-/

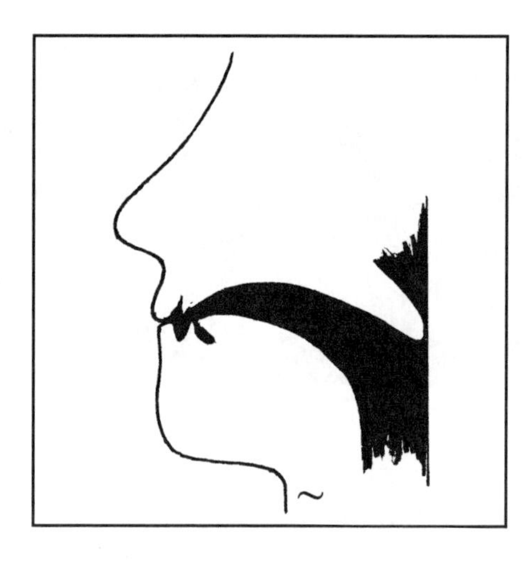

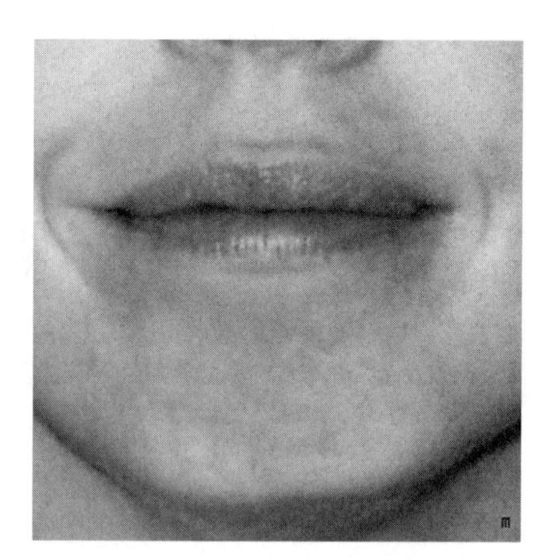

Lips are shut, air dammed, and lips opened abruptly with voicing. The articulation can be seen. Voicing can be felt on the throat. A low mid frequency sound. A Lissajous pattern clarifies the acoustic clues. The explosive release can be seen by either the Lissajous pattern, the rapid movement of the end of a paper strip held in front of the mouth, or the needle of a sound level meter.

Prosodic Drill

bæbæbæ bæ**bæ**bæ bæbæ**bæ**

bæbæbæbæ bæ**bæ**bæbæ bæbæ**bæ**bæ

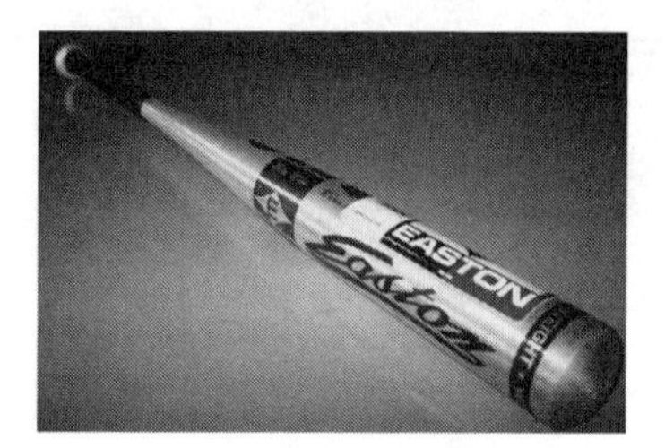

bat

Swing the ________.

beet bit bait bet boot boat bought but

bag bug bake bike back

Lesson 16 /-b/

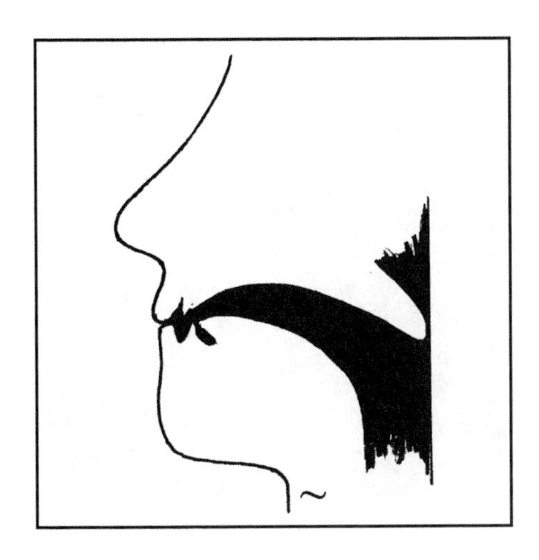

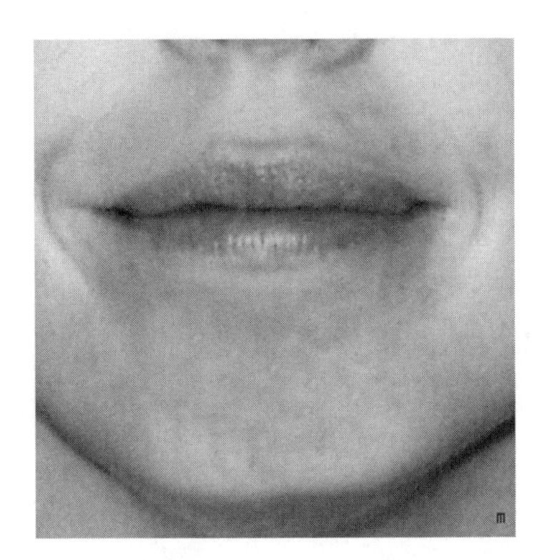

Air dammed behind shut lips, held without release, or released lightly with voicing. The articulation can be seen. Voicing can be felt on the throat. A low mid frequency sound. The explosive release can be seen by either the Lissajous pattern, the rapid movement of a paper strip held in front of the mouth, or the needle of a sound level meter.

Prosodic Drill

ɪbɪbɪb ɪb**ɪb**ɪb ɪbɪb**ɪb**

ɪbɪbɪbɪb ɪb**ɪb**ɪbɪb ɪbɪb**ɪb**ɪb

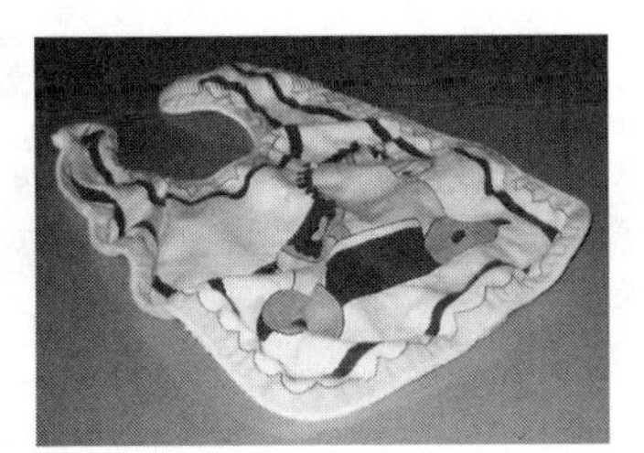

bib

It is a baby's ________.

cab dab hub lab nab tab

cob lob mob knob sob

Lesson 17 /p-/

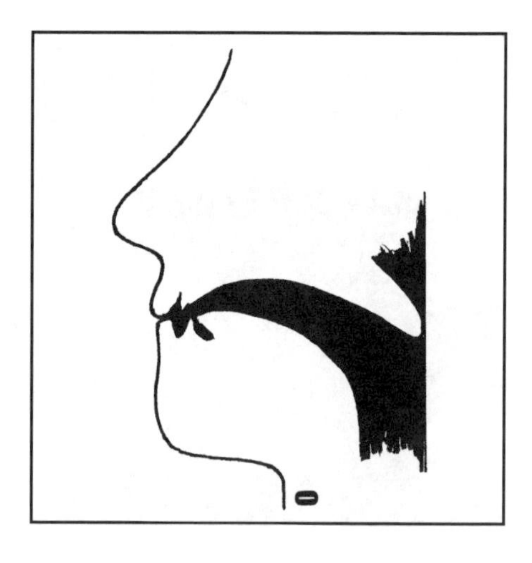

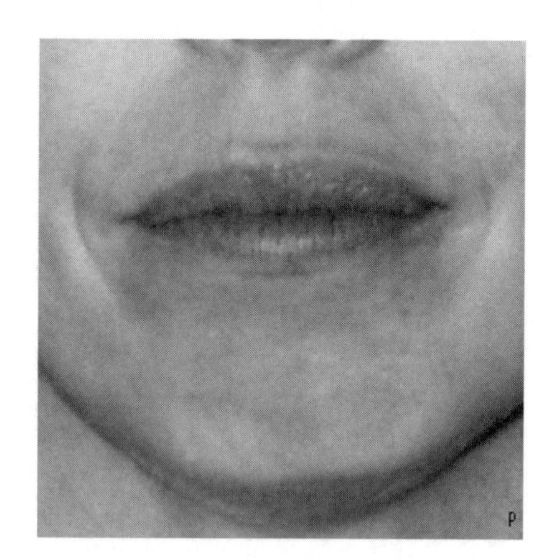

Lips are shut, air dammed, and lips opened abruptly with audible aspiration of air. The articulation can be seen. An explosive and long release can be seen either by the Lissajous pattern, the rapid movement of the end of a paper strip held in front of the mouth, or the needle of a sound level meter.

Prosodic Drill

pɛpɛpɛ pɛ**pɛ**pɛ pɛpɛ**pɛ**

pɛpɛpɛpɛ pɛ**pɛ**pɛpɛ pɛpɛ**pɛ**pɛ

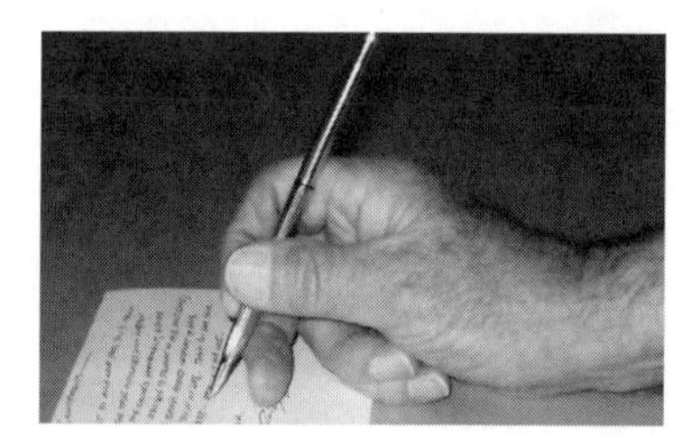

pen

Write with a ________.

peach pick pole pig pie pearl

path pan pail pear pipe pile

Lesson 18 /-p/

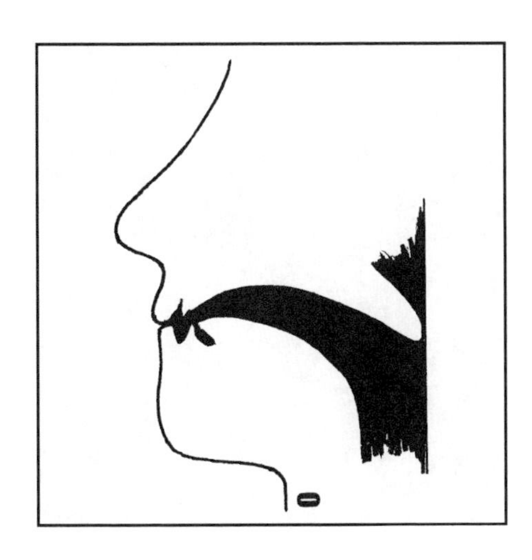

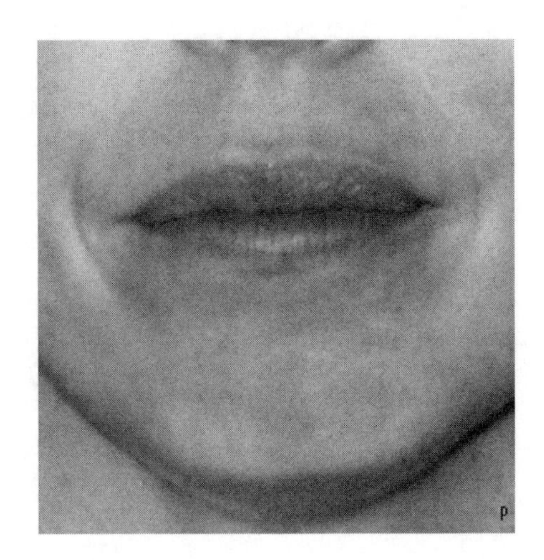

Lips are shut, air dammed and released abruptly with audible aspiration. The articulation can be seen. An explosive release can be seen either by a Lissajous pattern, the rapid movement of a paper strip held in front of the mouth, or the needle of a sound level meter.

Prosodic Drill

opopop op**op**op opop**op**

opopopop op**op**opop opop**op**op

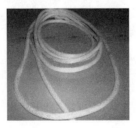

rope

Throw the ________.

lip lap deep hoop cape

chop sleep cape clap stop

Lesson 19 /w-/

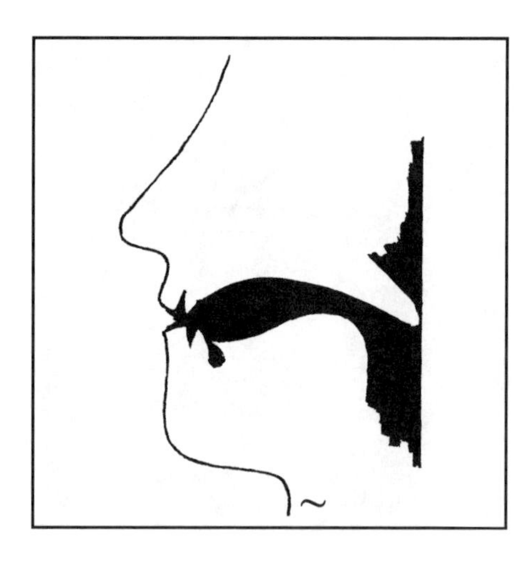

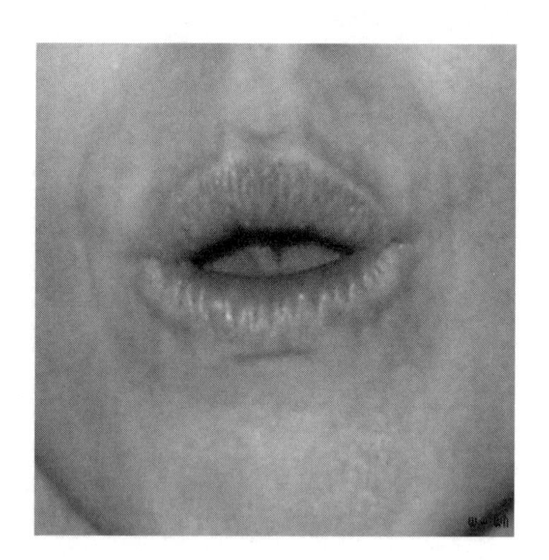

Lips pursed and separated, back of tongue high, voice passes through. Lips can be seen but not the tongue. Voicing may be felt. A low frequency sound. A Lissajous pattern clarifies the acoustic clues.

Prosodic Drill

waɪwaɪwaɪ waɪ**waɪ**waɪ waɪwaɪ**waɪ**

waɪwaɪwaɪwaɪ waɪ**waɪ**waɪwaɪ waɪwaɪ**waɪ**waɪ

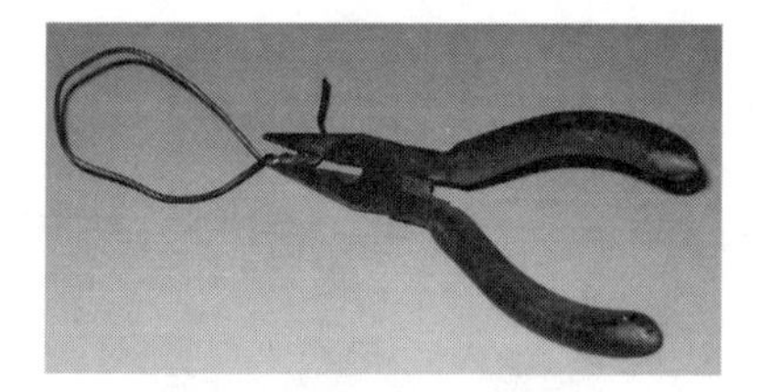

wire

Twist the ________.

wig worm web weave world

wasp wealth woods witch wash

Lesson 20 /ʍ-/

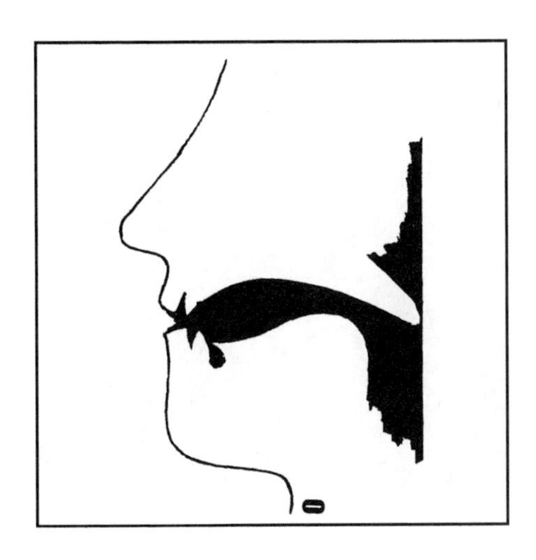

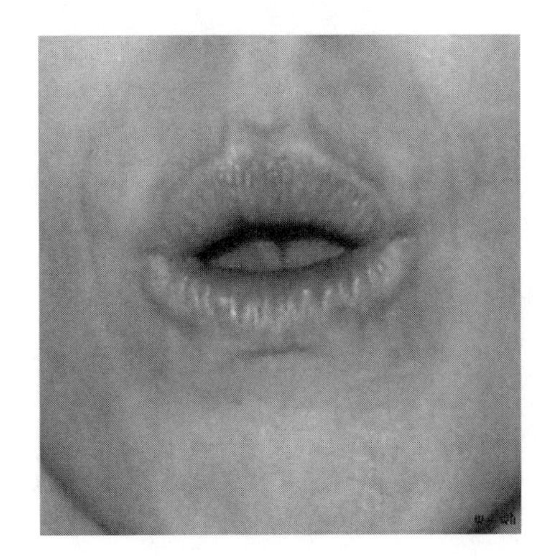

Lips pursed and separated, back of tongue high, breath passes through. Lips can be seen but not the tongue. Breath flow can be seen either by the Lissajous pattern, the rapid movement of a paper strip held in front of the mouth, or the needle of a sound level meter.

Prosodic Drill

ʍiʍiʍi ʍi**ʍi**ʍi ʍiʍi**ʍi**

ʍiʍiʍiʍi ʍi**ʍi**ʍiʍi ʍiʍi**ʍi**ʍi

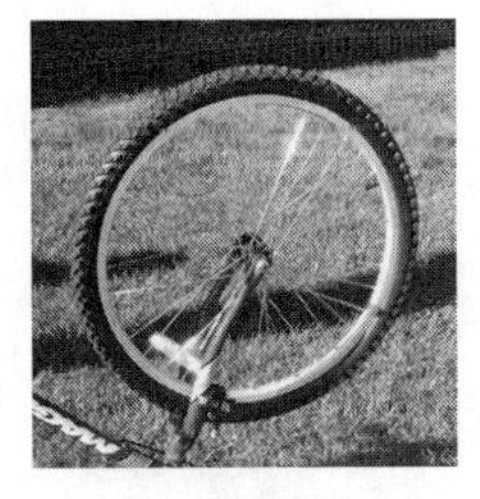

wheel

Turn the ________.

whelp whirl while when

where why while which

Lesson 21 /f-/

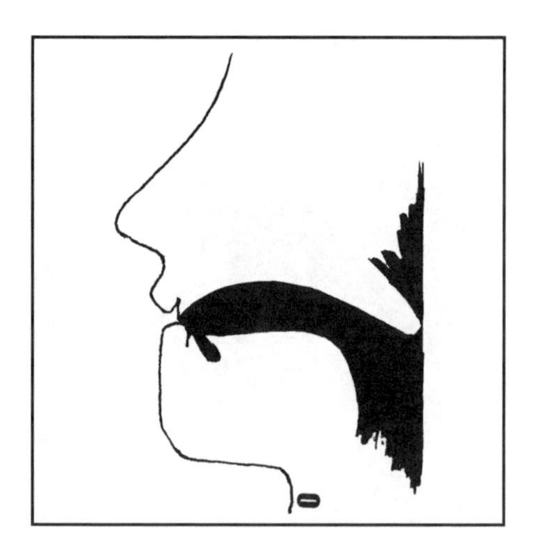

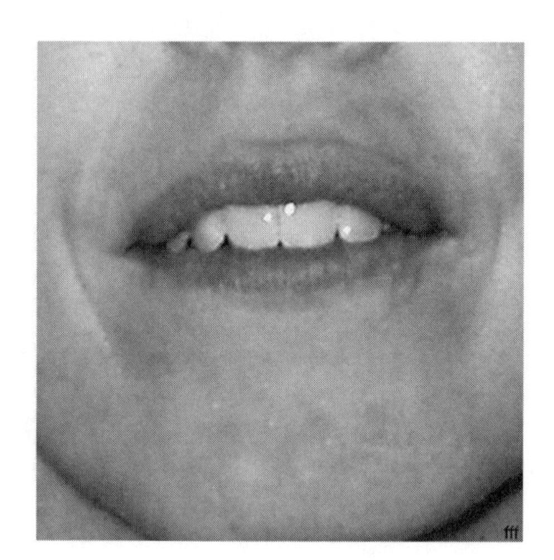

Lower lip touches upper teeth and breath passes through this articulation with audible friction (no voice). The articulation can be seen. The sound is high frequency. Evidence of it is indicated either by the Lissajous pattern, the movement of the end of a paper strip held in front of the mouth, or the needle of a sound level meter.

Prosodic Drill

fɪfɪfɪ   fɪ**fɪ**fɪ   fɪfɪ**fɪ**

fɪfɪfɪfɪ   fɪ**fɪ**fɪfɪ   fɪfɪ**fɪ**fɪ

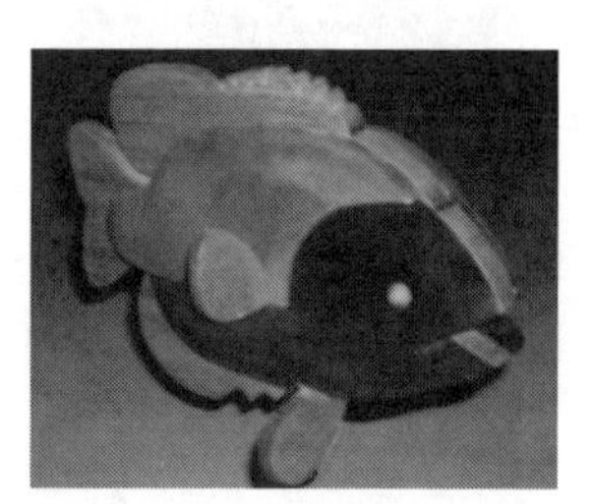

fish

Eat the ________.

phone   file   fire   fern   food

fill   fold   fan   fast   feel   fell

Lesson 22 /-f/

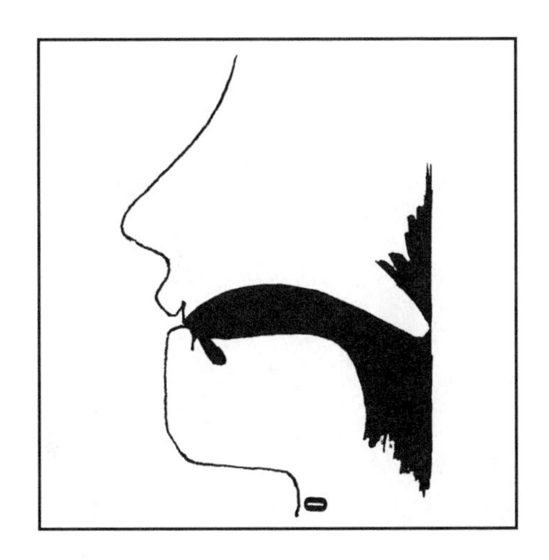

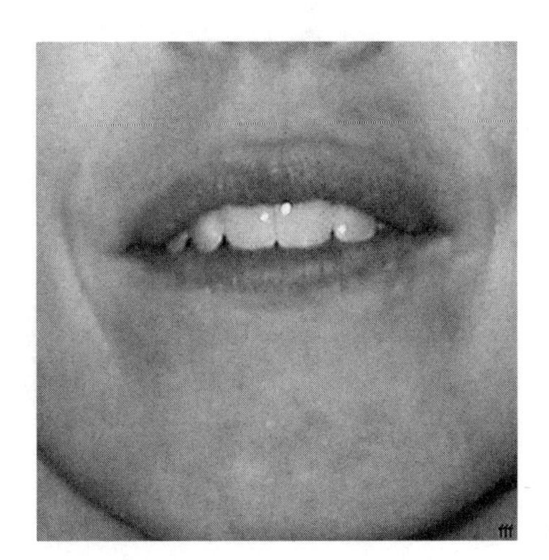

Lower lip touches upper teeth and breath passes through this articulation with audible friction (no voice). The articulation can be seen. The sound is high frequency. Evidence of it is indicated by the Lissajous pattern, the movement of a paper strip held in front of the mouth, or the needle of a sound level meter.

Prosodic Drill

aɪfaɪfaɪf   aɪf**aɪf**aɪf   aɪfaɪf**aɪf**

aɪfaɪfaɪfaɪf   aɪf**aɪf**aɪfaɪf   aɪfaɪf**aɪf**aɪf

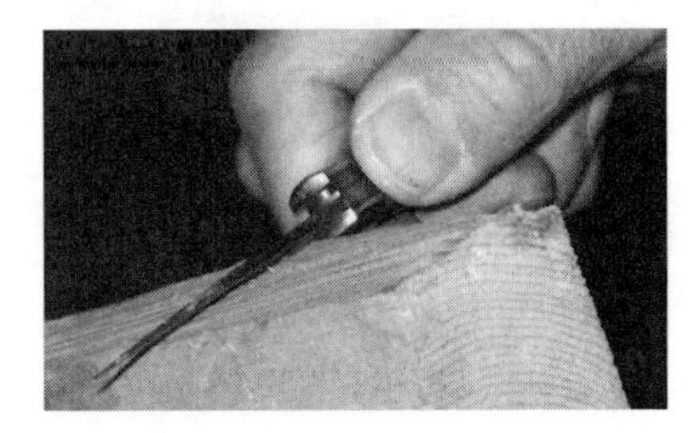

knife

Cut with a ________.

cough   muff   cuff   stuff   tough

puff   rough   loaf   off   chief

Lesson 23 /v-/

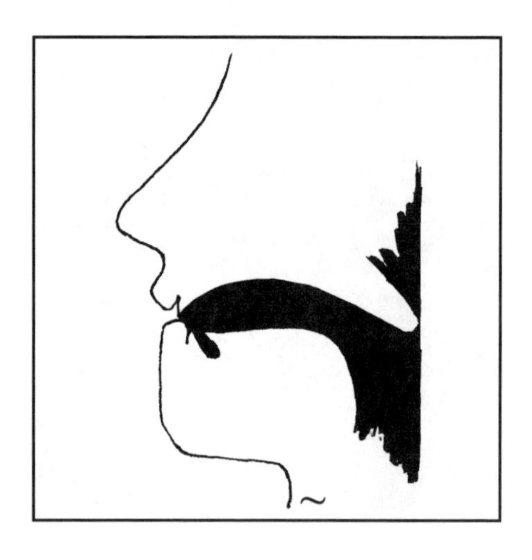

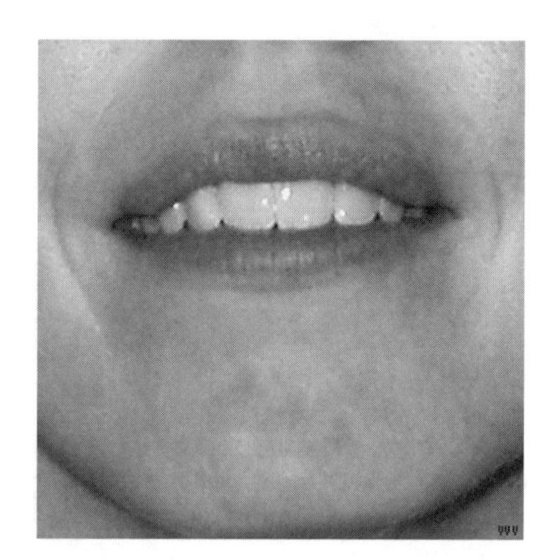

Lower lip touches upper teeth and voice passes through this articulation with audible friction. The lower lip vibrates. The articulation can be seen. The sound is low frequency and high frequency. Evidence of the sound is indicated by the Lissajous pattern, the movement of a paper strip, or the needle of a sound level meter.

Prosodic Drill

veveve veve**ve**ve veve**ve**

vevevevee veve**ve**veve veveve**ve**ve

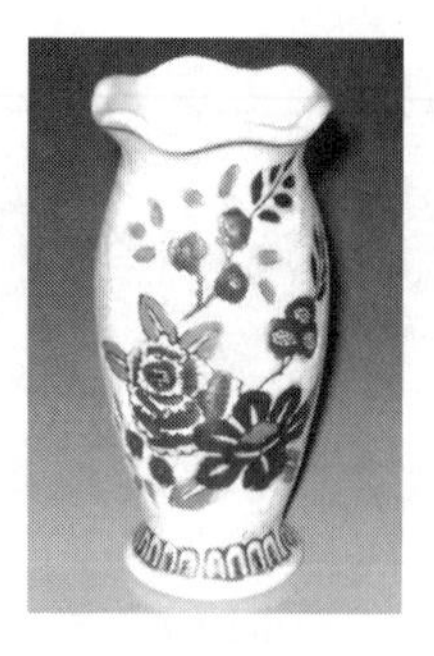

vase

Fill the ________.

vest veil vine vault view vat

veer vest voice viper void vote

Lesson 24 /-v/

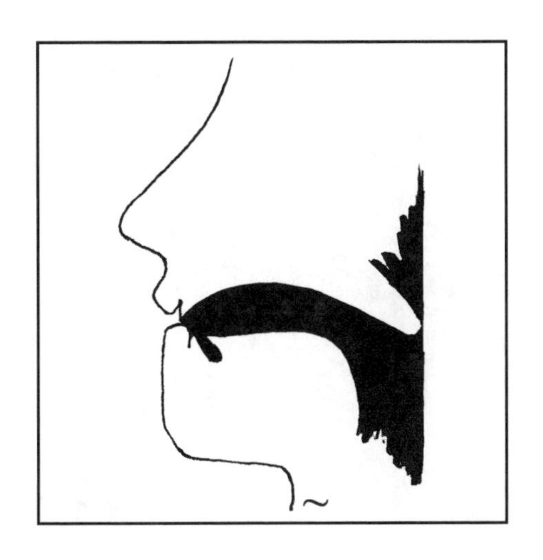

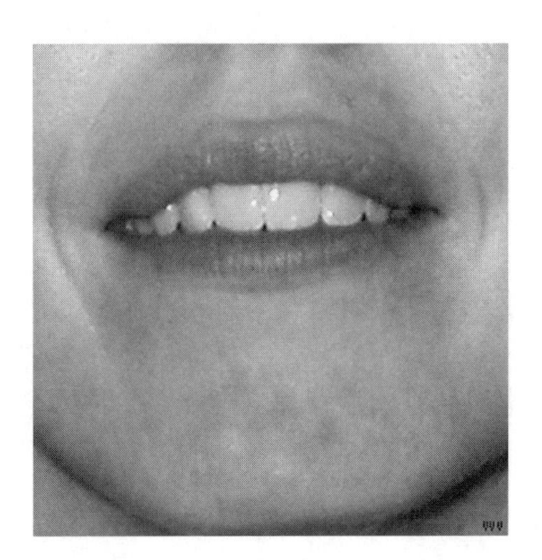

Lower lip touches upper teeth and voice passes through this articulation with audible friction. The lower lip vibrates. The articulation can be seen. The sound is low frequency and high frequency. Evidence of the sound is indicated by the Lissajous pattern, the movement of a paper strip, or the needle of a sound level meter.

Prosodic Drill

ʌvəvəv ʌv**ʌv**əv əvəv**ʌv**

ʌvəvəvəv əv**ʌv**əvəv əvəv**ʌv**əv

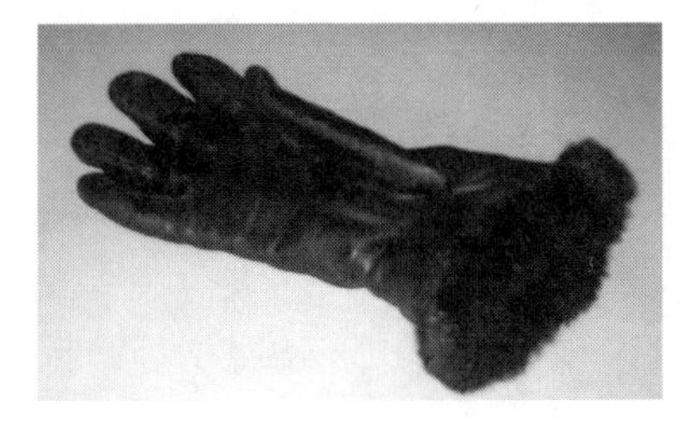

glove

Put on the ________.

weave groove stove shove five

give hive save pave dive

Lesson 25 /θ-/

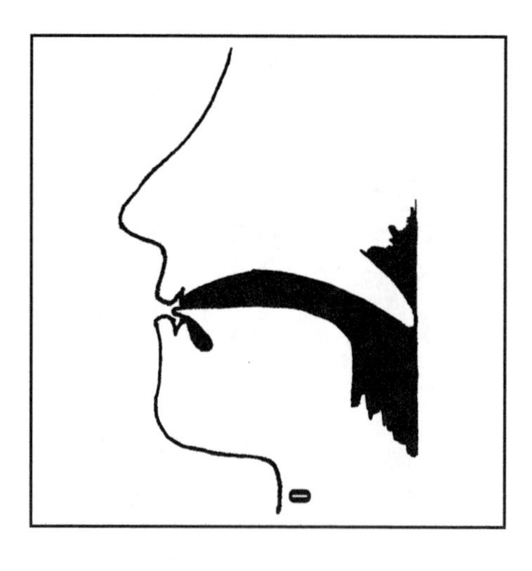

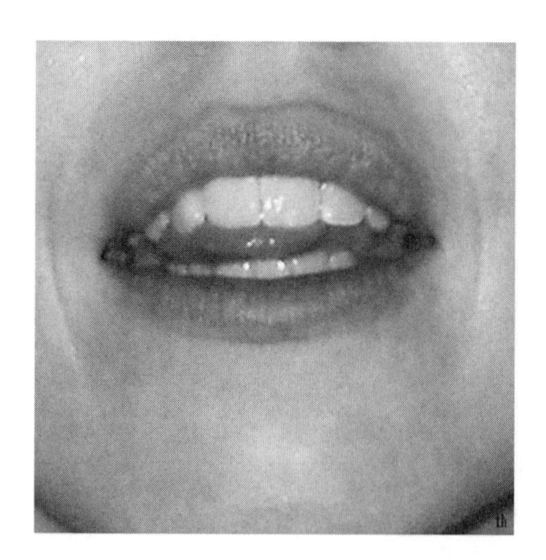

Tongue tip between the upper and lower teeth and breath passes between this articulation with audible friction (no voice). The articulation can be seen. The sound is high frequency. Evidence of the sound is indicated by the Lissajous pattern, the movement of a paper strip, or the needle of a sound level meter.

Prosodic Drill

θʌθəθə θə**θʌ**θə θəθə**θʌ**

θʌθəθəθə θə**θʌ**θəθə θəθə**θʌ**θə

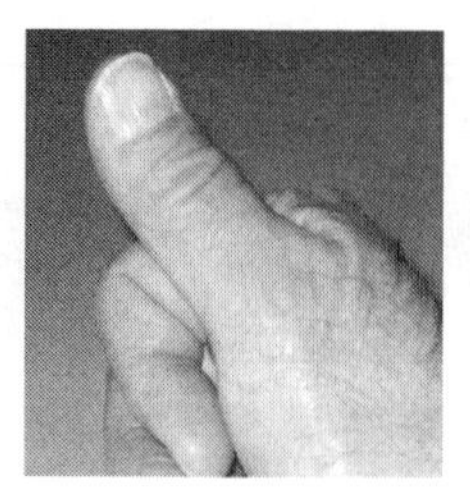

thumb

thistle think thing thimble

thorn thorax thong thought

Lesson 26 /-θ/

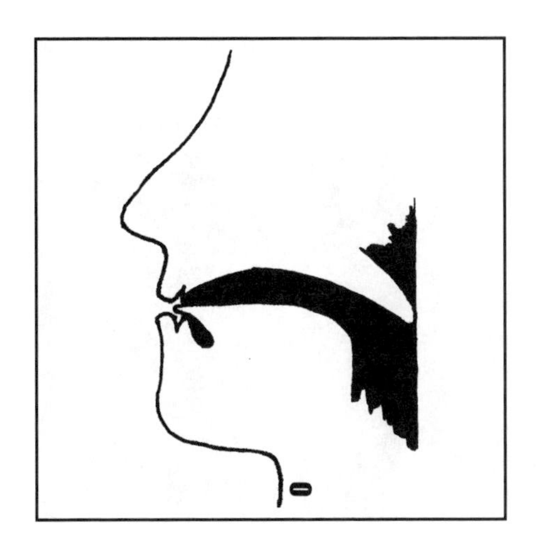

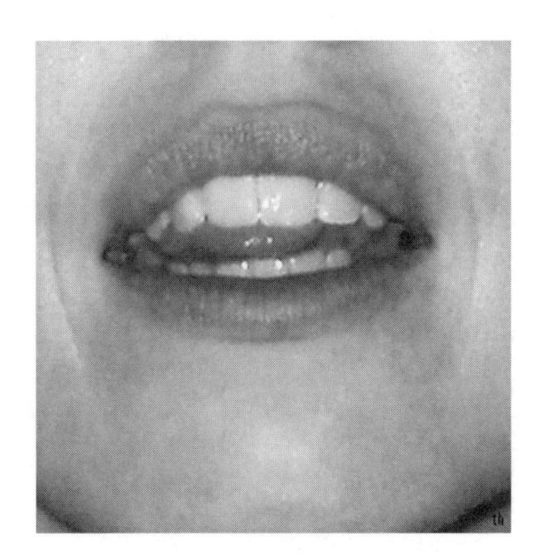

Tongue tip between the upper and lower teeth and breath passes between this articulation with audible friction (voiceless). The articulation can be seen. The sound is high frequency. Evidence of the sound is indicated by the Lissajous pattern, the movement of a paper strip, or the needle of a sound level meter.

Prosodic Drill

iθiθiθ iθ**iθ**iθ iθiθ**iθ**

iθiθiθiθ iθ**iθ**iθiθ iθiθ**iθ**iθ

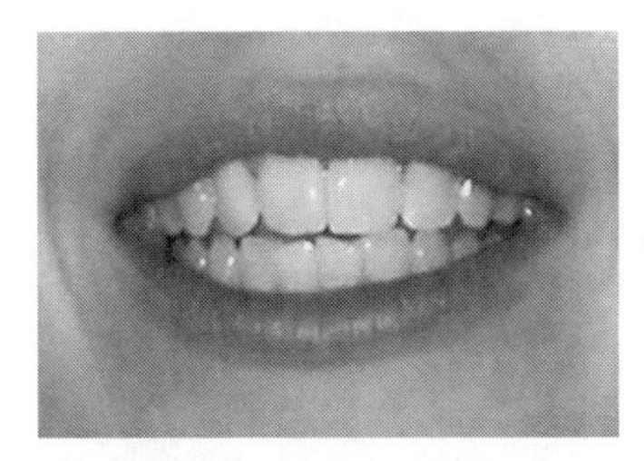

teeth

Brush your ________.

path bath math breath

moth cloth tooth

Lesson 27 / ð-/

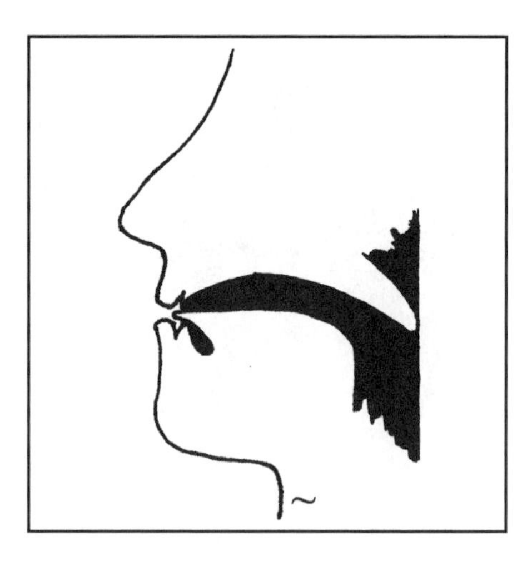

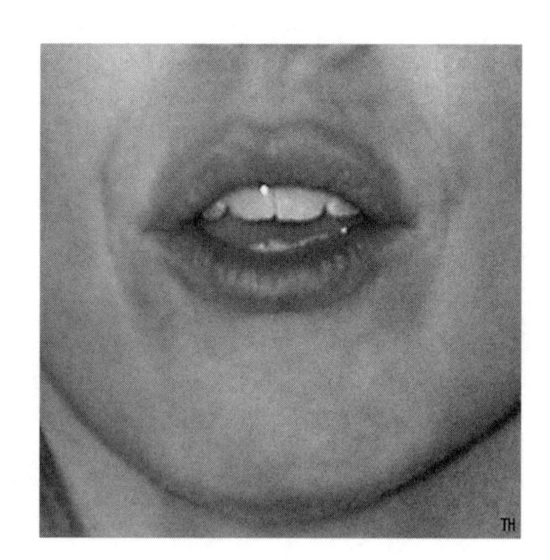

Tongue tip between the upper and lower teeth and voice passes between this articulation with audible friction. The tongue tip vibrates. The articulation can be seen. The sound is low, mid, and high frequency. Evidence of the sound is indicated by the Lissajous pattern, the movement of a paper strip, or the needle of a sound level meter.

Prosodic Drill

ðɛðɛðɛ ðɛ**ðɛ**ðɛ ðɛðɛ**ðɛ**

ðɛðɛðɛðɛ ðɛ**ðɛ**ðɛðɛ ðɛðɛ**ðɛ**ðɛ

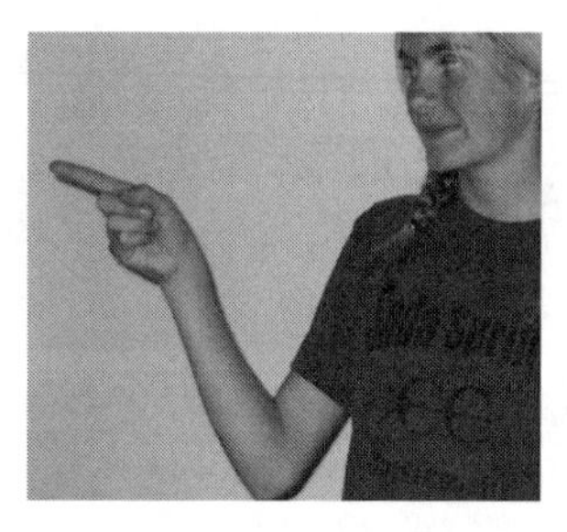

there

Point over ________.

the these those them then than

Lesson 28 /-ð/

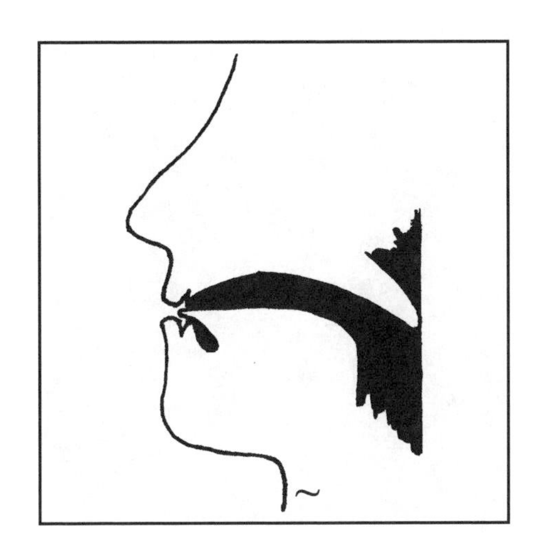

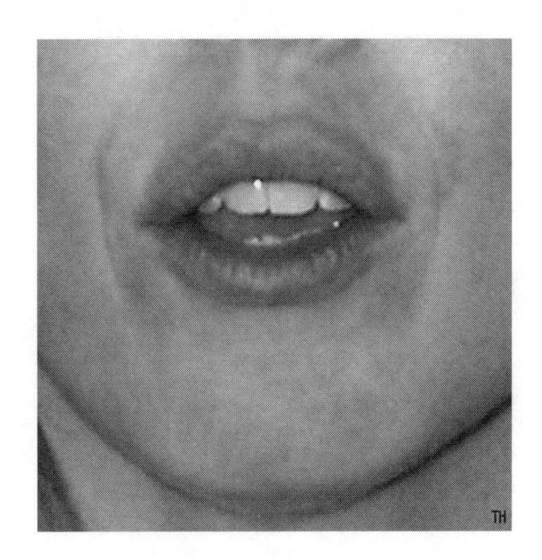

Tongue tip between upper and lower teeth and voice passes between this articulation with audible friction. The tongue tip vibrates. The articulation can be seen. The sound is low, mid, and high frequency. Evidence of the sound is indicated by the Lissajous pattern, the movement of a paper strip, or the needle of a sound level meter.

Prosodic Drill

eðeðeð eð**eð**eð eðeð**eð**

eðeðeðeð eð**eð**eðeð eðeð**eð**eð

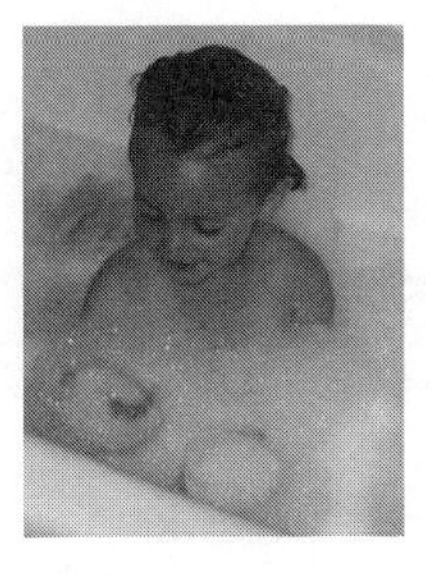

bathe

See him ________

lathe breathe clothe soothe smooth

Lesson 29 /h-/

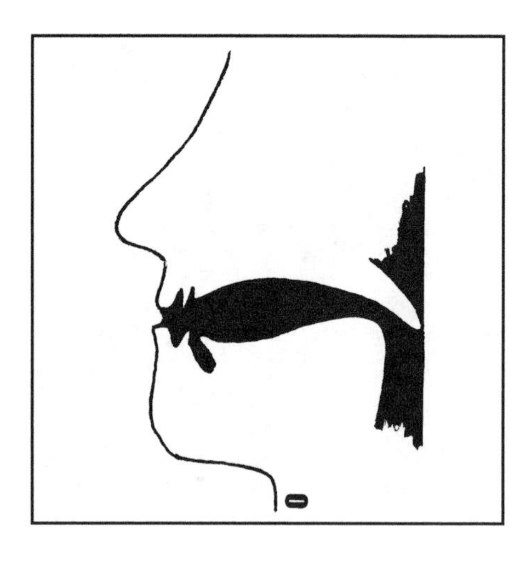

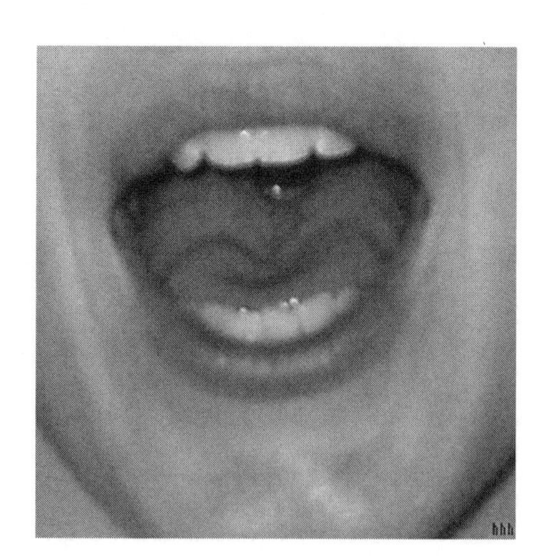

Breath passes through the mouth with audible friction. Tongue, mouth, and mandible positions determined by the preceding and succeeding vowel or diphthong. No voice. A place of articulation cannot be seen. There is a mid frequency clue. Evidence of the sound is indicated by the Lissajous pattern, the movement of a paper strip, or the needle of a sound level meter.

Prosodic Drill

hʊhʊhʊ hʊ**hʊ**hʊ hʊhʊ**hʊ**

hʊhʊhʊhʊ hʊ**hʊ**hʊhʊ hʊhʊ**hʊ**hʊ

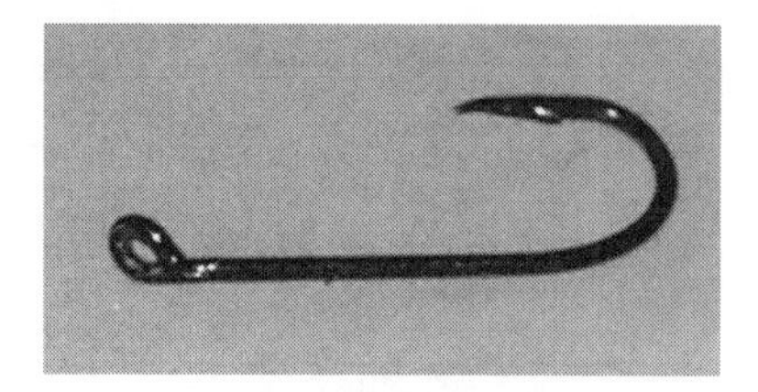

hook

Bait the ________.

he heat hit hedge help hair

hub hump heart hind hound

Lesson 30 /m-/

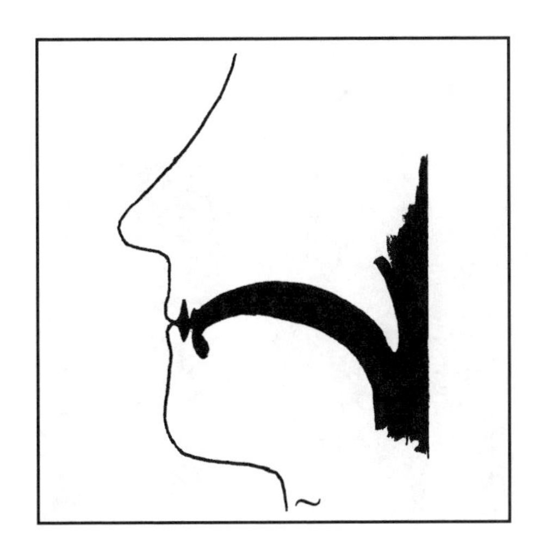

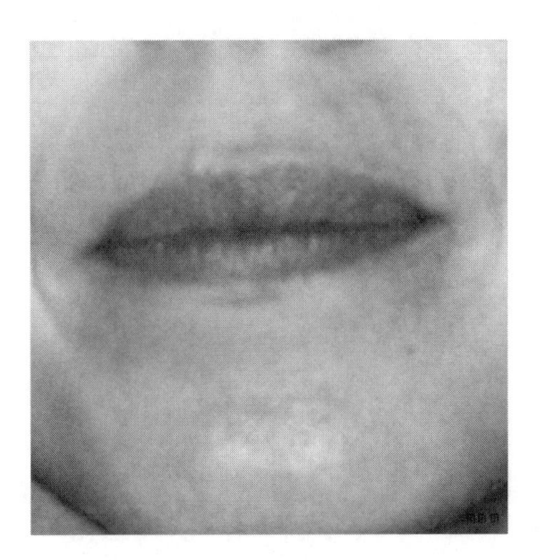

The lips are shut, the velopharyngeal port is open, and voice passes through the nose. Voicing may be felt on the throat, and nasality on the nose. A low frequency sound. Evidence of the sound is indicated by the Lissajous pattern, the movement of a paper strip, or the needle of a sound level meter.

Prosodic Drill

mæmæmæ mæ**mæ**mæ mæmæ**mæ**

mæmæmæmæ mæ**mæ**mæmæ mæmæ**mæ**mæ

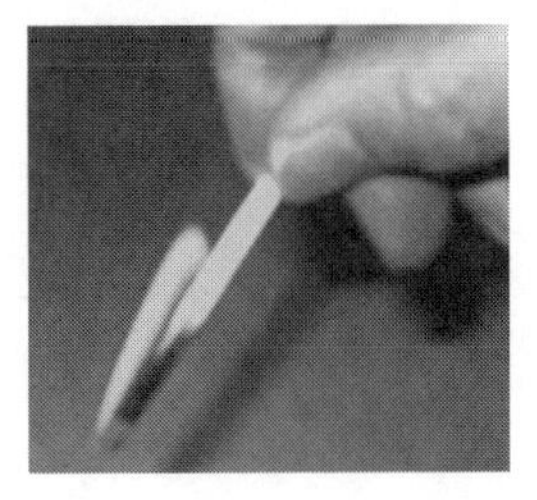

match

Light a ________.

milk men man mask muff

mug moon mop mouse mouth

Lesson 31 /-m/

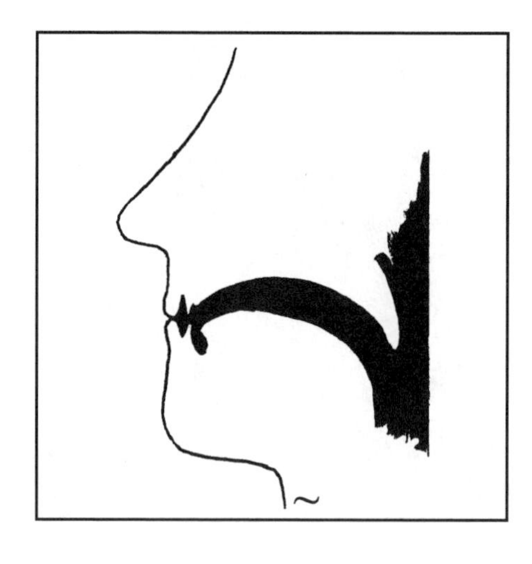

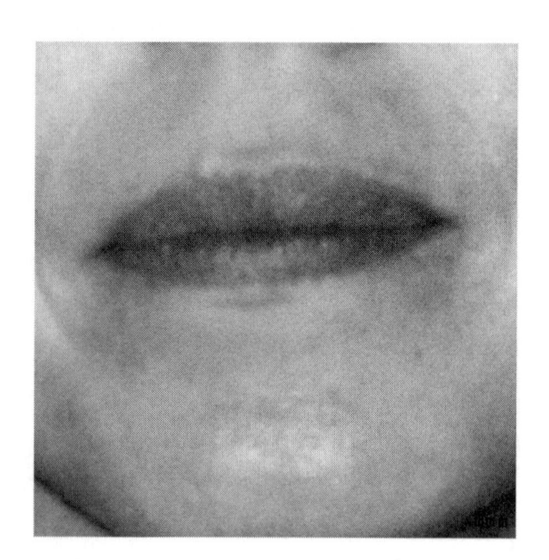

The lips are shut, the velopharyngeal port is open, and voice passes through the nose. Voicing may be felt on the throat, and nasality on the nose. A low frequency sound. Evidence of the sound is indicated by the Lissajous pattern, the movement of a paper strip, or the needle of a sound level meter.

Prosodic Drill

ʌməməm əm**ʌm**əm əməm**ʌm**

ʌməməməm əm**ʌm**əməm əməm**ʌm**əm

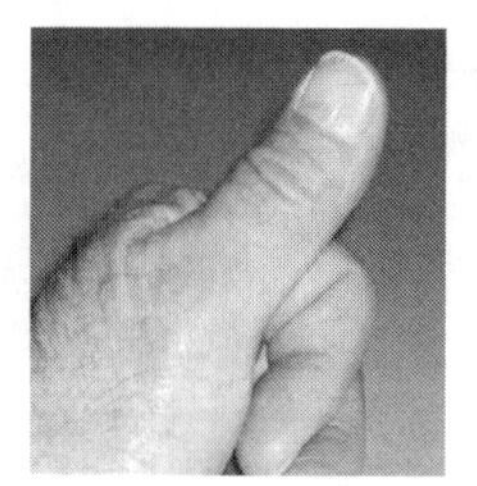

thumb

Show me your ________.

beam seam game same dam

gum dumb dome comb farm charm

Lesson 32 /d-/

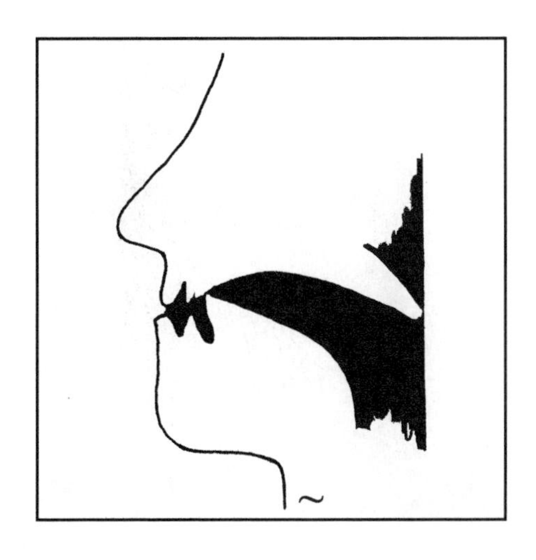

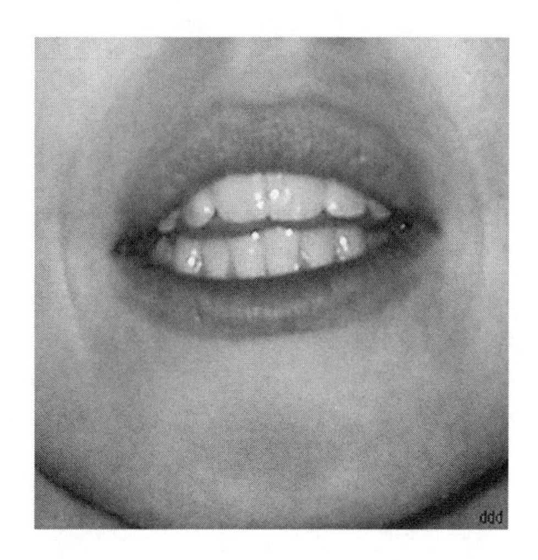

The tongue tip against the alveolar ridge momentarily shuts off the air stream. Air dams and is explosively released with voice as the tongue tip separates from the ridge. Voicing may be felt on the throat. The articulation position and release can be seen when the mouth is open and the head tilted back. A low-mid frequency sound. The sound is indicated either by the Lissajous pattern, the movement of a paper strip, or the needle of a sound level meter.

Prosodic Drill

dododo do**do**do dodo**do**

dodododo do**do**dodo dodo**do**do

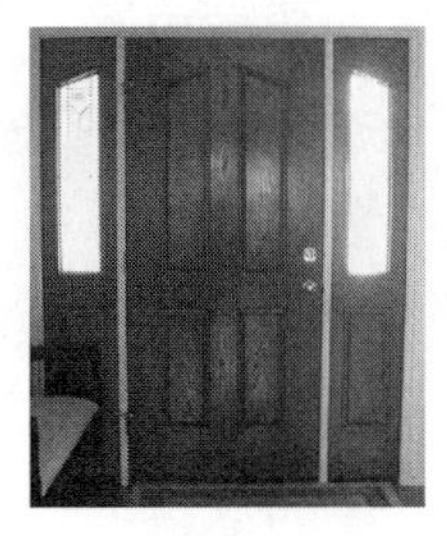

door

Shut the ________.

deep deer deck dam dump

dirt doom dome doll dime down

Lesson 33 /-d/

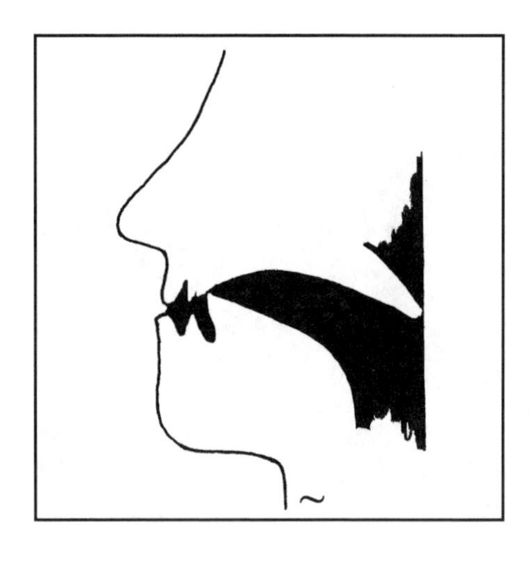

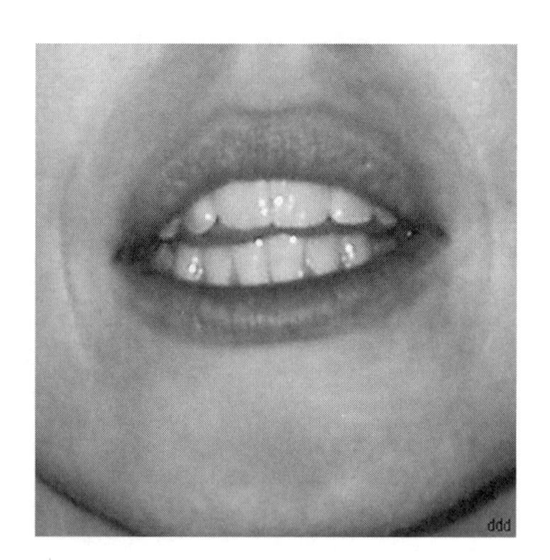

The tongue tip against the alveolar ridge momentarily shuts off the air stream. Air dams and is released slightly with voicing. The articulation position and slight release can be seen when the mouth is open and the head tilted back. A low-mid frequency sound. The sound is indicated either by a Lissajous pattern, the movement of a paper strip, or the needle of a sound level meter.

Prosodic Drill

ɛdɛdɛd ɛd**ɛd**ɛd ɛdɛd**ɛd**

ɛdɛdɛdɛd ɛd**ɛd**ɛdɛd ɛdɛd**ɛd**ɛd

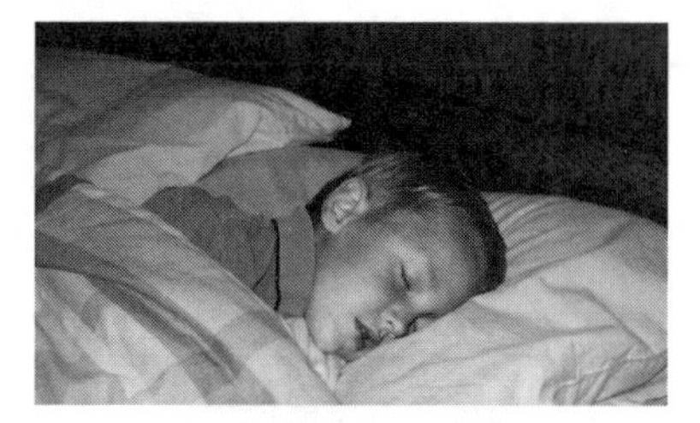

bed

Sleep in a ________.

bead feed lid head dead bad lad

mud heard food road pod blade died

Lesson 34 /t-/

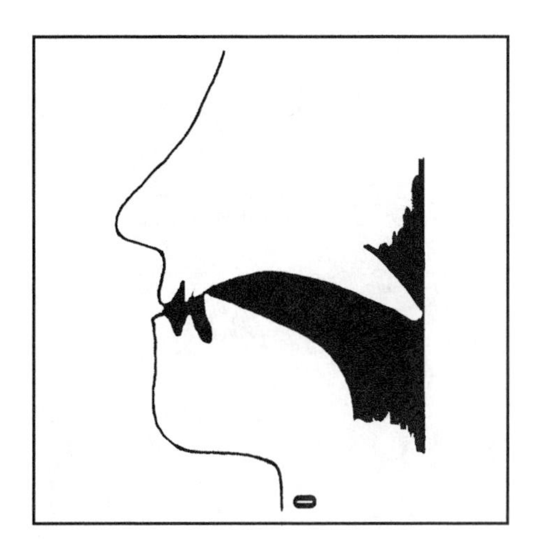

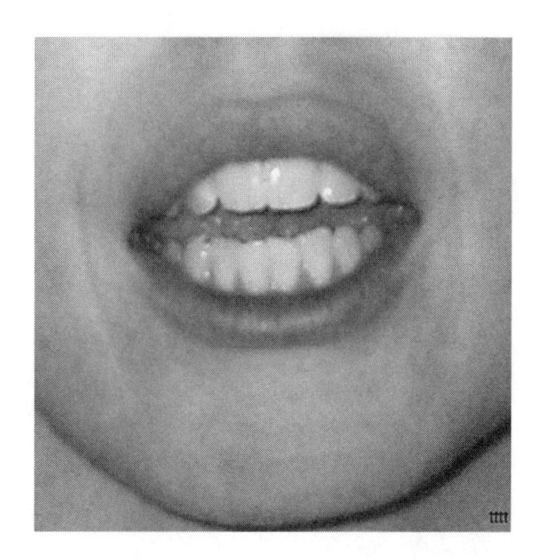

The tongue tip against the alveolar ridge momentarily shuts off the air stream. Air dams and is explosively released as the tongue separates from the ridge. The articulation position and release can be seen when the mouth is open and the head tilted back. A low-mid frequency sound. The sound is indicated either by a Lissajous pattern, the movement of a paper strip, or the needle of a sound level meter.

Prosodic Drill

tetete te**te**te tete**te**

tetetete te**te**tete tete**te**te

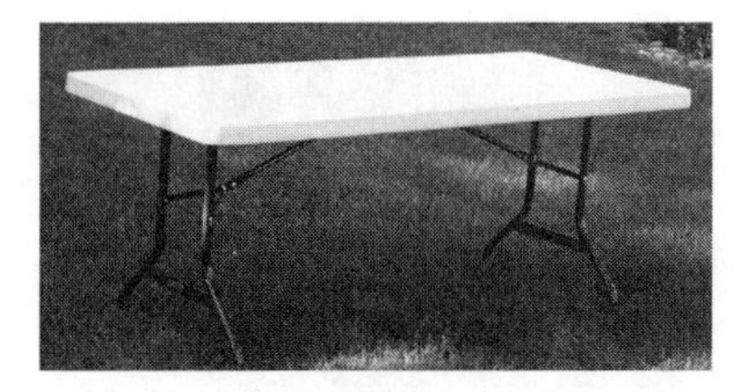

table

Eat at the ________.

teeth tip tail ten tab tub

turtle tooth toe top towel tie

Lesson 35 /-t/

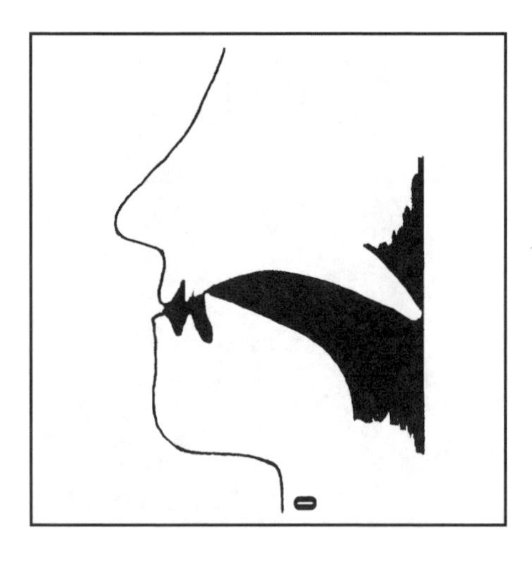

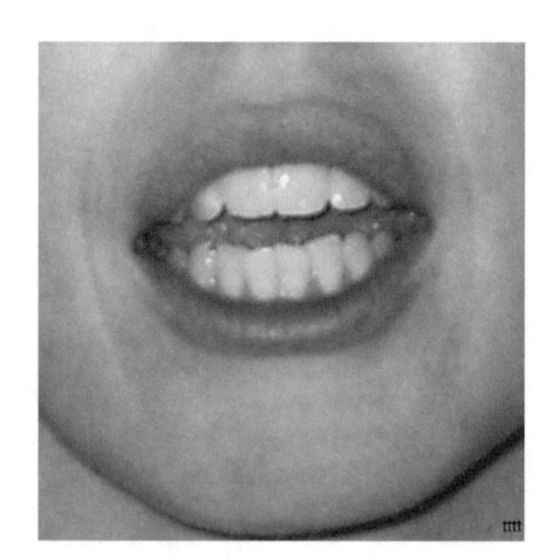

The tongue tip against the alveolar ridge momentarily shuts off the air stream. Air dams and is explosively released as the tongue separates from the ridge. The articulation position and release can be seen when the mouth is open and the head tilted back. A low-mid frequency sound is indicated either by a Lissajous pattern, the movement of a paper strip, or the needle of a sound level meter.

Prosodic Drill

ɪtɪtɪt   ɪt**ɪt**ɪt   ɪtɪt**ɪt**

ɪtɪtɪtɪt   ɪt**ɪt**ɪtɪt   ɪtɪt**ɪt**ɪt

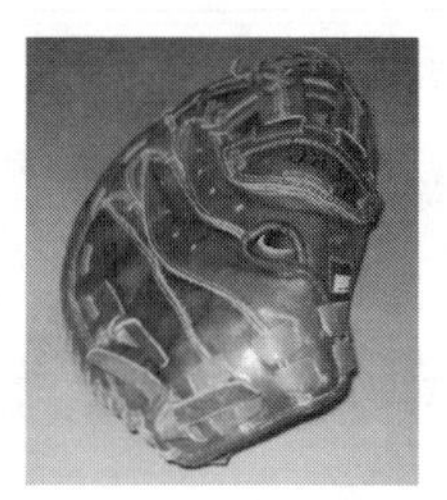

mitt

It's a baseball ________.

meet   met   mate   mat   mutt   dirt

boot   coat   cot   bout   bite

Lesson 36 /ʃ-/

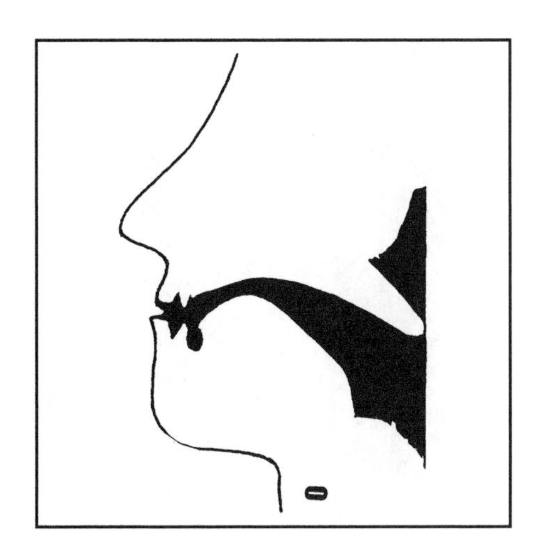

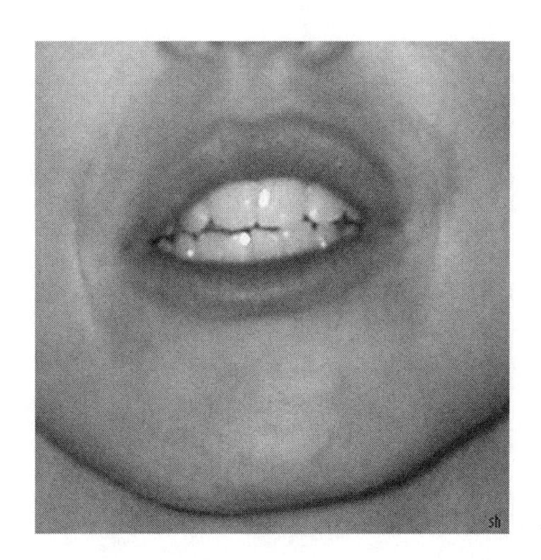

Front of tongue is raised, forming a broad central aperture. Breath passes through this aperture and strikes nearly shut teeth with audible friction. Lips are squared. The broad tongue position can be seen by opening the mouth and spreading the lips. When the lips are squared and the sound produced, which is mid-high frequency, the tongue cannot be seen. The sound is indicated either by a Lissajous pattern, the movement of a paper strip, or the needle of a sound level meter.

Prosodic Drill

ʃuʃuʃu ʃu**ʃu**ʃu ʃuʃu**ʃu**

ʃuʃuʃuʃu ʃu**ʃu**ʃuʃu ʃuʃu**ʃu**ʃu

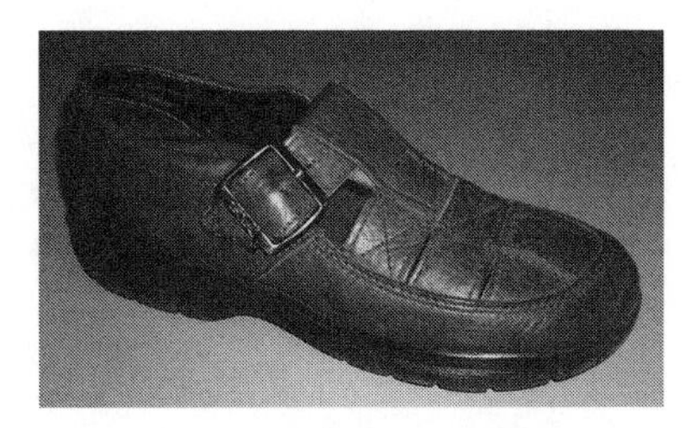

shoe

Put on the ________.

sheep ship shape shell shut shirt

shoe show shot shout shy

Lesson 37 /-ʃ/

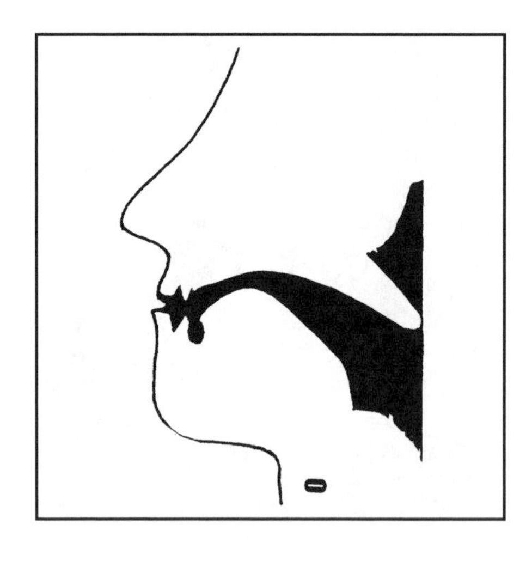

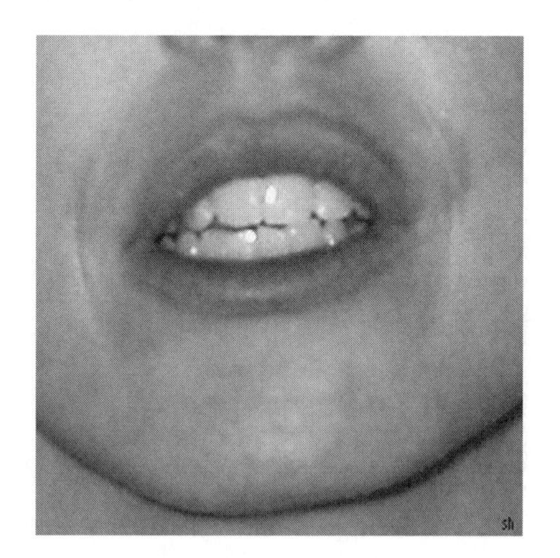

Front of tongue is raised, forming a broad central aperture. Breath passes through this aperture and strikes nearly shut teeth with audible friction. Lips are squared. The broad tongue position can be seen by opening the mouth and spreading the lips. When the lips are squared and the sound produced, which is mid-high frequency, the tongue cannot be seen. The sound is indicated by a Lissajous pattern, the movement of a paper strip, or the needle of a sound level meter.

Prosodic Drill

ɪʃɪʃɪʃ ɪʃ**ɪʃ**ɪʃ ɪʃɪʃ**ɪʃ**

ɪʃɪʃɪʃɪ ɪʃ**ɪʃ**ɪʃɪʃ ɪʃɪʃ**ɪʃ**ɪʃ

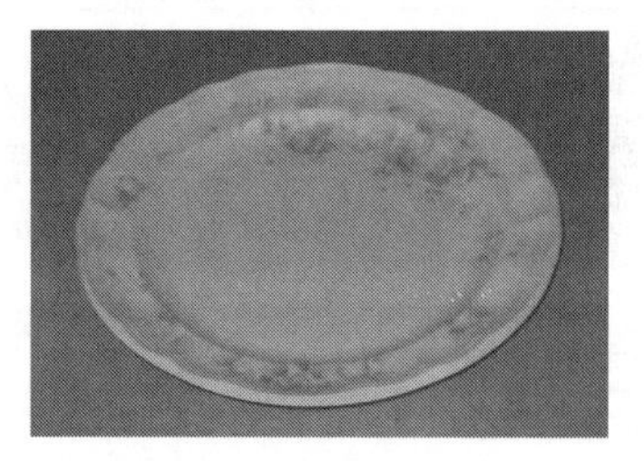

dish

Eat on a ________.

fish mesh mash sash mush

hush crush push bush posh

Lesson 38 /-ʒ/

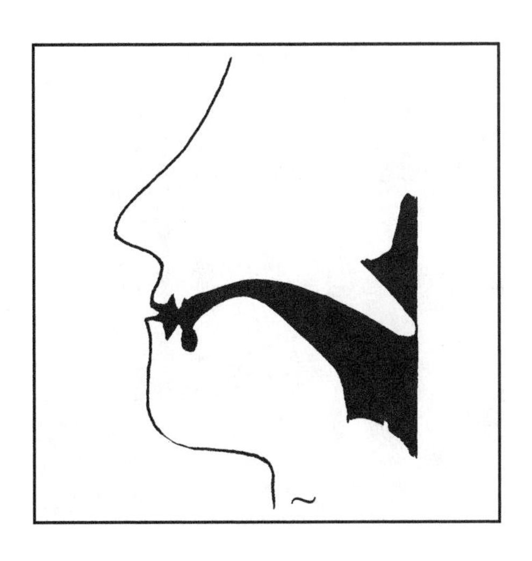

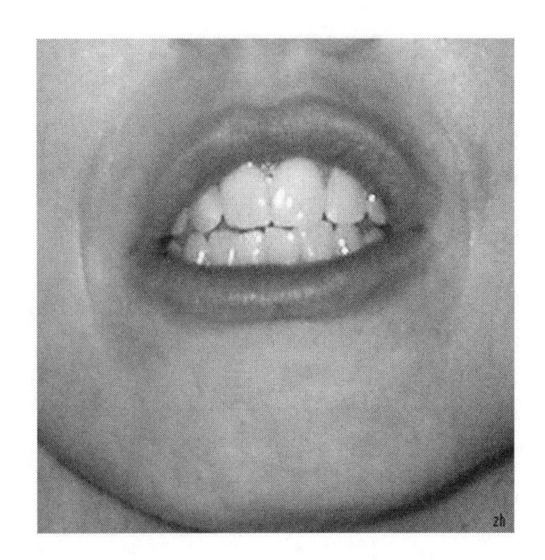

Front view of tongue is raised, forming a broad central aperture. Voice passes through this aperture and strikes nearly shut teeth with audible friction. Lips are squared. The broad tongue position can be seen by opening the mouth and spreading the lips. When the lips are squared and the sound produced, which is a low-mid-high frequency buzz, the tongue cannot be seen. The sound is indicated by a Lissajous pattern, the movement of a paper strip, or the needle of a sound level meter.

Prosodic Drill

ɪʒɪʒɪʒ ɪʒ**ɪʒ**ɪʒ ɪʒɪʒ**ɪʒ**

ɪʒɪʒɪʒɪʒ ɪʒ**ɪʒ**ɪʒɪʒ ɪʒɪʒ**ɪʒ**ɪʒ

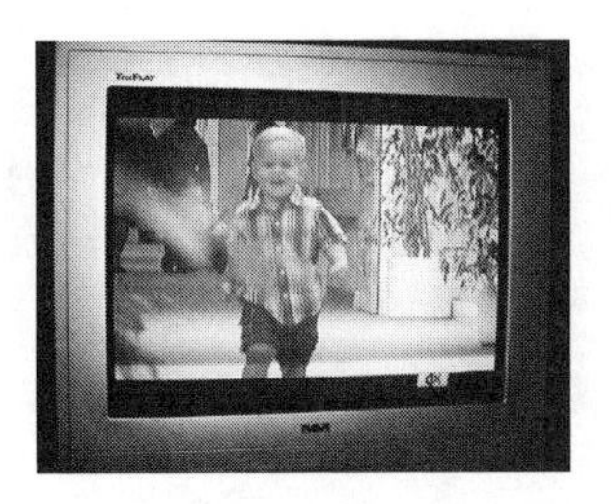

television

Watch ________.

measure pleasure vision Asian

Persian adhesion aversion

Lesson 39 /s-/

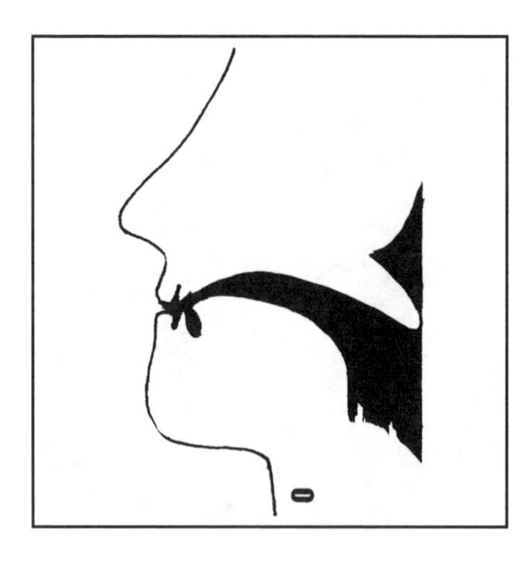

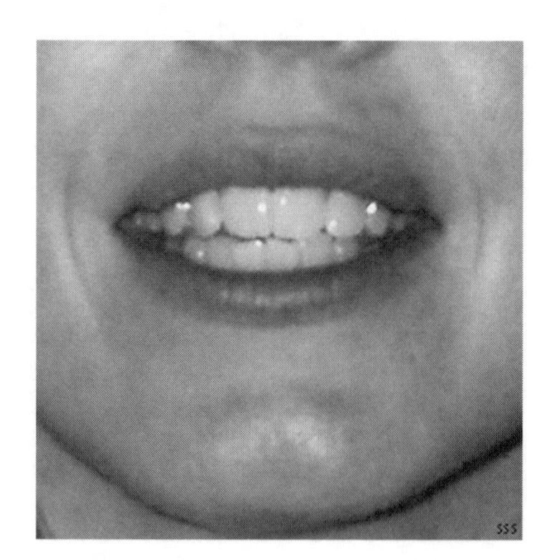

Front of tongue is raised high, forming a narrow central aperture. Breath passes through it striking nearly shut teeth with audible high frequency friction. The high tongue articulation ordinarily cannot be seen because the teeth are nearly closed. It can be seen if the mouth is opened. The sound is indicated by a Lissajous pattern, the movement of a paper strip, or the needle of a sound level meter.

Prosodic Drill

sososo so**so**so sososo**so**

sosososo so**so**soso soso**so**so

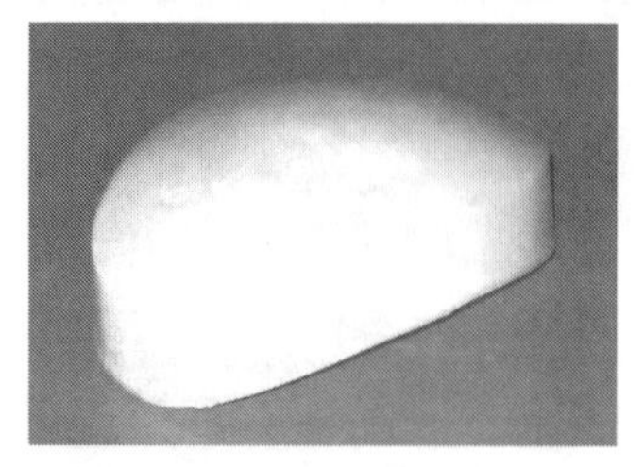

soap

Wash with ________.

seep sick sing set sash sad

soup suit sore suck sock side

Lesson 40 /-s/

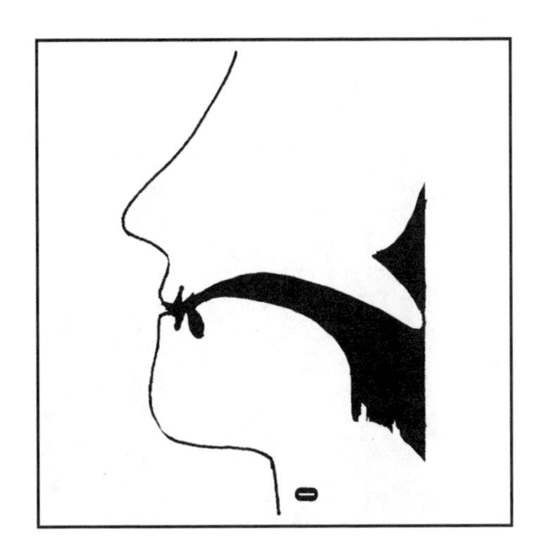

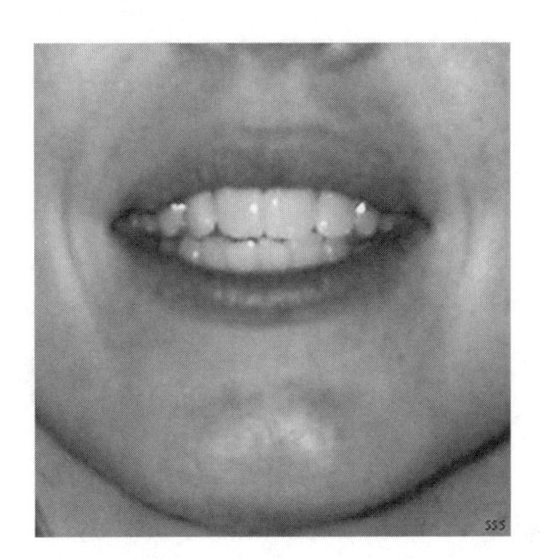

Front of tongue is raised high, forming a narrow central aperture. Breath passes through it striking nearly shut teeth with audible high frequency friction. The high tongue articulation ordinarily cannot be seen because the teeth are nearly closed. It can be seen if the mouth is open. The sound is indicated by a Lissajous pattern, the movement of a paper strip, or the needle of a sound level meter.

Prosodic Drill

ʌSəsəs əs**ʌS**əs əsəs**ʌS**

ʌSəsəsəs əs**ʌS**əsəs əsəs**ʌS**əs

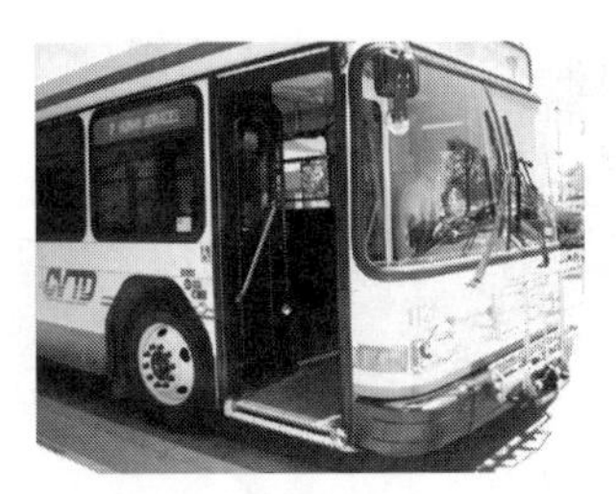

bus

Ride the ________.

geese miss kiss mess gas

fuss goose boss mouse mice

Lesson 41 /z-/

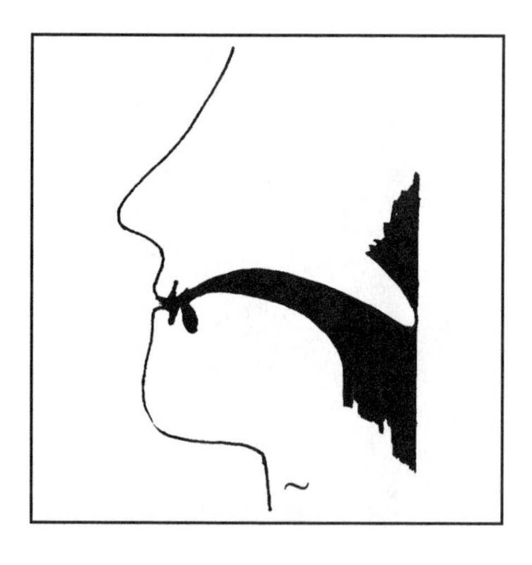

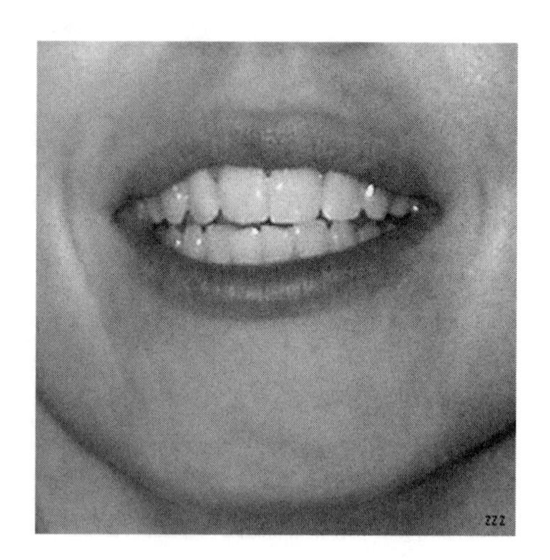

Front of tongue is raised high, forming a narrow central aperture. Voice passes through it striking nearly closed teeth with audible low and high frequency friction. The high tongue articulation ordinarily cannot be seen because the teeth are nearly closed. It can be seen if the mouth is open. Voicing can be felt on the throat. Tongue tip vibration can be felt. The sound is indicated by either a Lissajous pattern, the movement of a paper strip, or the needle of a sound level meter.

Prosodic Drill

ZIZIZI ZI**ZI**ZI ZIZI**ZI**

ZIZIZIZI ZI**ZI**ZIZI ZIZI**ZI**ZI

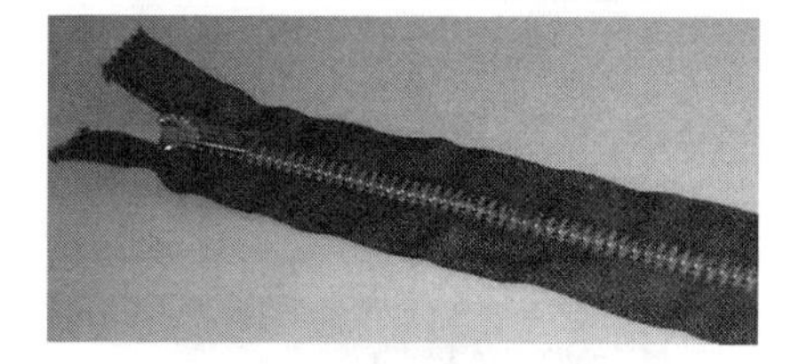

zipper

That's a ________.

zeal zip zit zest zap zoo zone

Lesson 42 */-z/*

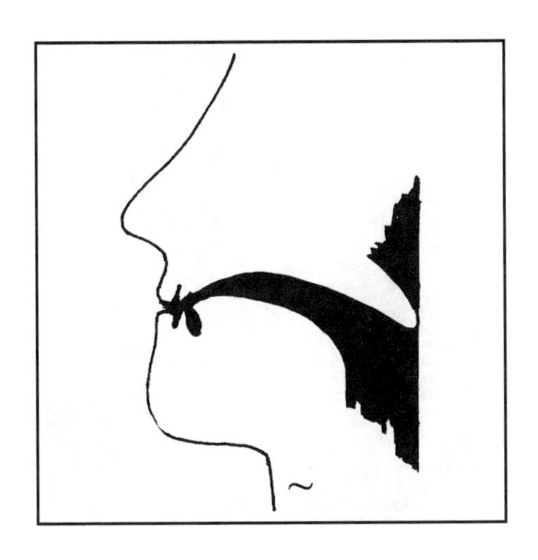

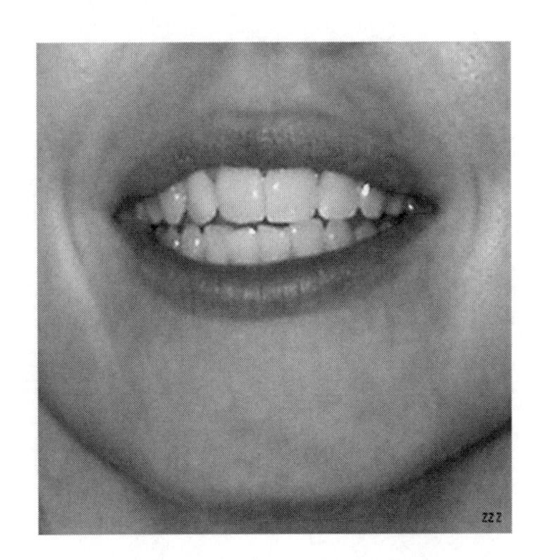

Front of tongue is raised high, forming a narrow central aperture. Voices passes through it striking nearly closed teeth with audible low and high frequency friction. The high tongue articulation ordinarily cannot be seen because the teeth are nearly closed. It can be seen if the mouth is open. Voicing can be felt on the throat. Tongue tip vibration can be felt. The sound is indicated by either a Lissajous pattern, the movement of a paper strip, or the needle of a sound level meter.

Prosodic Drill

aɪzaɪzaɪz aiz**aɪz**aɪz aɪzaɪz**aɪz**

aɪzaɪzaɪzaɪz aiz**aɪz**aɪzaɪz aizaɪz**aiz**aɪz

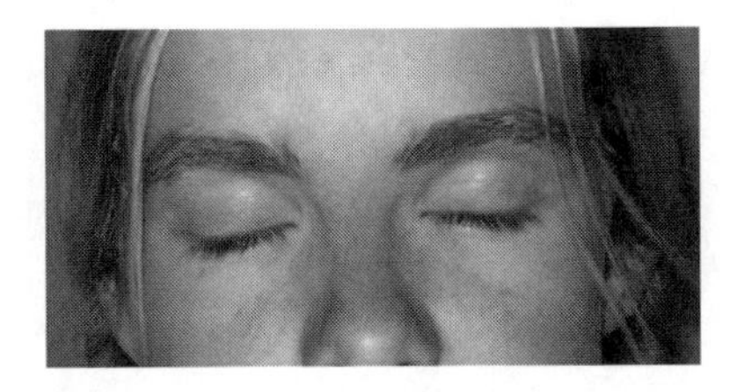

eyes

Close your ________.

bees is pigs beds eggs has

was buzz lose pose pause cows

Lesson 43 /n-/

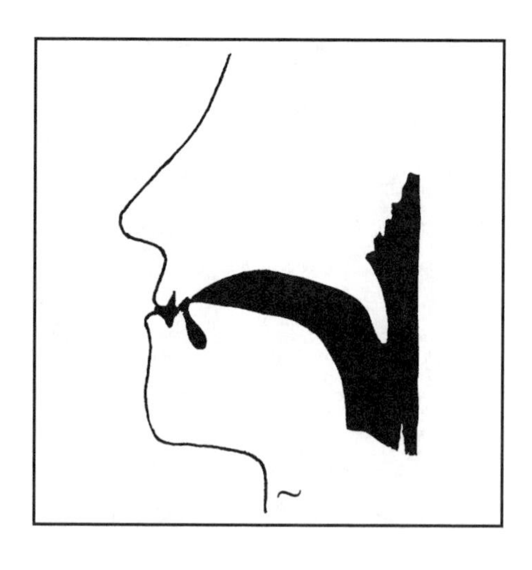

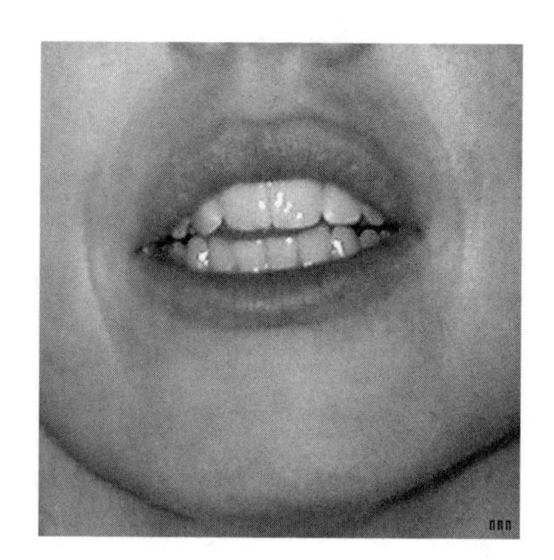

Tongue tip is to the alveolar ridge, velopharyngeal port is open, and voice passes through the nose. The tongue tip ordinarily cannot be seen. It can be seen if the mouth is open and the head tilted back. Voicing may be felt on the throat. Nasality may be felt on the nose. The sound is low frequency. The sound is indicated by either a Lissajous pattern, the movement of a paper strip, or the needle of a sound level meter.

Prosodic Drill

naɪnaɪnaɪ naɪ**naɪ**naɪ naɪnaɪ**naɪ**

naɪnaɪnaɪnaɪ naɪ**naɪ**naɪnaɪ naɪnaɪ**naɪ**naɪ

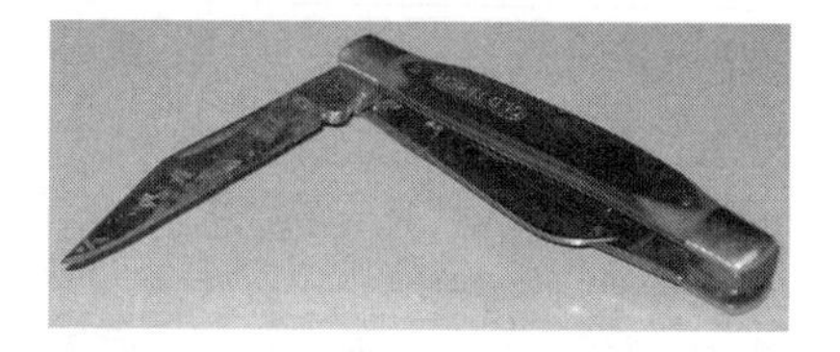

knife

Close the ________.

knee knit net nail nap nut

noose nose not now night

Lesson 44 /-n/

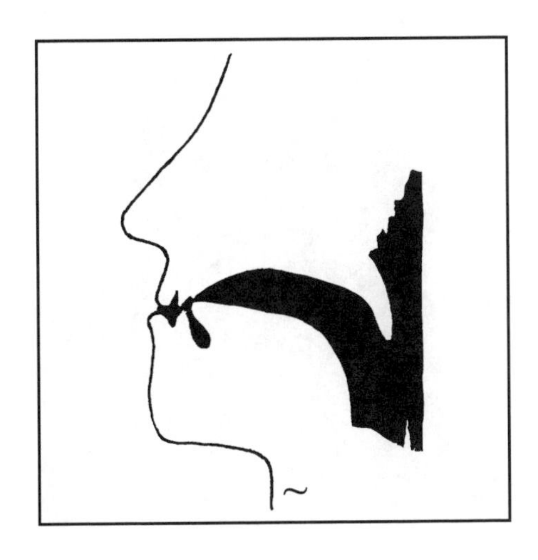

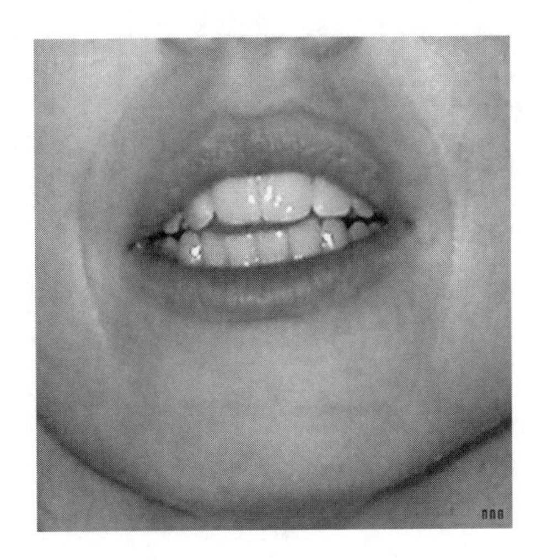

Tongue tip is to the alveolar ridge, velopharyngeal port is open, and voice passes through the nose. The tongue tip ordinarily cannot be seen. It can be seen if the mouth is open and the head tilted back. Voicing may be felt on the throat. Nasality may be felt on the nose. The sound is low frequency. It is indicated by a Lissajous pattern, the movement of a paper strip, or the movement of the sound level meter needle.

Prosodic Drill

ænænæn   æn**æn**æn   ænæn**æn**

ænænænæn   æn**æn**ænæn   ænæn**æn**æn

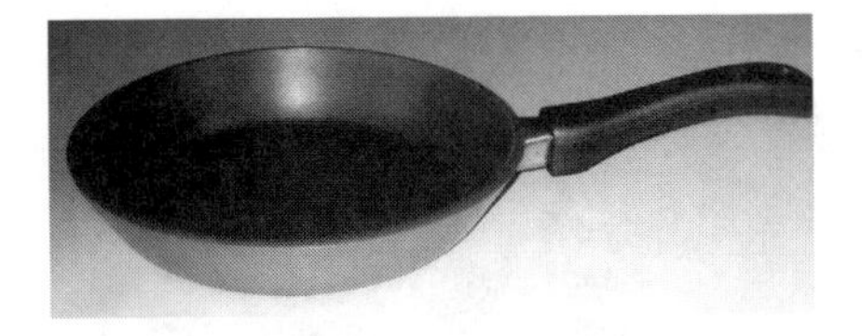

pan

Heat the ________.

bean   pin   pen   man   fun

boon   bone   phone   lawn   town   pine

Lesson 45 /l-/

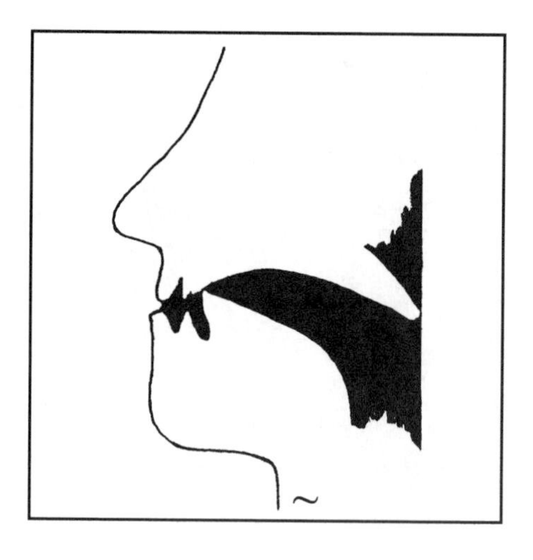

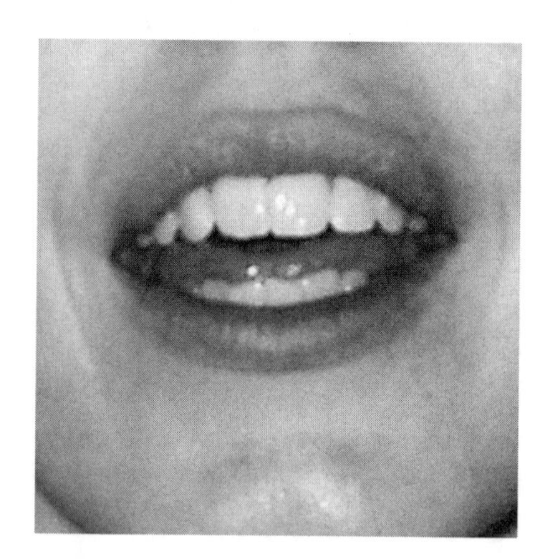

Tongue tip is to the alveolar ridge, sides of the tongue are lowered, and voice passes laterally through the mouth. The tongue tip can be seen if the mouth is open and the head tilted back. The sides of the tongue cannot be seen. Voicing may be felt on the throat. The sound is low frequency. It is indicated by a Lissajous pattern, a paper strip movement, or a sound level meter needle movement. It may help to place the tongue blade on the upper lip to make the sound, and then pull it back to its normal location.

Prosodic Drill

lalala la**la**la lala**la**

lalalala la**la**lala lala**la**la

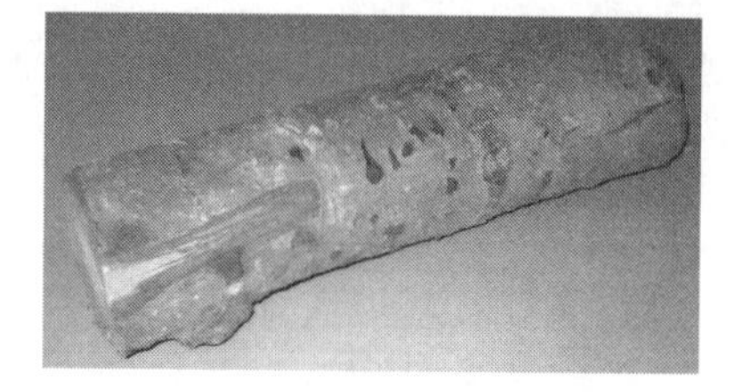

log

Chop the ________.

leaf lick leg lake laugh luck

loose lobe lob loud like

Lesson 46 /-l/

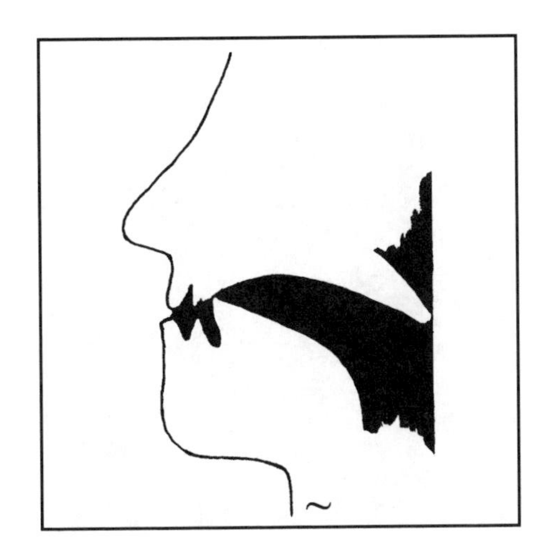

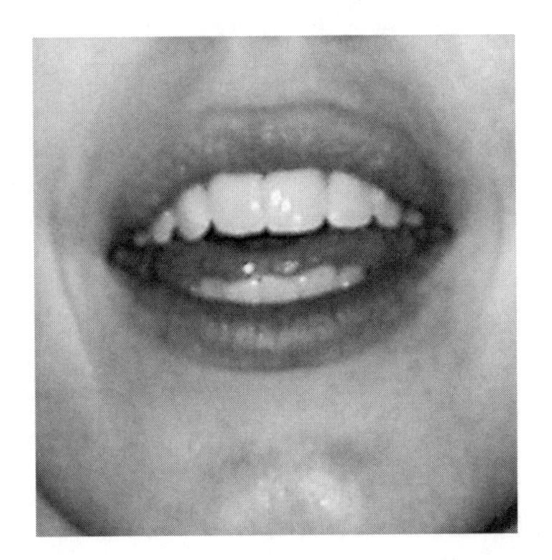

Tongue tip is to the alveolar ridge, sides of the tongue are lowered, and voice passes laterally through the mouth. The tongue tip can be seen if the mouth is open and the head tilted back. The sides of the tongue cannot be seen. Voicing may be felt on the throat. The sound is low frequency. The sound is indicated by a Lissajous pattern, a paper strip movement, or a sound level meter needle movement. It may help to place the tongue blade on the upper lip to make the sound, and then pull it back to its normal location.

Prosodic Drill

elelel el**el**el elel**el**

elelelel el**el**elel elel**el**el

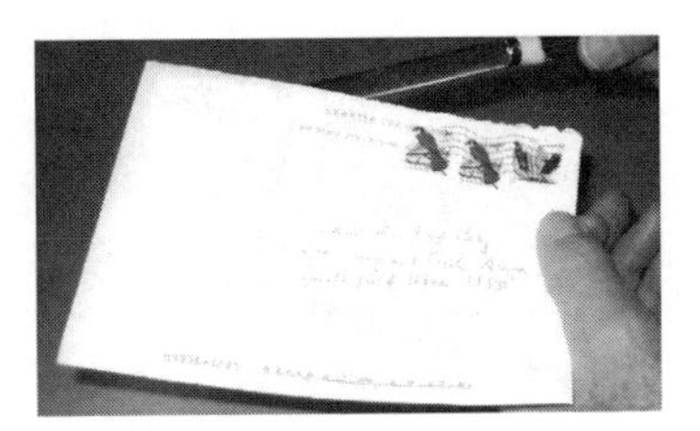

mail

Open the ________.

peal pill pell pail pal pull

pool pole pall towel tile

Lesson 47 /g-/

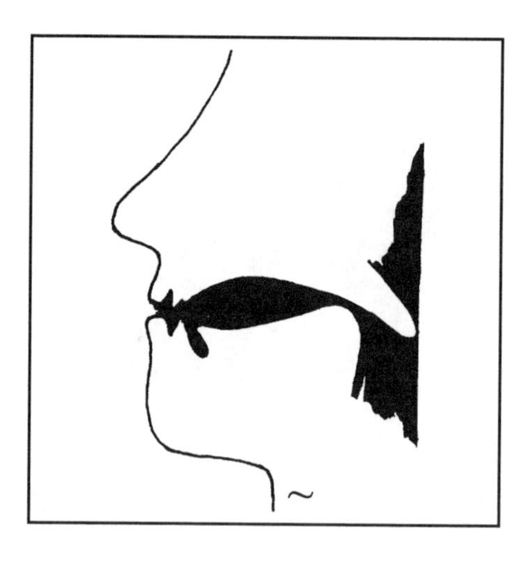

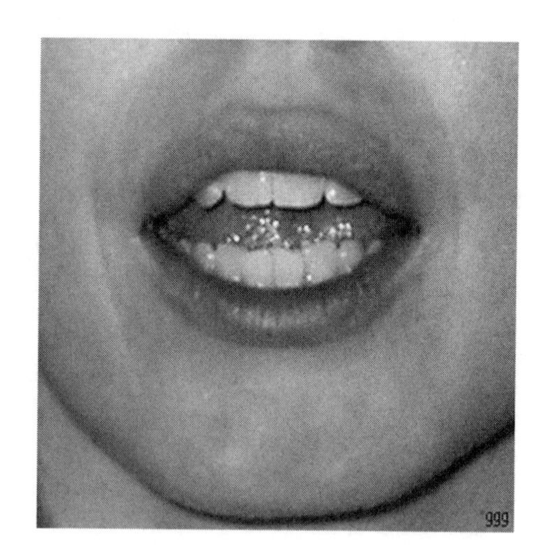

Back of the tongue against the velum shuts off the voiced air stream. Air dams up, and then the back of the tongue explosively separates from the velum, releasing the voice. The sound is low and high frequency. Voicing and quick release may be felt by placing a finger tip on the skin covering the thyroid cartilage. The original tongue position can be seen by opening the mouth and tilting back the head while using a flashlight and looking into a mirror. The sound is indicated by a Lissajous pattern, a paper strip movement, or a sound level meter needle movement.

Prosodic Drill

gægægæ gæ**gæ**gæ gægæ**gæ**

gægægægæ gæ**gæ**gægæ gægæ**gæ**gæ

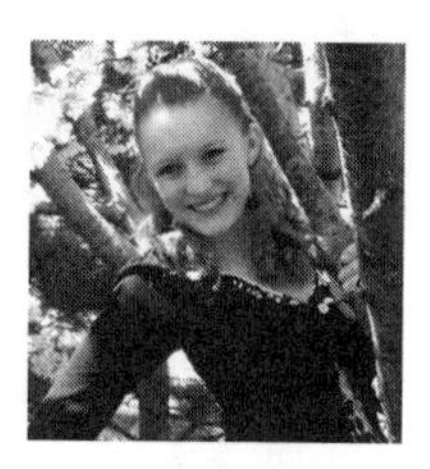

gal

She is a ________.

geese gill gale gull girl

goose ghost gob gout guile

Lesson 48 /-g/

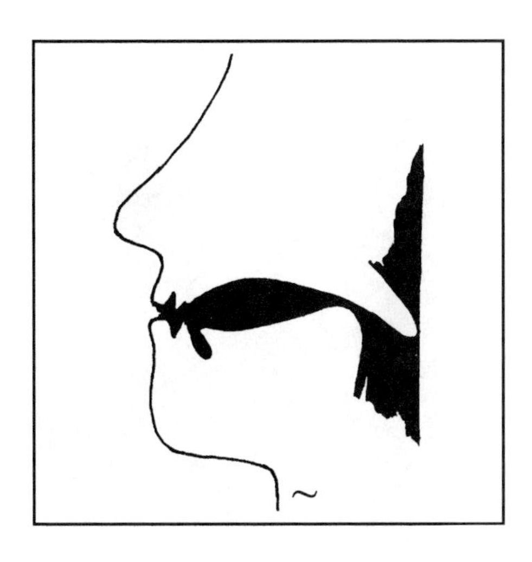

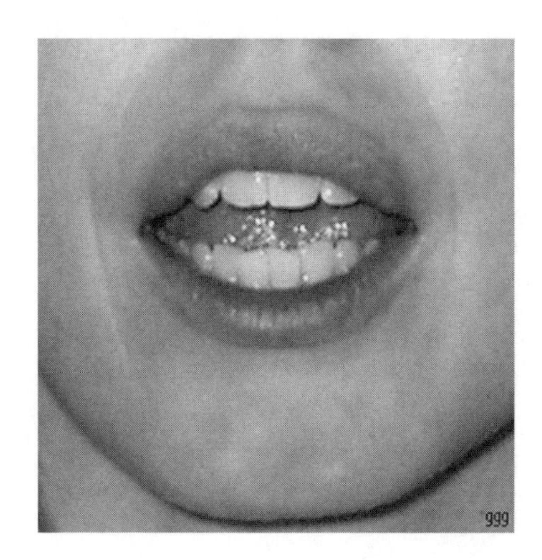

Back of tongue against velum momentarily shuts off the air stream. Air dams up and is released slightly with voicing. The articulation position and slight release can be seen when the mouth is open and the head tilted back. A low-high frequency sound. It is indicated either by a Lissajous pattern, the movement of a paper strip, or the needle of a sound level meter.

Prosodic Drill

ægægæg   æg**æg**æg   ægæg**æg**

ægægægæg   æg**æg**ægæg   ægæg**æg**æg

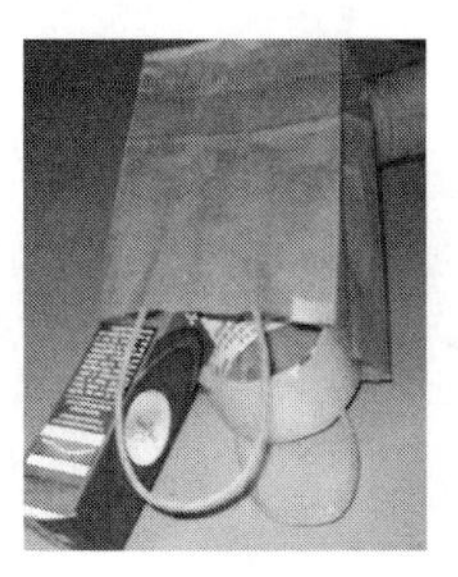

bag

Empty the ________.

pig   big   wig   egg   leg   tag

bug   dug   lug   bog   dog   fog   hog

Lesson 49 /k-/

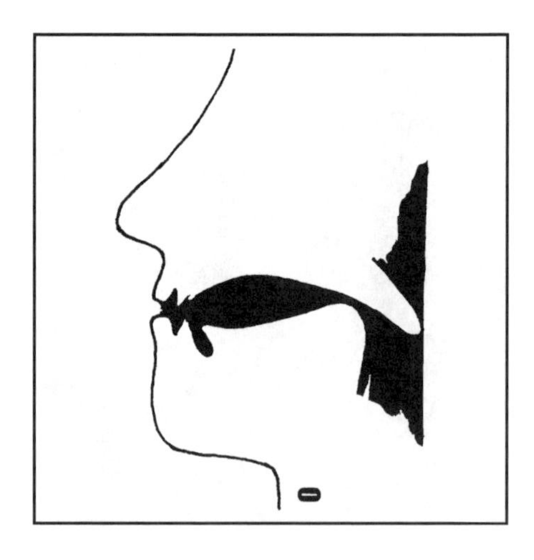

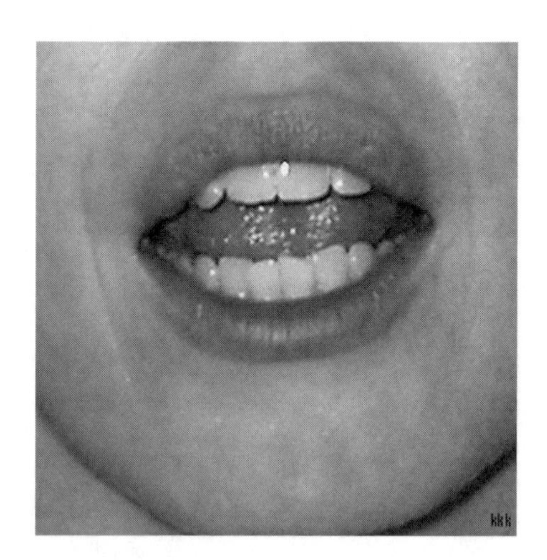

Back of tongue against velum momentarily shuts off the air stream. Air dams up and then the back of the tongue is separated from the velum with audible friction. The articulation can be seen by opening the mouth and tilting back the head. Also use a flashlight and even a mirror. Voicing is absent. The explosive release can be seen by a Lissajous pattern, the movement of a paper strip, or the needle of a sound level meter. The sound is low and high frequency.

Prosodic Drill

kokoko ko**ko**ko koko**ko**

kokokoko ko**ko**koko koko**ko**ko

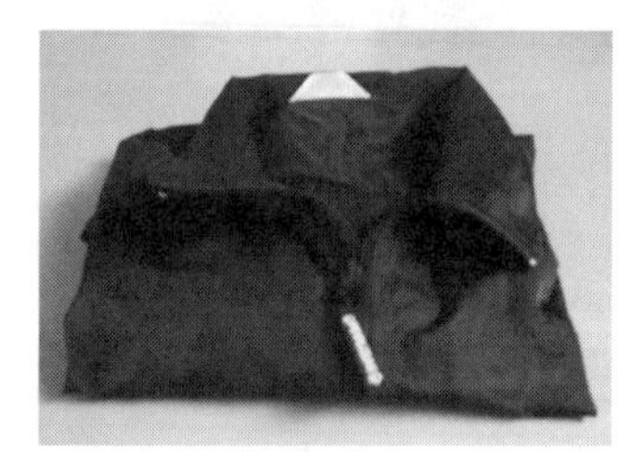

coat

Put on the ________.

key kiss cane cap cab can cup

cool coon cone coal call cow kite

Lesson 50 /-k/

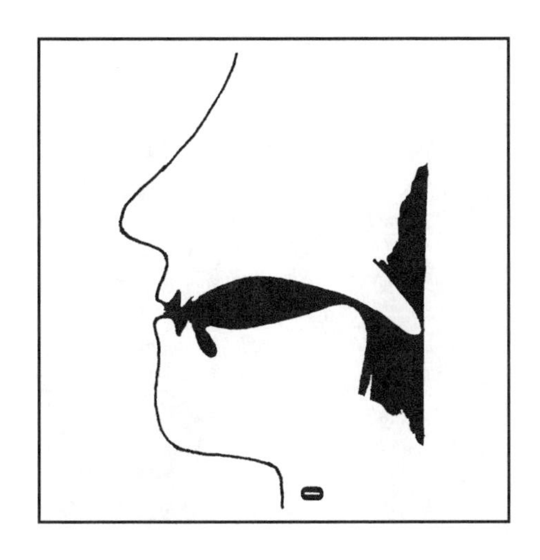

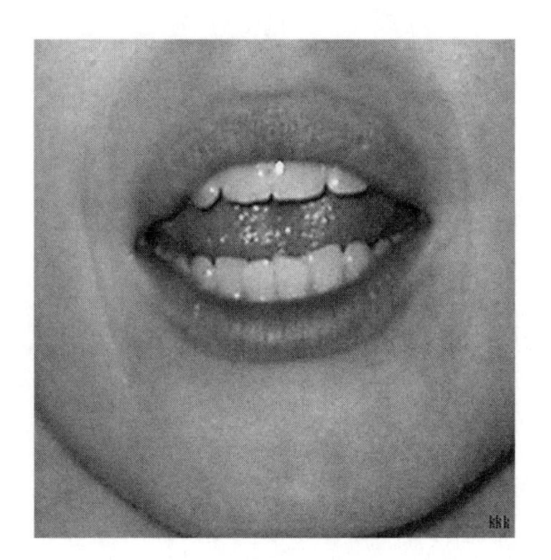

Back of tongue against velum momentarily shuts off the air stream. Air dams up and then the back of the tongue is slightly separated from the velum. The articulation can be seen by opening the mouth and tilting back the head. Also use a flashlight and even a mirror. Voicing is absent. The slight release can be seen by a Lissajous pattern, the movement of a paper strip, or the needle of a sound level meter. The sound is low and high frequency.

Prosodic Drill

ʊkʊkʊk ʊk**ʊk**ʊk ʊkʊk**ʊk**

ʊkʊkʊkʊk ʊk**ʊk**ʊkʊk ʊkʊk**ʊk**ʊk

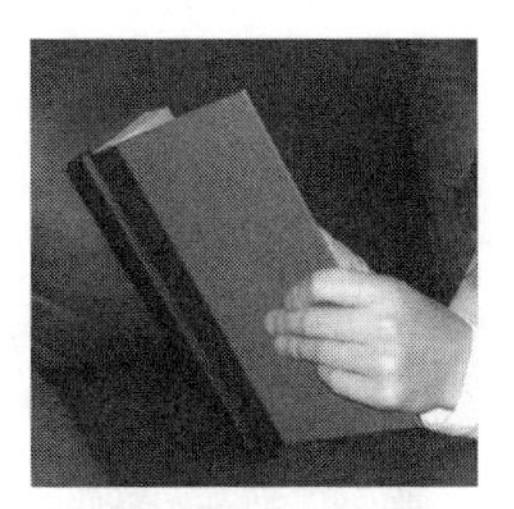

book

Read the ________.

beak pick deck bake back buck

poke soak sock dock lock like

Lesson 51 /tʃ-/

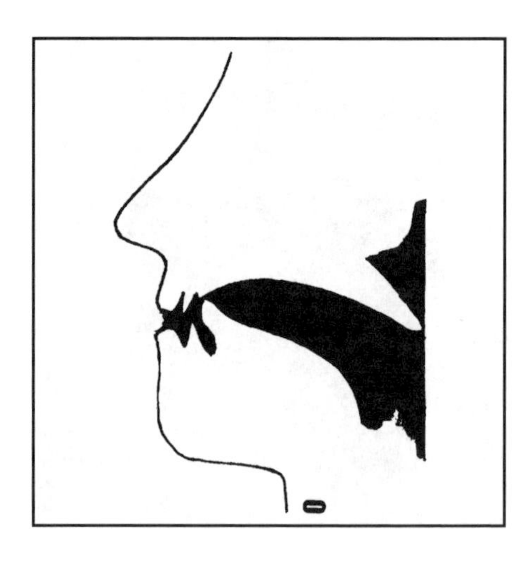

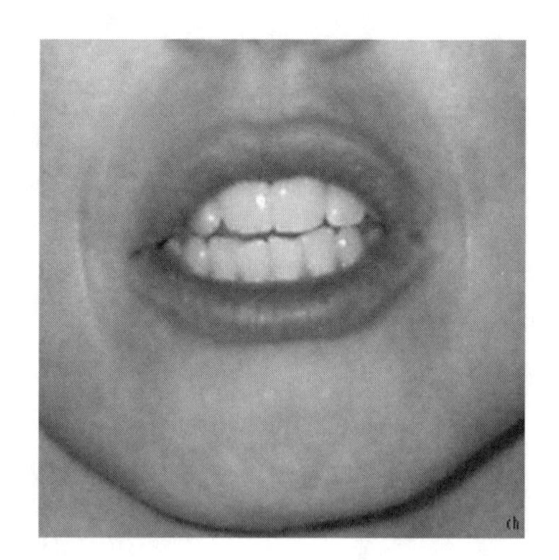

Tongue tip is to the alveolar ridge as for the /t/ and separated through the /ʃ/ articulation with an audible explosion of breath. Teach this sound after teaching the /t/ and /ʃ/ sounds. Say the two sound in succession, faster and faster, until a /tʃ/ occurs. The square mouth opening and /t/ articulation can be seen. The sound is low and high frequency. Voicing is absent. The pronounced explosive release can be seen by a Lissajous pattern, the movement of a paper strip, or the needle movement of a sound level meter.

Prosodic Drill

tʃɛtʃɛtʃɛ tʃɛ**tʃɛ**tʃɛ tʃɛtʃɛ**tʃɛ**

tʃɛtʃɛtʃɛtʃɛ tʃɛ**tʃɛ**tʃɛtʃɛ tʃɛtʃɛ**tʃɛ**tʃɛ

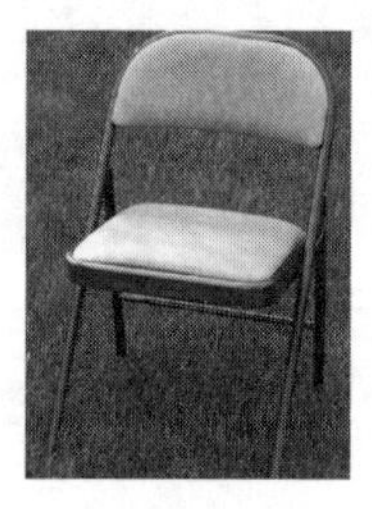

chair

Sit on the ________.

chief chip check chase church

choose chose chaw chow chive

Lesson 52 /-tʃ/

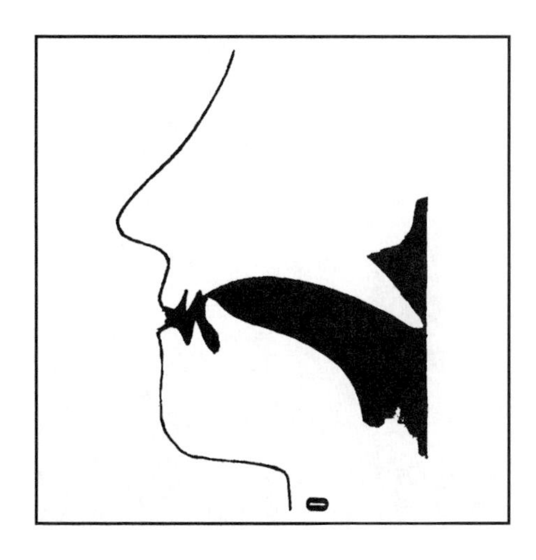

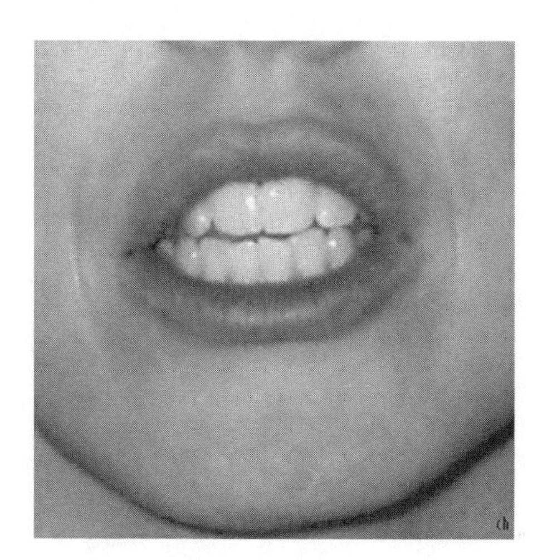

Tongue tip is to the alveolar ridge as for /t/ and separated through the /ʃ/ articulation with an audible explosion of breath. Teach this sound after teaching the /t/ and /ʃ/ sounds. Say the two sounds in succession, faster and faster, until a /tʃ/ occurs. The square mouth opening and /t/ articulation can be seen. The sound is low and high frequency. Voicing is absent. The explosive release can be seen by a Lissajous pattern, the movement of a paper strip, or the needle movement of a sound level meter.

Prosodic Drill

ætʃætʃætʃ ætʃ**ætʃ**ætʃ ætʃætʃ**ætʃ**

ætʃætʃætʃætʃ ætʃ**ætʃ**ætʃætʃ ætʃætʃ**ætʃ**ætʃ

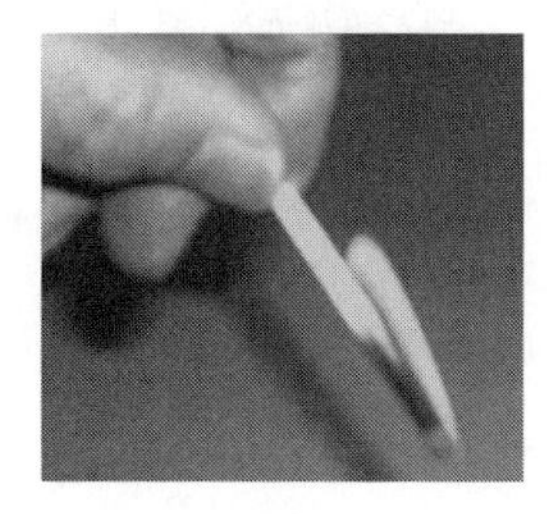

match

Light a ________.

peach pitch wretch catch much

mooch poach botch vouch

Lesson 53 /dʒ-/

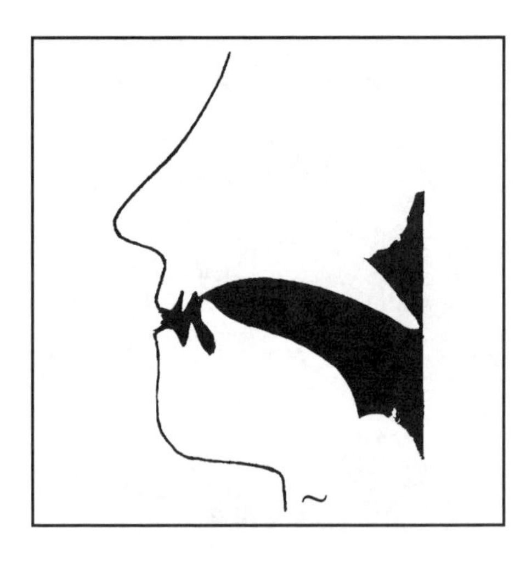

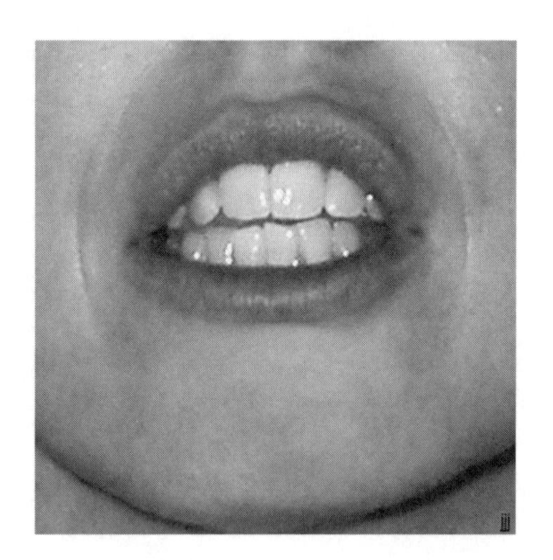

Tongue tip is to the alveolar ridge as for /d/ and separated through the /ʒ/ articulation with an audible explosion of voice. Teach this sound after teaching the /d/ and /ʒ/ sounds. Say the two sounds in succession, faster and faster, until a /dʒ/ occurs. The square mouth opening and the /d/ articulation can be seen. The explosive release can be seen by a Lissajous pattern, the movement of a paper strip, or the needle movement of a sound level meter.

Prosodic Drill

dʒædʒædʒæ dʒæ**dʒæ**dʒæ dʒædʒæ**dʒæ**

dʒædʒædʒædʒæ dʒæ**dʒæ**dʒædʒæ dʒædʒæ**dʒæ**dʒæ

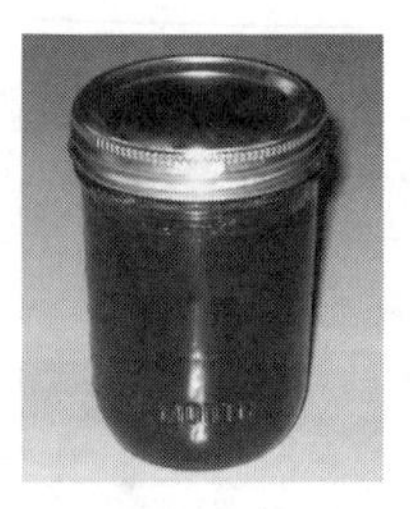

jam

That's a bottle of ________.

jeep gyp jest jail jack jump

jewel joke jaw joust jail

Lesson 54 /-dʒ/

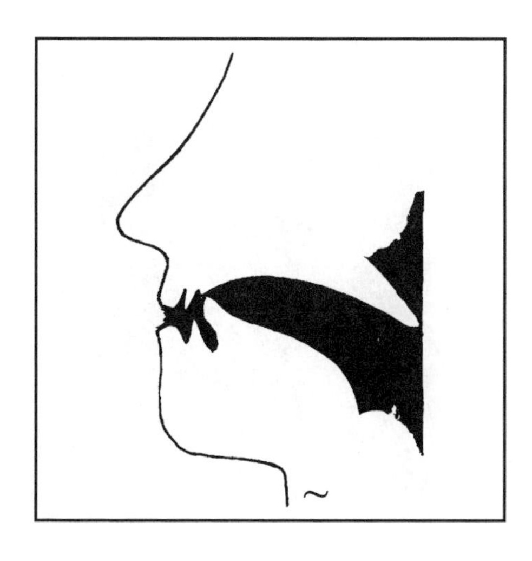

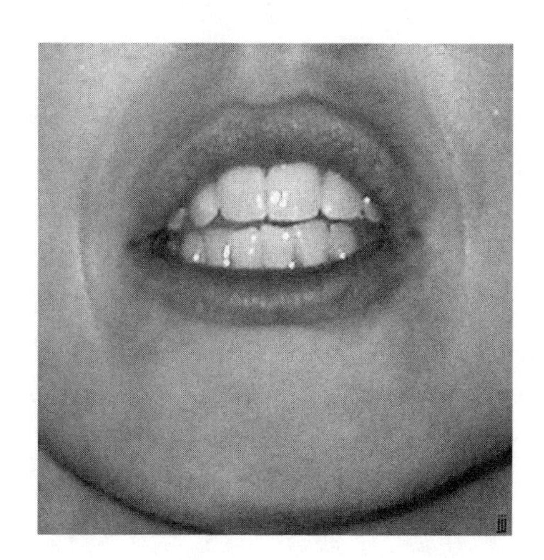

Tongue tip is to the alveolar ridge as for /d/ and separated through the /ʒ/ articulation with an audible explosion of voice. Teach this sound after teaching the /d/ and /ʒ/ sounds. Say the two sounds in succession, faster and faster, until a /dʒ/ occurs. The square mouth opening and the /d/ articulation can be seen. The explosive release can be seen by a Lissajous pattern, the movement of a paper strip, or the needle movement of a sound level meter.

Prosodic Drill

ædʒædʒædʒ ædʒ**ædʒ**ædʒ ædʒædʒ**ædʒ**

ædʒædʒædʒædʒ ædʒ**ædʒ**ædʒædʒ ædʒædʒ**ædʒ**ædʒ

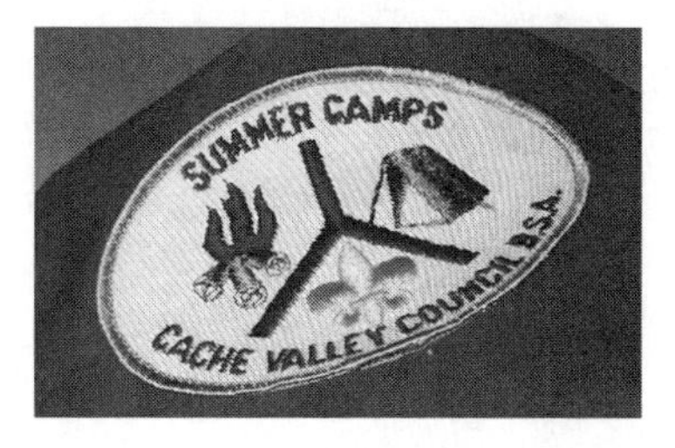

badge

That's a scout ________.

bridge edge ledge cage page

sage rage budge fudge

Lesson 55 /-ŋ/

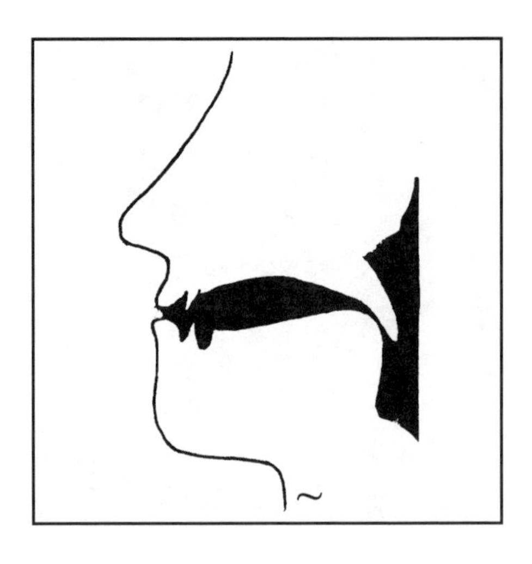

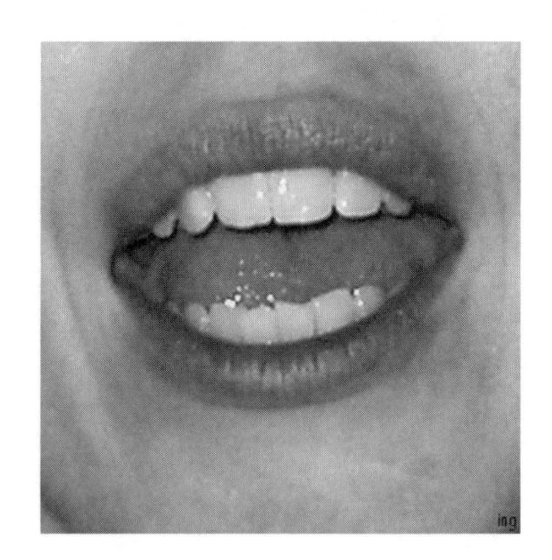

Back of tongue is to the velum and voice passes through the nose. This articulation can be seen by opening the mouth and tilting back the head. The velopharyngeal port is open. Voicing may be felt on the throat. Nasality may be felt on the nose. This low frequency sound is indicated by a Lissajous pattern or the needle movement of a sound level meter.

Prosodic Drill

ɪŋɪŋɪŋ ɪŋ**ɪŋ**ɪŋ ɪŋɪŋ**ɪŋ**

ɪŋɪŋɪŋɪŋ ɪŋ**ɪŋ**ɪŋɪŋ ɪŋɪŋ**ɪŋ**ɪŋ

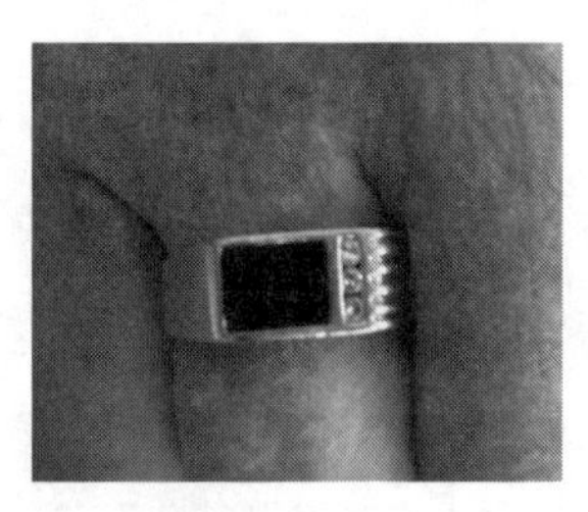

ring

Wear the ________.

ding sing pang bang fang

tongue lung bong thong long

Lesson 56 /r-/

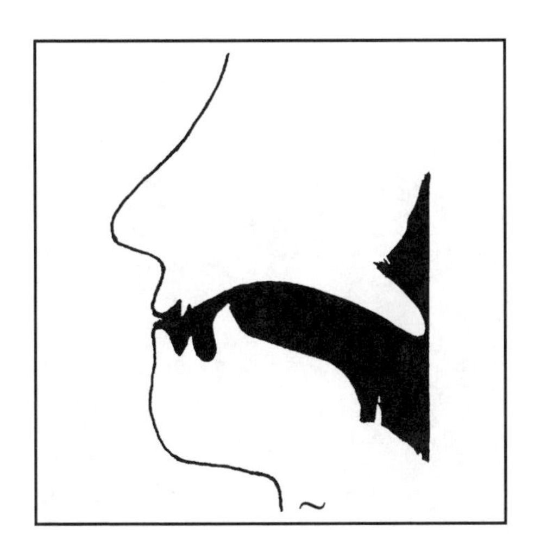

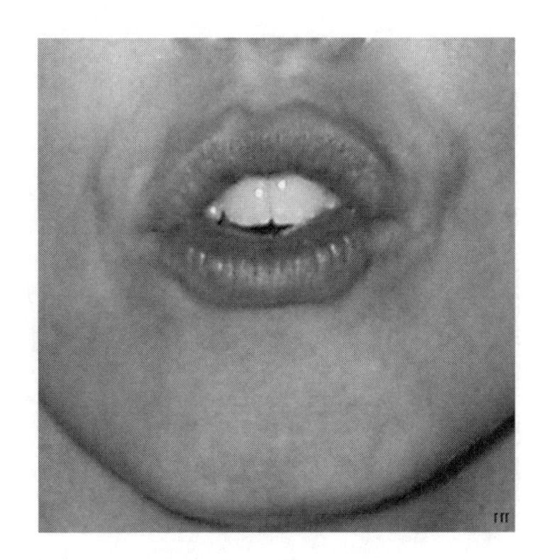

Front of tongue is high, tip up (can be retroflex) or down. Sides of tongue against upper molars. Lips squared. Voice passes between the tongue and palate and out of the mouth. The retroflex tongue articulation cannot be seen while in the mouth. It can be seen if retroflexed out of the mouth. This low frequency sound is indicated by a Lissajous pattern or by the needle movement of a sound level meter.

Prosodic Drill

rarara **ra**ra ...

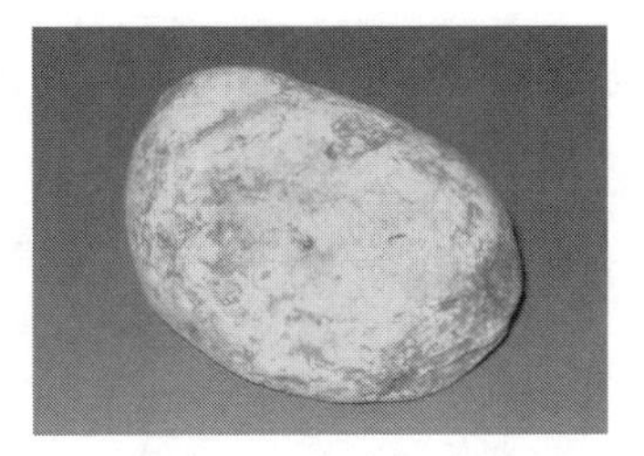

rock

Pick up the ________.

reef rip rib wreck rain ran rug

room roll raw round write

Lesson 57 /-r/

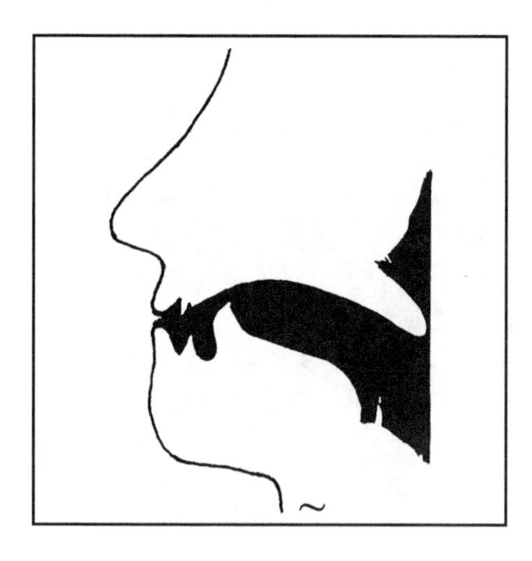

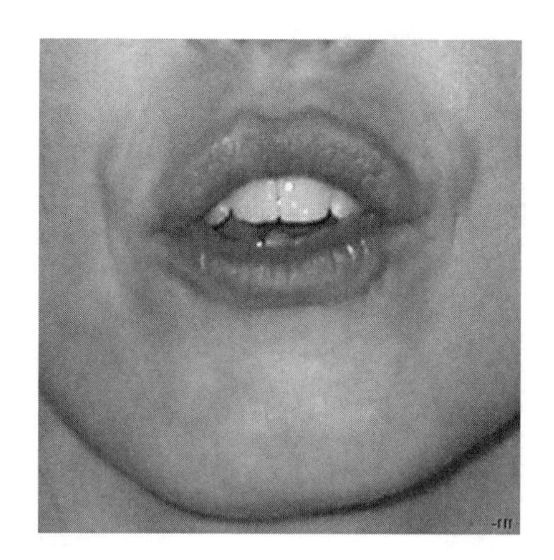

Front of tongue is high, tip up (can be retroflex) or down. Sides of tongue against upper molars. Lips squared. Voice passes between the tongue and palate and out of the mouth. The retroflex tongue articulation cannot be seen while in the mouth. It can be seen if retroflexed out of the mouth. This low frequency sound is indicated by a Lissajous pattern or by the needle movement of a sound level meter.

Prosodic Drill

ororor   or**or**or   oror**or**

orororor   or**or**oror   oror**or**or

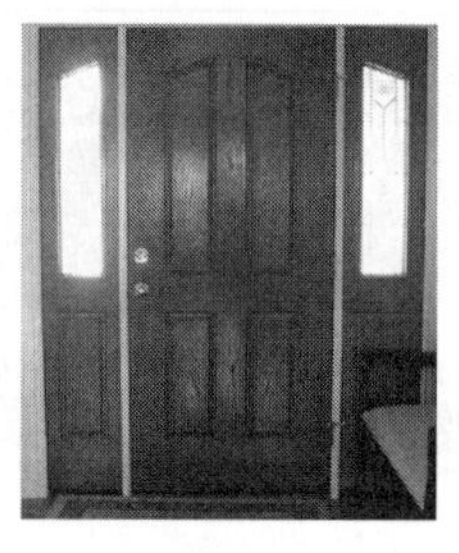

door

Open the ________.

hear   tear   bear   pear   cur

poor   bore   for   car   far

Lesson 58 /sm-/

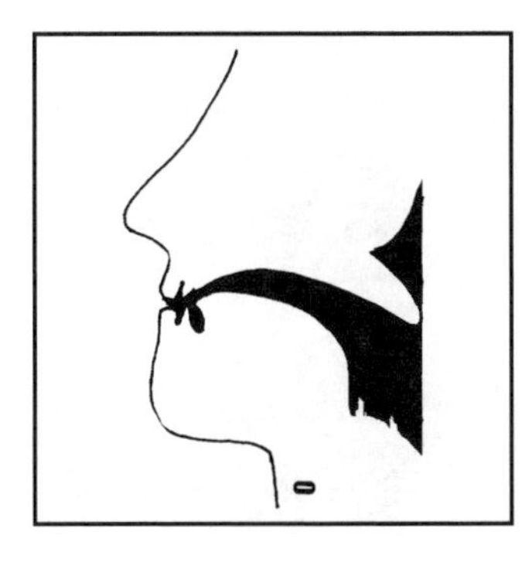
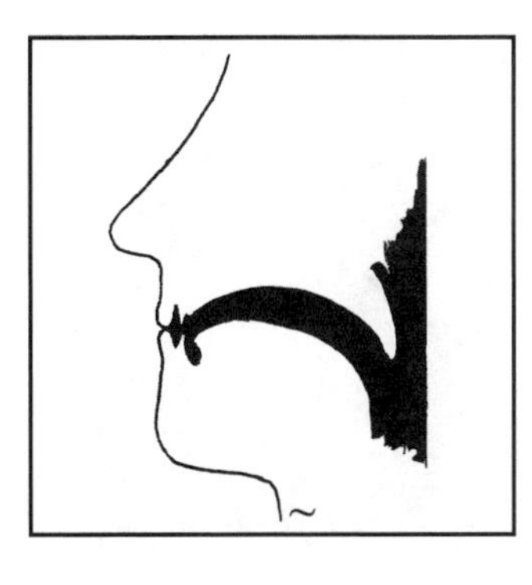
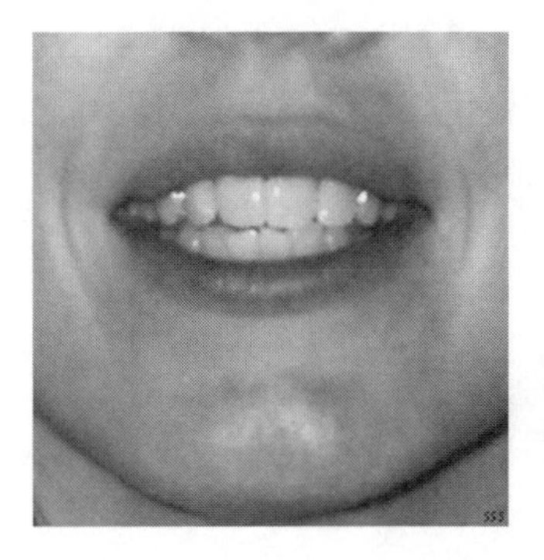
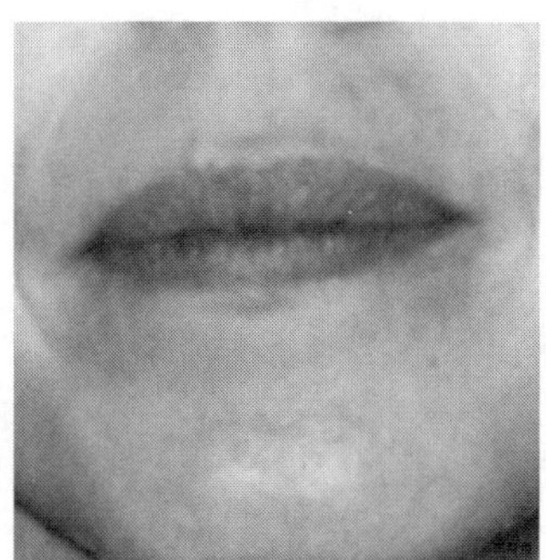

Teach this consonant blend after teaching the /s/ and /m/ sounds. Say the two sounds in succession, faster and faster, until /sm-/ occurs. The first sound is voiceless, orally produced, and high frequency. The second sound is voiced, nasally produced, and low frequency. The successive parts of this blend are indicated by Lissajous patterns, paper strip movement, and needle movement of the sound level meter.

Prosodic Drill

smɛsmɛsmɛ   smɛ**smɛ**smɛ   smɛsmɛ**smɛ**

smɛsmɛsmɛsmɛ   smɛ**smɛ**smɛsmɛ   smɛsmɛ**smɛ**smɛ

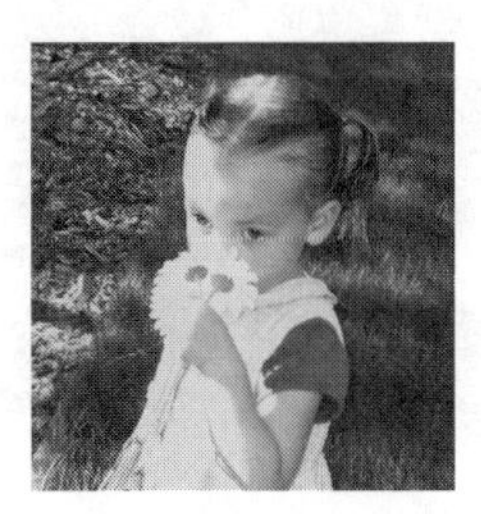

smell

The flowers ________.

smear   smash   smut   smudge

smirk   smooth   small   smart

Lesson 59 /sp-/

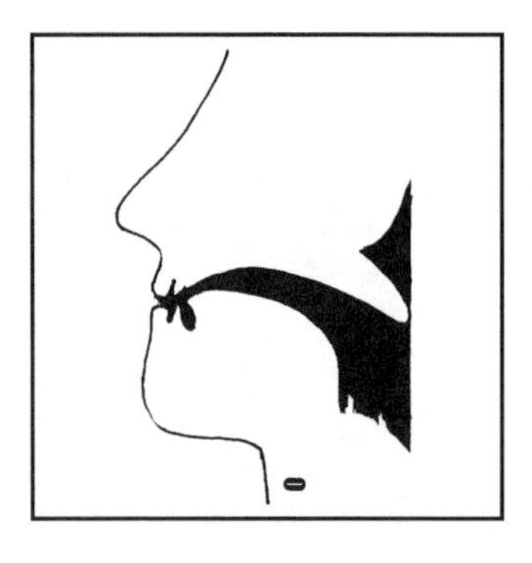

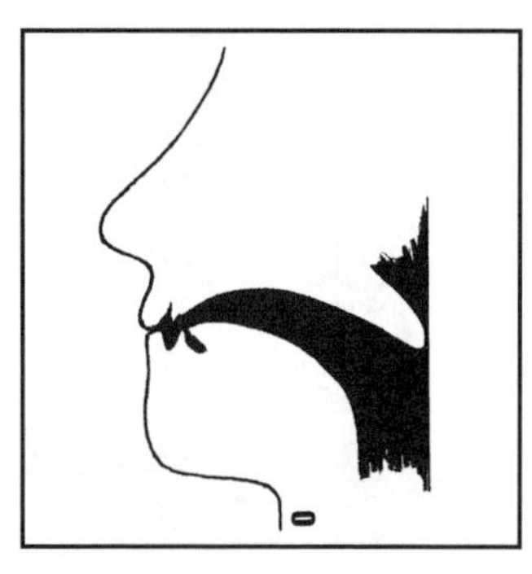

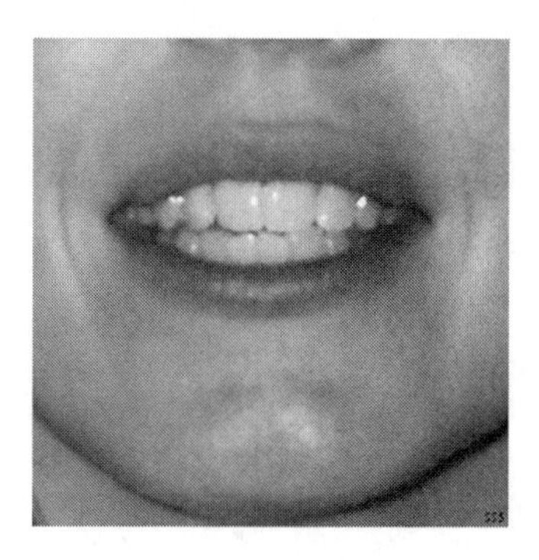

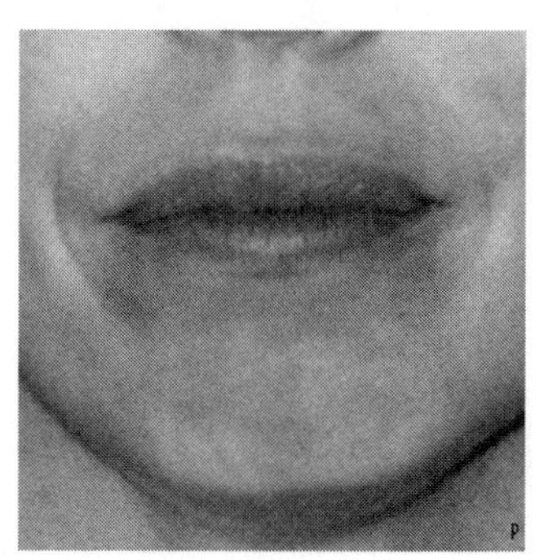

Teach this consonant blend after teaching the /s/ and /p/ sounds. Say the two sounds in succession, faster and faster, until /sp-/ occurs. Both sounds are voiceless, the first high frequency and the second low frequency. The successive parts of this blend are indicated by Lissajous patterns and paper strip movements.

Prosodic Drill

spɪspɪspɪ spɪ**spɪ**spɪ spɪspɪ**spɪ**

spɪspɪspɪspɪ spɪ**spɪ**spɪspɪ spɪspɪ**spɪ**spɪ

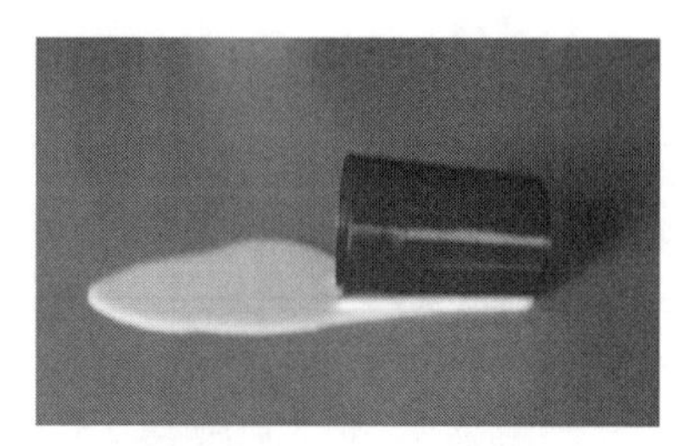

spill

It's a milk ________.

speak speed spin spell spade spat

spud spool spoke spot spider

Lesson 60 /sw-/

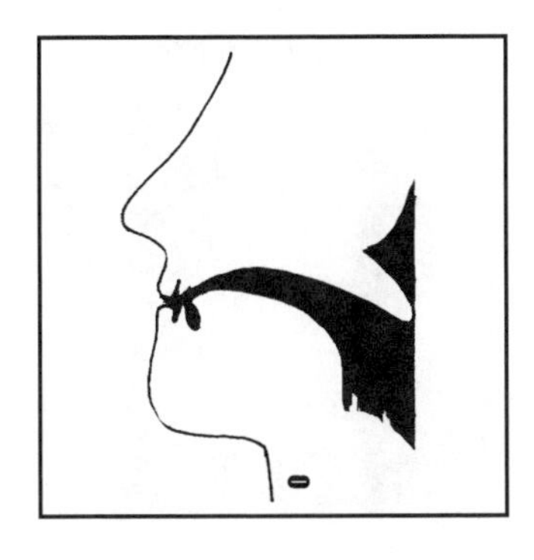
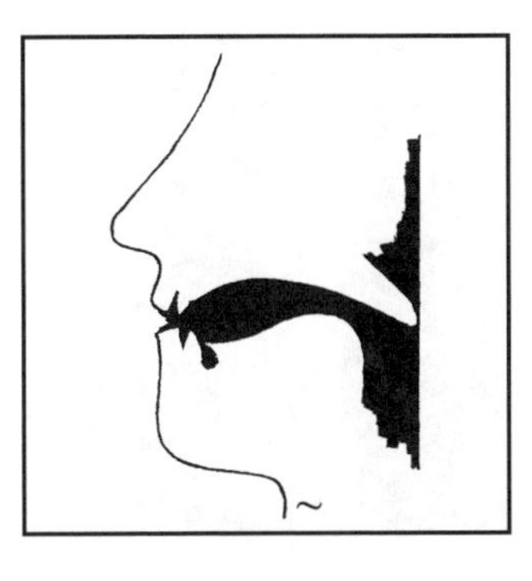
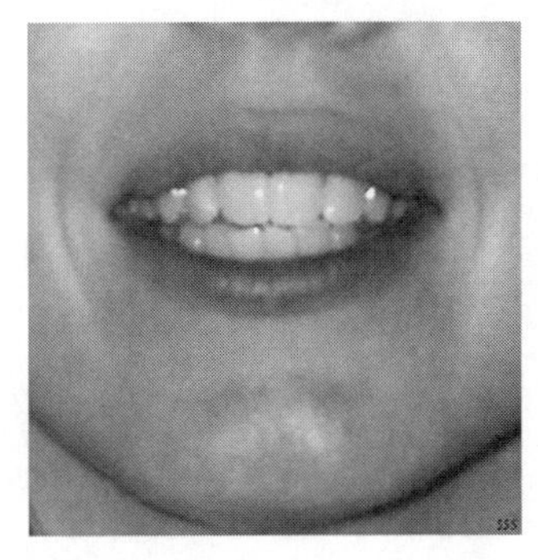
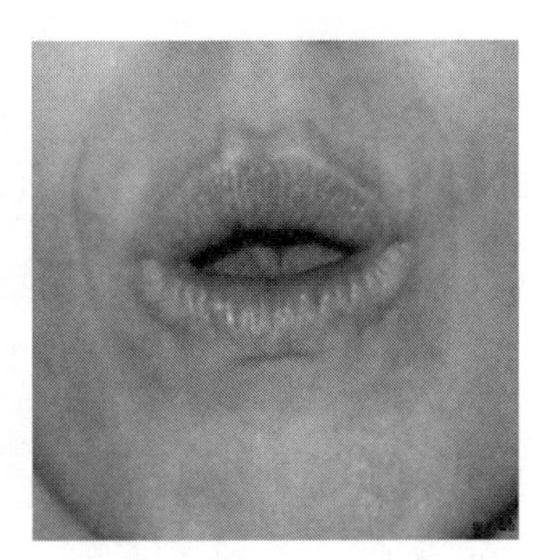

Teach this consonant blend after teaching the /s/ and /w/ sounds. Say the two sounds in succession, faster and faster, until /sw-/ occurs. The first sound is voiceless and high frequency, the second voiced and low frequency. Both sounds are produced through the mouth. The successive parts of this blend are indicated by Lissajous patterns and paper strip and meter needle movements.

Prosodic Drill

swiswiswi swi**swi**swi swiswi**swi**

swiswiswiswi swi**swi**swiswi swiswi**swi**swi

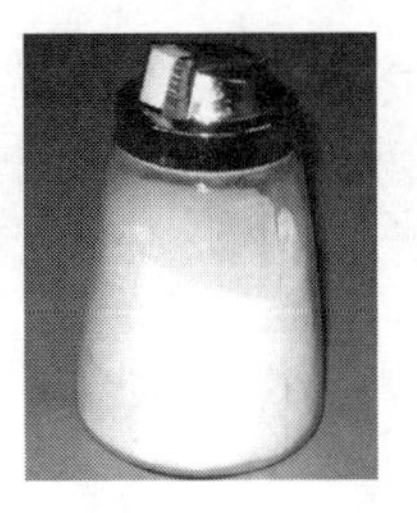

sweet

Sugar is ________.

swing swell suede swap

swoop swoon swarm swipe

Lesson 61 /sk-/

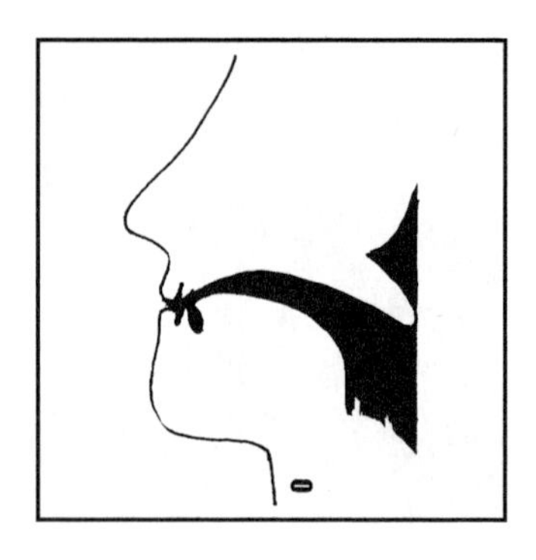
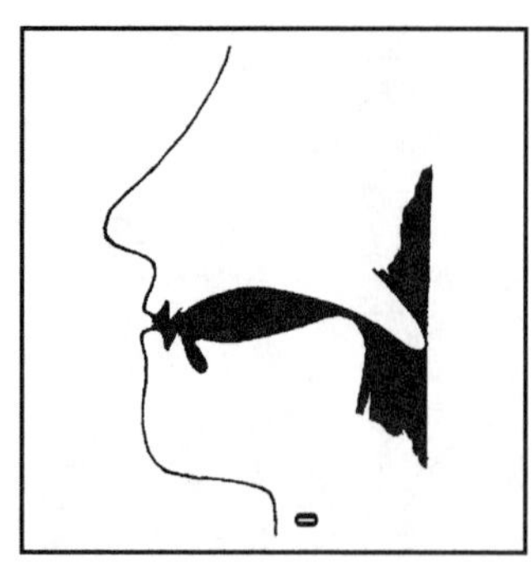
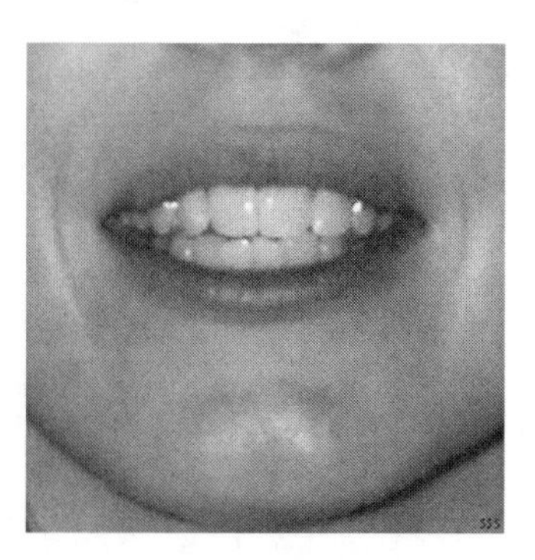
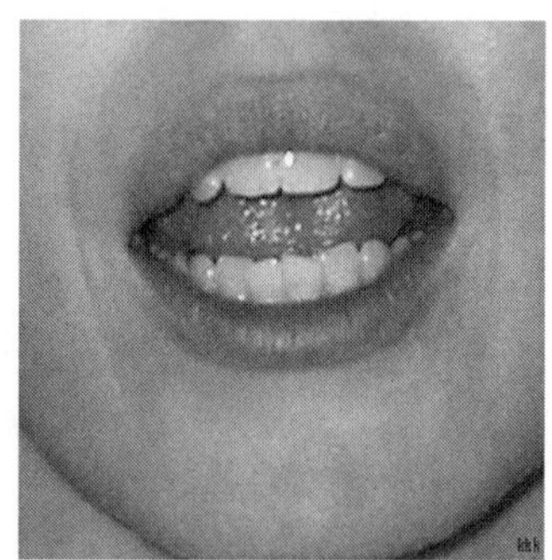

Teach this consonant blend after teaching the /s/ and /k/ sounds. Say the two sounds in succession, faster and faster, until /sk-/occurs. Both sounds are voiceless and high frequency. The successive parts of this blend are indicated by Lissajous patterns and paper strip movements.

Prosodic Drill

skuskusku skus**ku**sku skusku**sku**

skuskuskusku sku**sku**skusku skusku**sku**sku

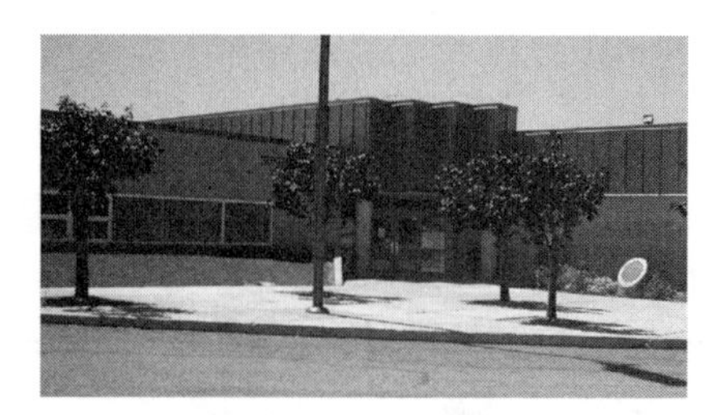

school

That's a ________.

ski skid sketch skate scat skull

skirt scoot scope scoff scout sky

Lesson 62 /sl-/

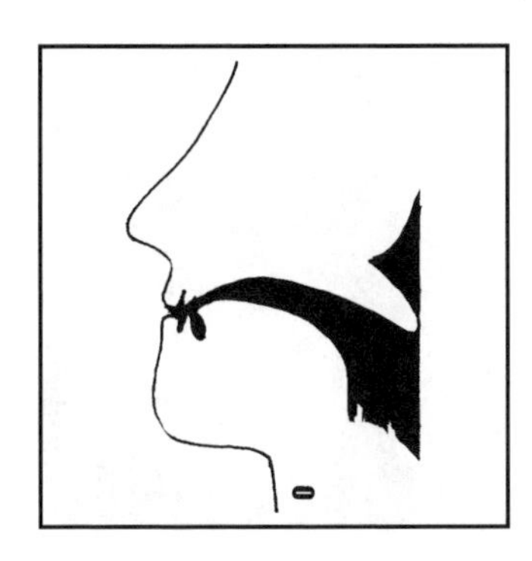
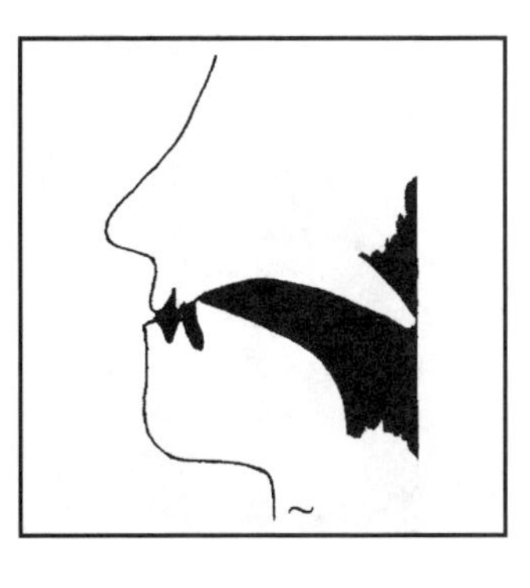
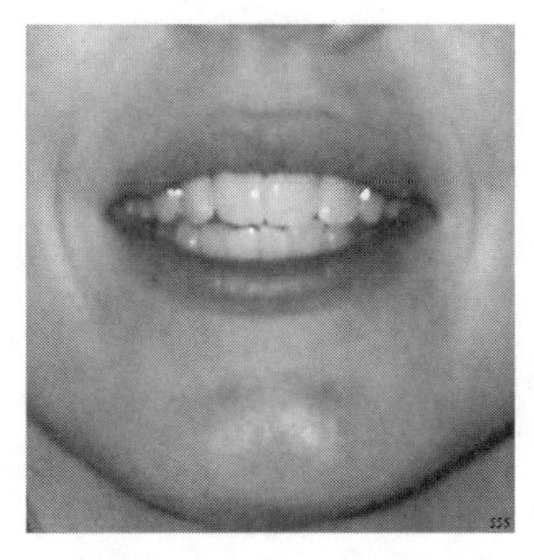
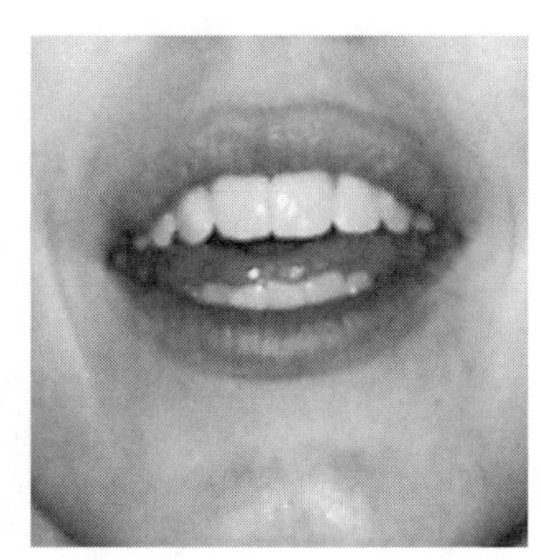

Teach this consonant blend after teaching the /s/ and /l/ sounds. Say the two sound in succession, faster and faster, until /sl-/ occurs. The first sound is voiceless and high frequency, the second voiced and low frequency. Both sounds are produced through the mouth. The successive parts of this blend are indicated by Lissajous patterns and paper strip and meter needle movements.

Prosodic Drill

slɛslɛslɛ   slɛ**slɛ**slɛ   slɛslɛ**slɛ**

slɛslɛslɛslɛ   slɛ**slɛ**slɛslɛ   slɛslɛ**slɛ**slɛ

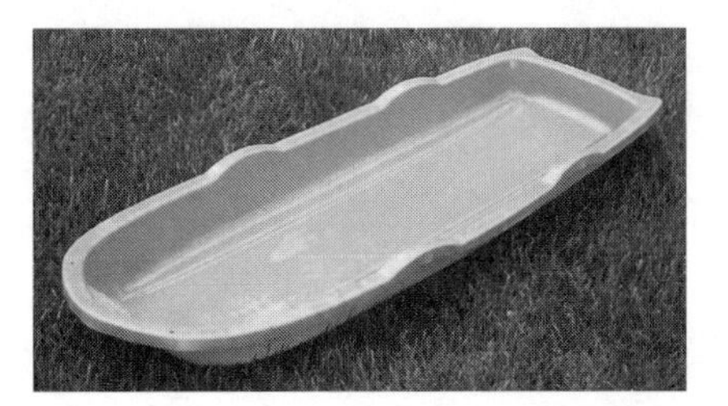

sled

Ride the ________.

sleep   slip   slept   slate   slap   slum

sloop   slope   slop   slot   slouch

Lesson 63 /sn-/

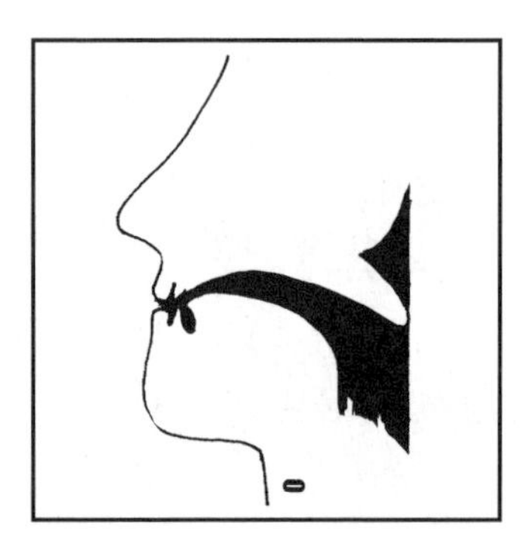

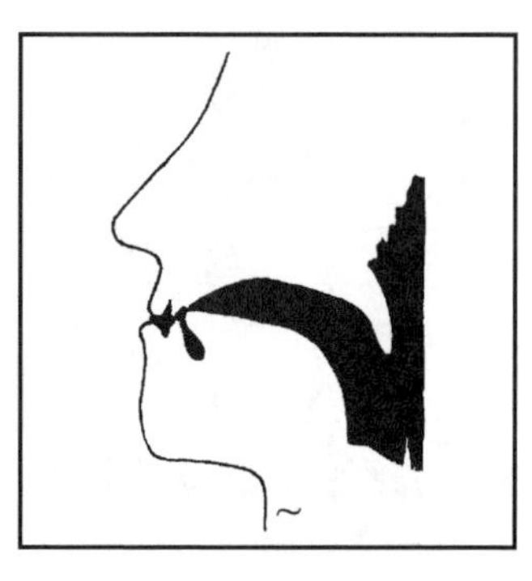

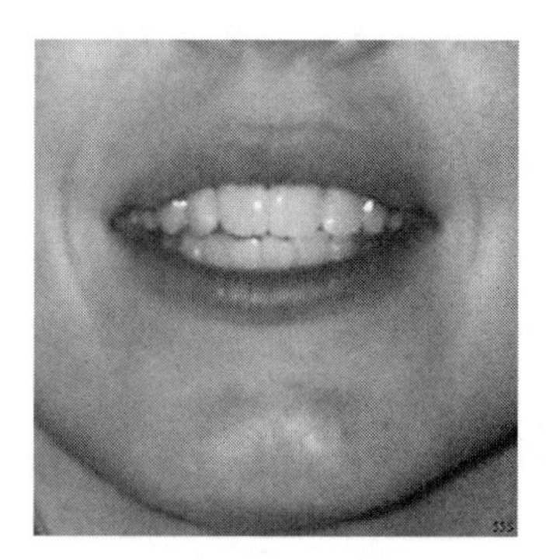

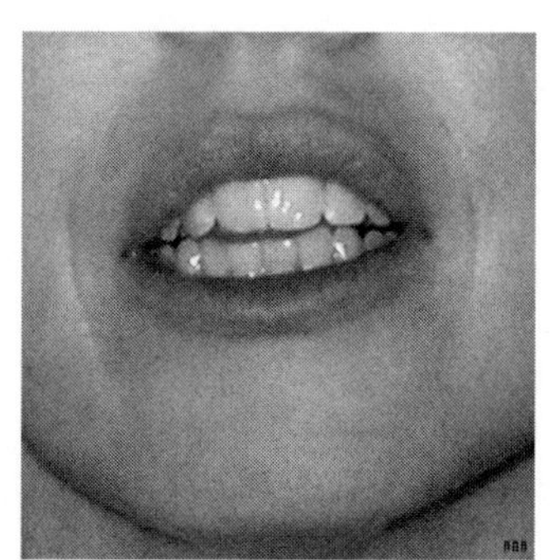

Teach this consonant blend after teaching the /s/ and /n/ sounds. Say the two sounds in succession, faster and faster, until /sn-/ occurs. The first sound is voiceless, high frequency, and orally produced. The second sound is voiced, low frequency, and nasally produced. The successive parts of this blend are indicated by Lissajous patterns and paper strip and meter needle movements.

Prosodic Drill

snesnesne snesnesne snesnesne (middle "sne" of the second and final "sne" of the third in bold)

snesnesnesne sne**sne**snesne snesne**sne**sne

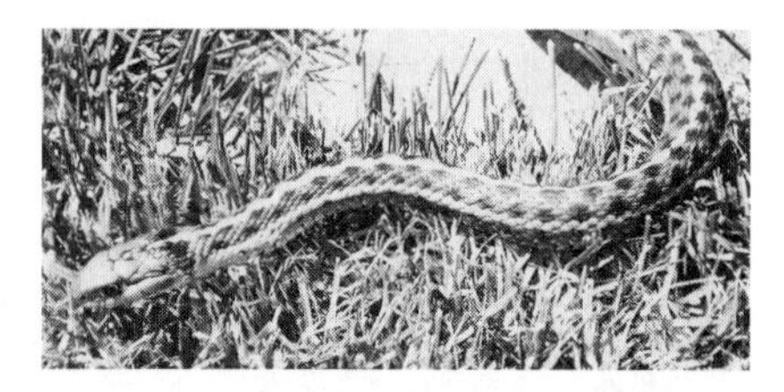

snake

That's a ________.

sneak snip snail snap snub

snoop snow snob snout snide

Lesson 64 /st-/

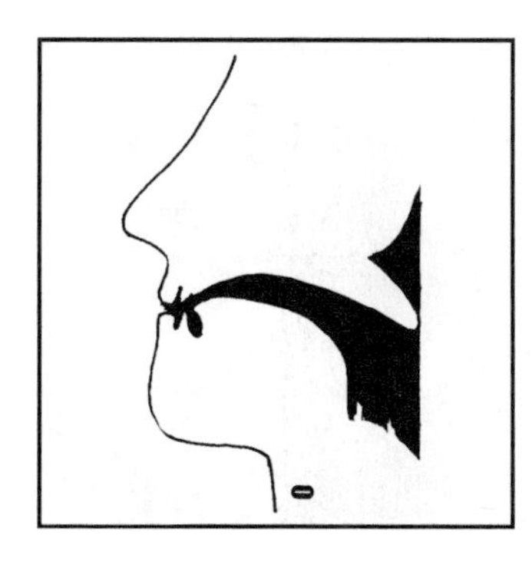

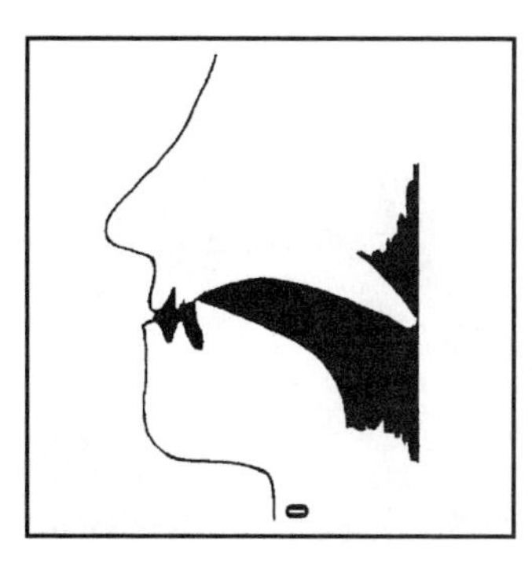

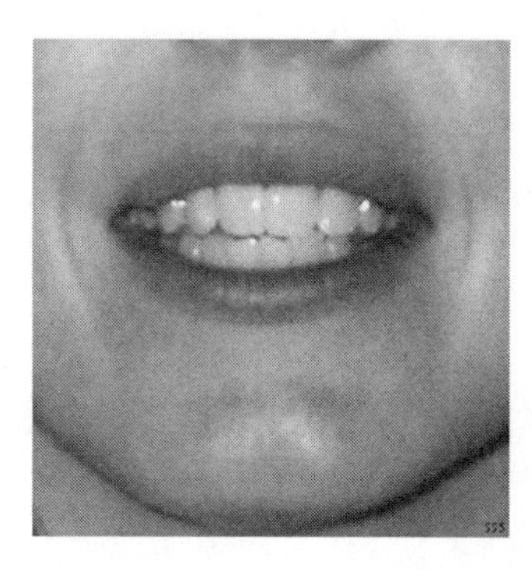

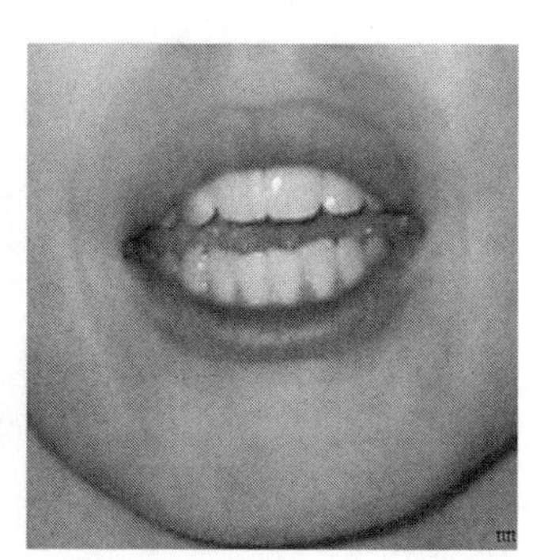

Teach this consonant blend after teaching the /s/ and /t/ sounds. Say the two sounds in succession, faster and faster, until /st-/ occurs. Both sounds are voiceless, high frequency, and orally produced. The successive parts of this blend are indicated by Lissajous patterns and paper strip and meter needle movements.

Prosodic Drill

stastasta stа**sta**sta stasta**sta**

stastastasta sta**sta**stasta stasta**sta**sta

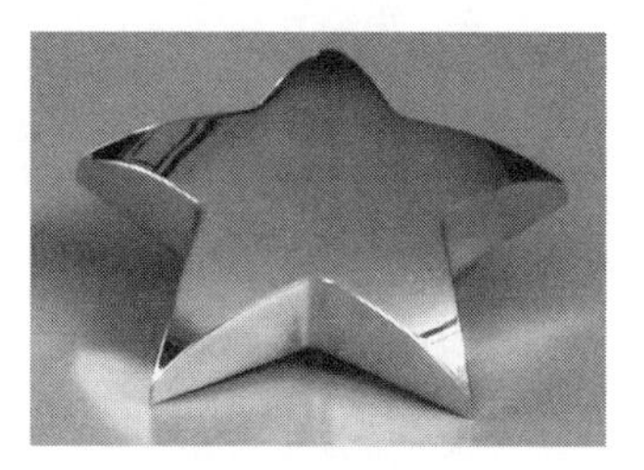

star

That's a ________.

steep stitch step stain stun stern

stool stove stop stout stifle

Lesson 65 /θr-/

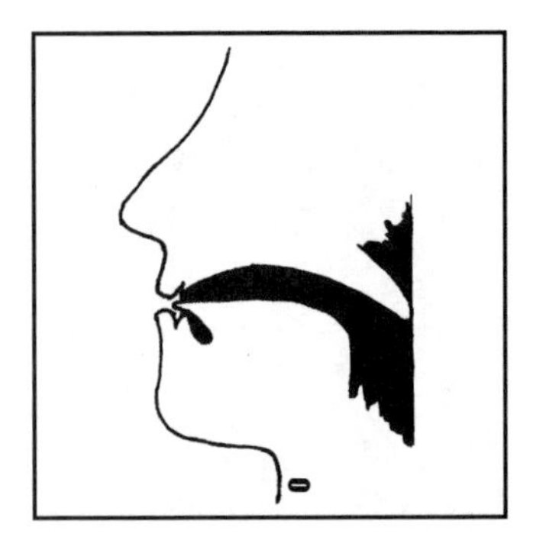
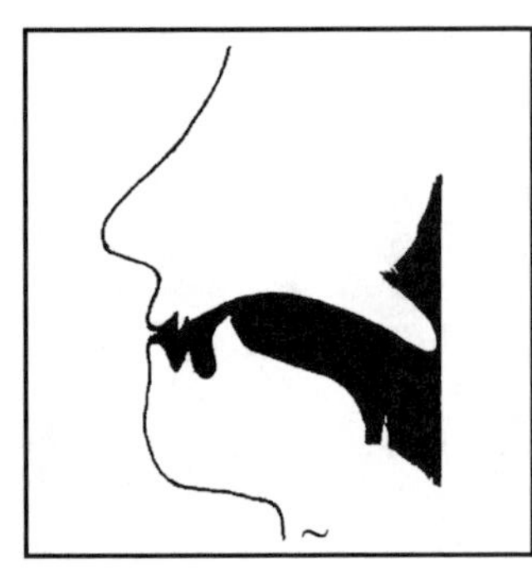
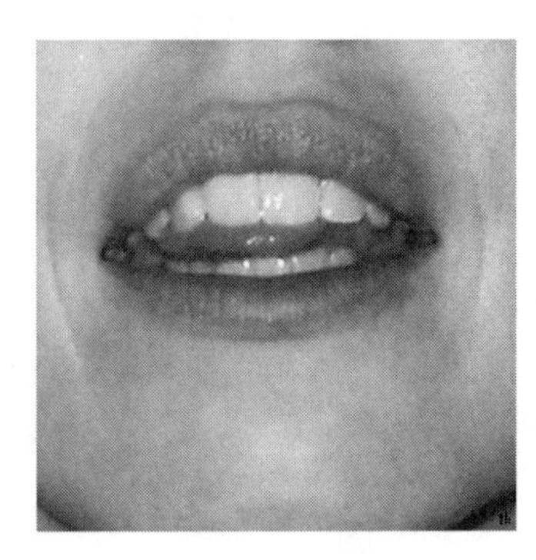
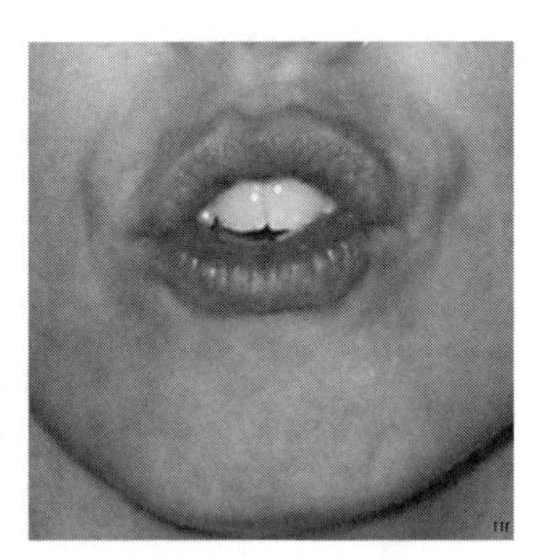

Teach this consonant blend after teaching the /θ/ and /r/ sounds. Says the two sounds in succession, faster and faster, until /θr-/ occurs. The first sound is voiceless, and the second voiced. Both are produced through the mouth. The successive parts of this blend are indicated by Lissajous patterns and paper strip and meter needle movements.

Prosodic Drill

θrɛθrɛθrɛ θrɛ**θrɛ**θrɛ θrɛθrɛ**θrɛ**

θrɛθrɛθrɛθrɛ θrɛ**θrɛ**θrɛθrɛ θrɛθrɛ**θrɛ**θrɛ

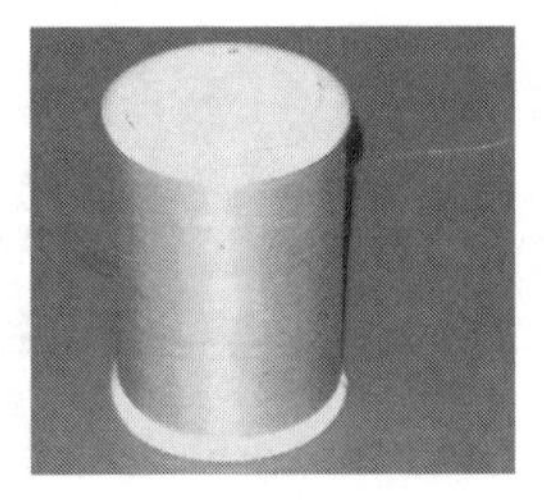

thread

It's a spool of ________.

three thrill threat thrush

through throw throat throb

Lesson 66 /bl-/

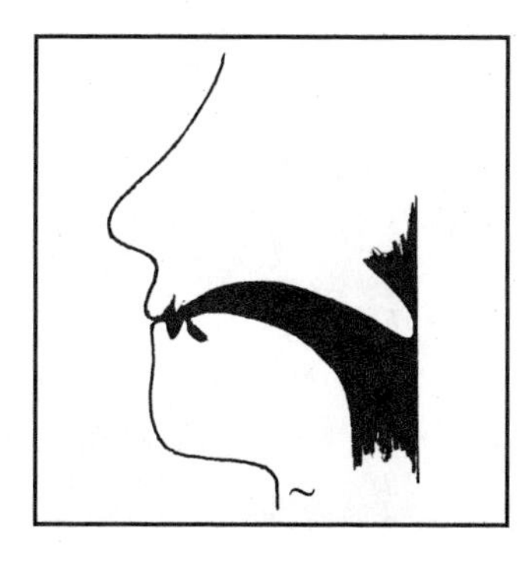
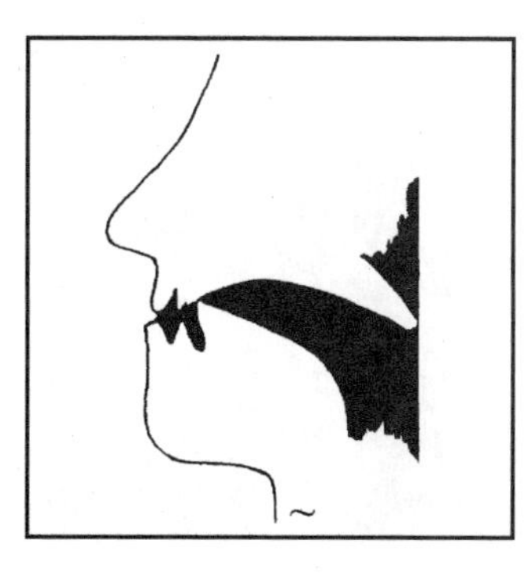
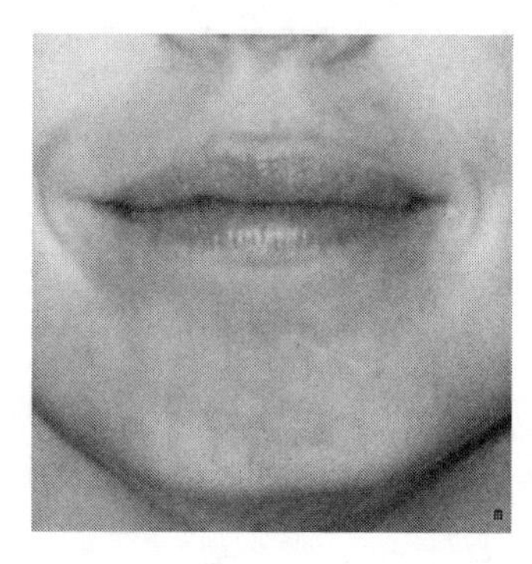
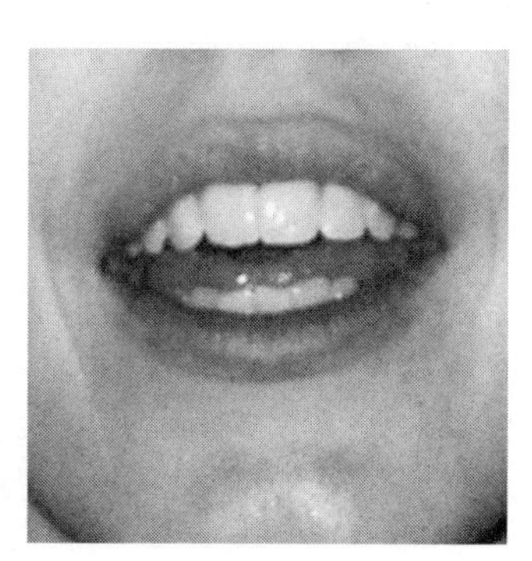

Teach this consonant blend after teaching the /b-/ and /l/ sounds. The articulation positions for the sounds are assumed simultaneously. The sounds are made together. A single Lissajous pattern, paper strip movement, or meter needle movement is indicative.

Prosodic Drill

blablabla bla**bla**bla blabla**bla**

blablablabla bla**bla**blabla blabla**bla**bla

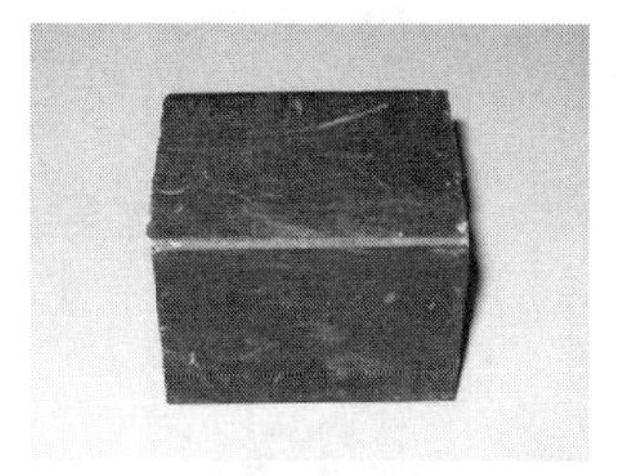

block

That's a ________.

bleed bliss bless blaze black

blood blurb blue blow blot

Lesson 67 /br-/

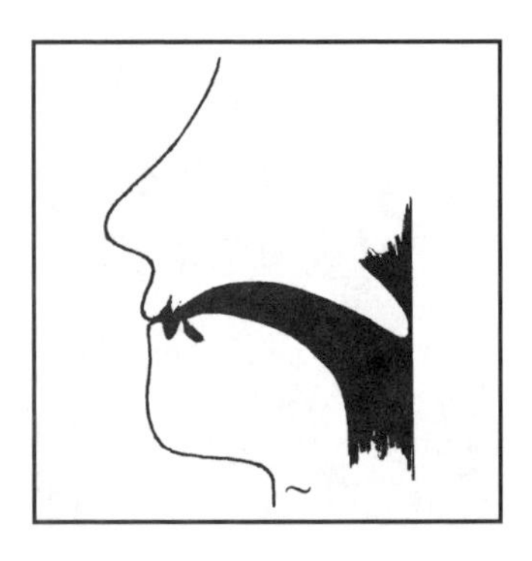
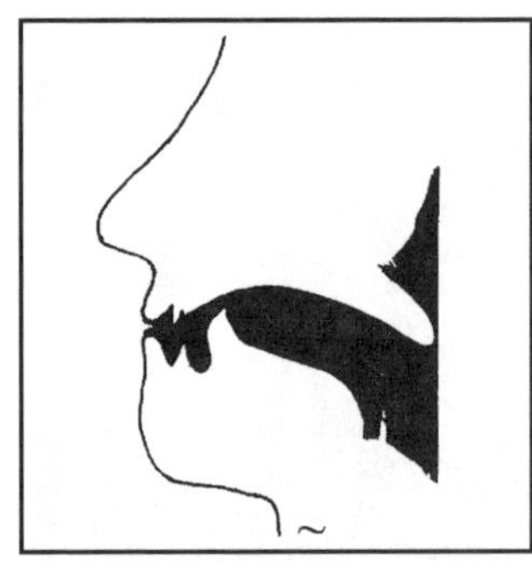
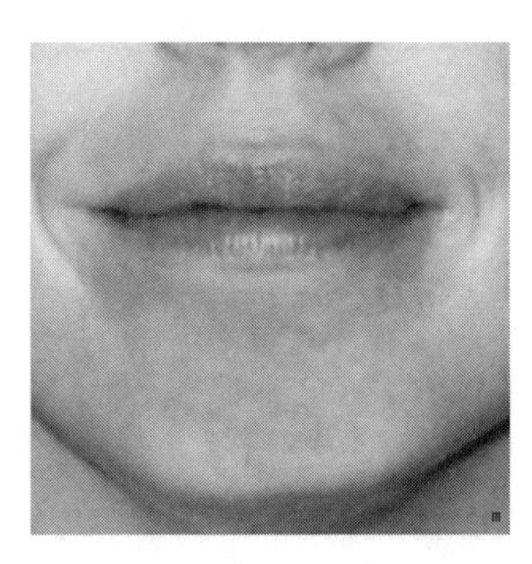
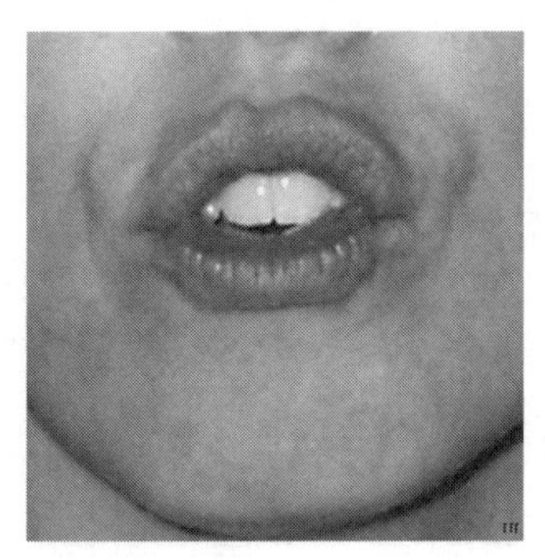

Teach this consonant blend after teaching the /b-/ and /r/ sounds. The articulation positions for the sounds are assumed simultaneously. The sounds are made together. A single Lissajous pattern, paper strip movement, or meter needle movement is indicative.

Prosodic Drill

brubrubru brு**bru**bru brubru**bru**

brubrubrubru bru**bru**brubru brubru**bru**bru

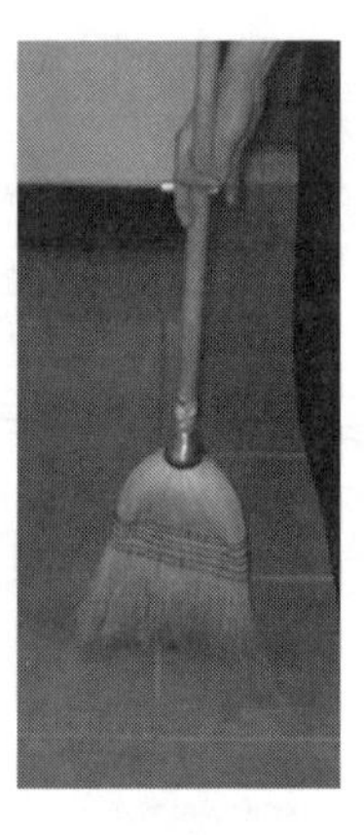

broom

Sweep with a ________.

breathe bridge bread brake brass brother

brood broke broad brow bride

Lesson 68 /fl-/

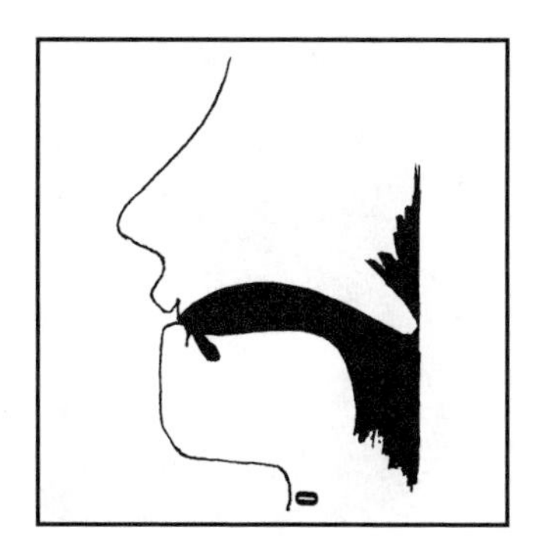
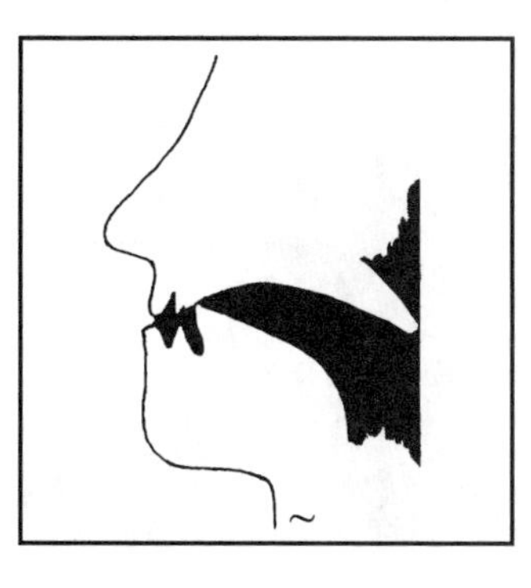
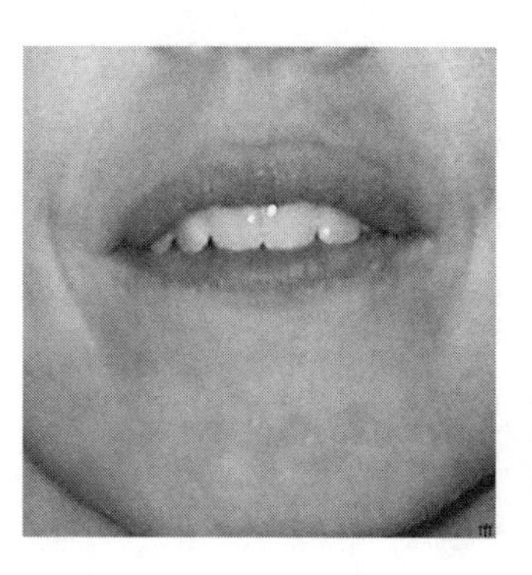
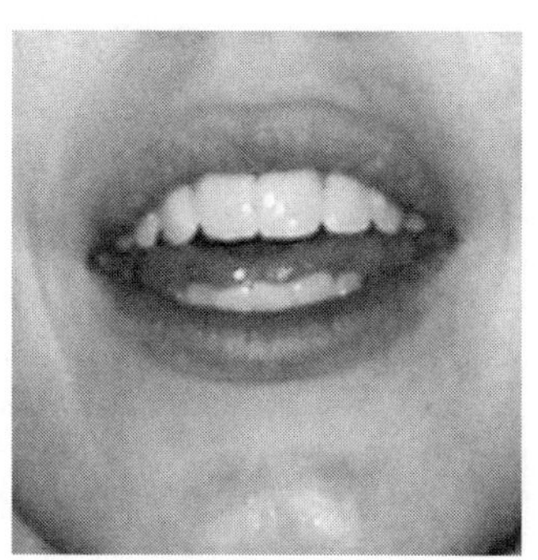

Teach this consonant blend after teaching the /f/ and /l/ sounds. The articulation positions for the sounds are assumed simultaneously. The sounds are made together. A single Lissajous pattern, paper strip movement, or meter needle movement is indicative.

Prosodic Drill

flofloflo flo**flo**flo floflo**flo**

floflofloflo flo**flo**floflo floflo**flo**flo

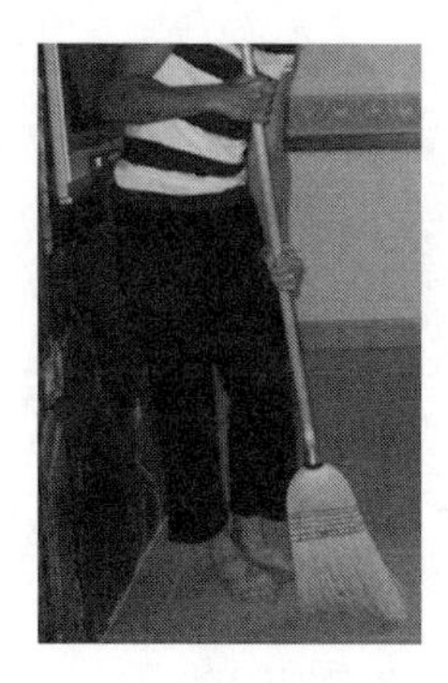

floor

Sweep the ________.

fleet flip fleck flake flack flub

flirt flew flow flop fly

Lesson 69 /fr-/

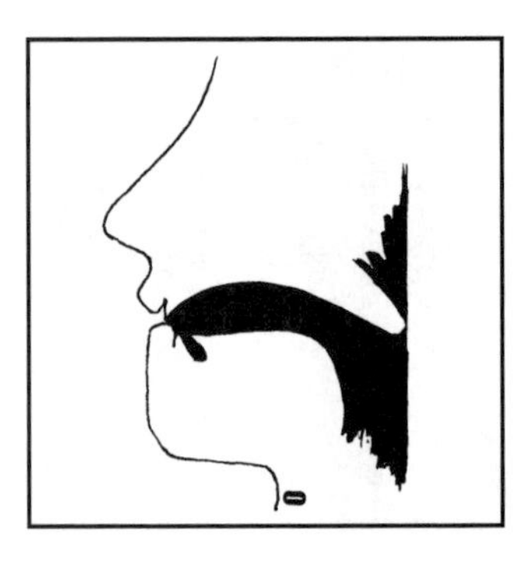
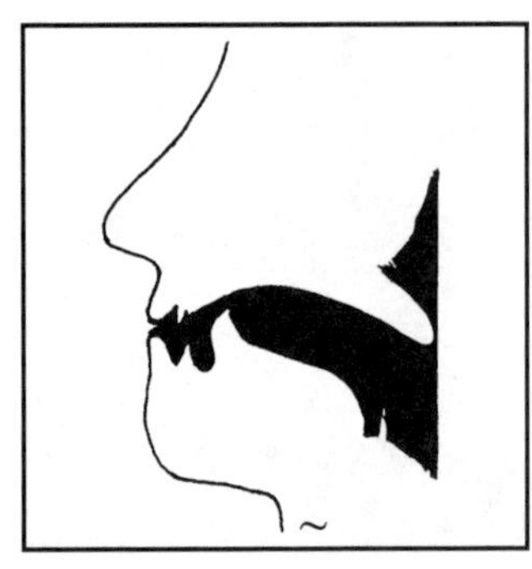
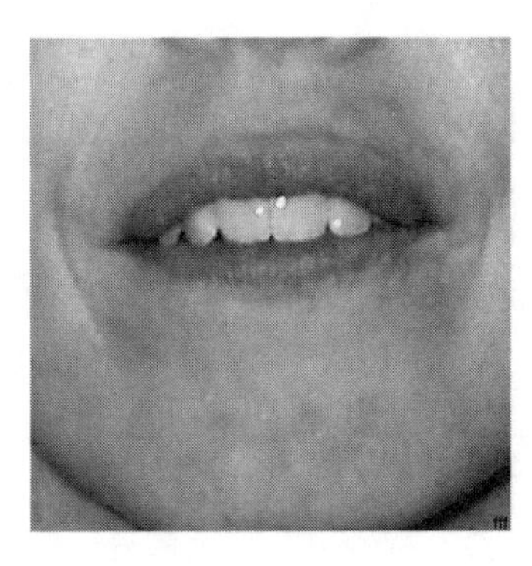
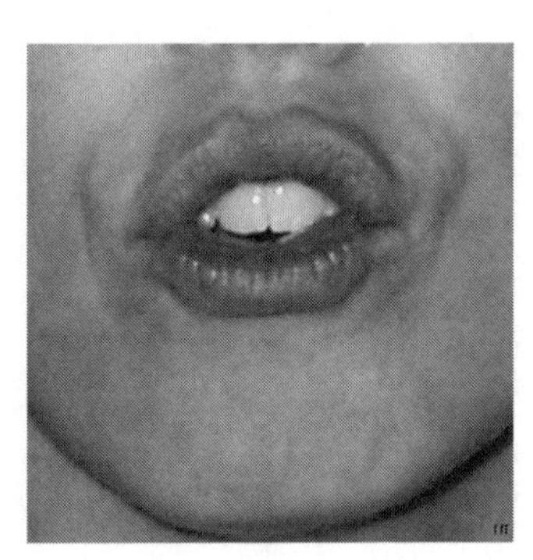

Teach this consonant blend after teaching the /f/ and /r/ sounds. The articulation positions for the sounds are assumed simultaneously. The sounds are made together. A single Lissajous pattern, paper strip movement, or meter needle movement is indicative.

Prosodic Drill

frefrefre frefrefre frefre**fre**

frefrefrefre fre**fre**frefre frefre**fre**fre

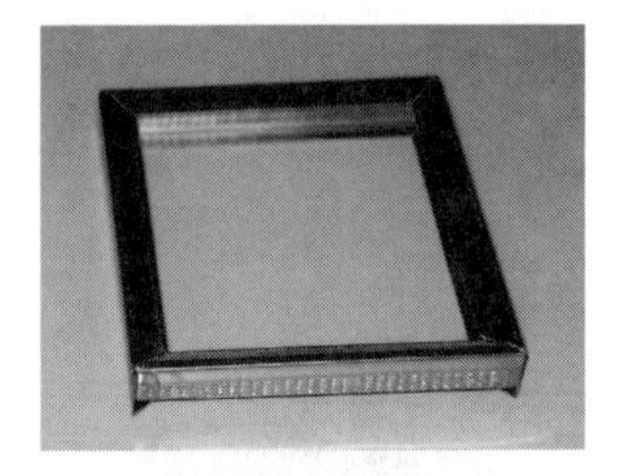

frame

That's a picture ________.

freeze frill friend frail frat

from fruit frost fright

Lesson 70 /kw-/

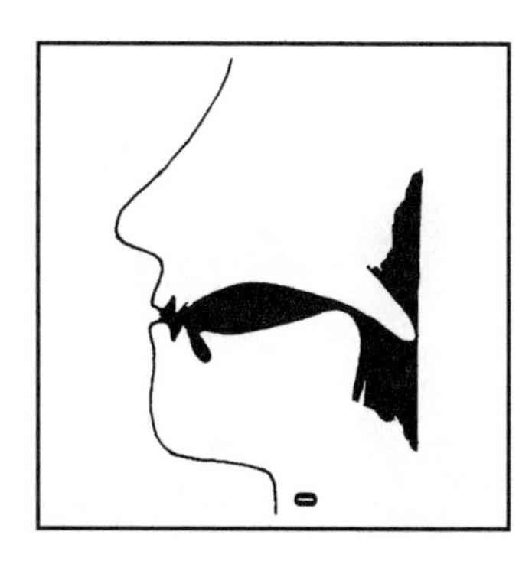
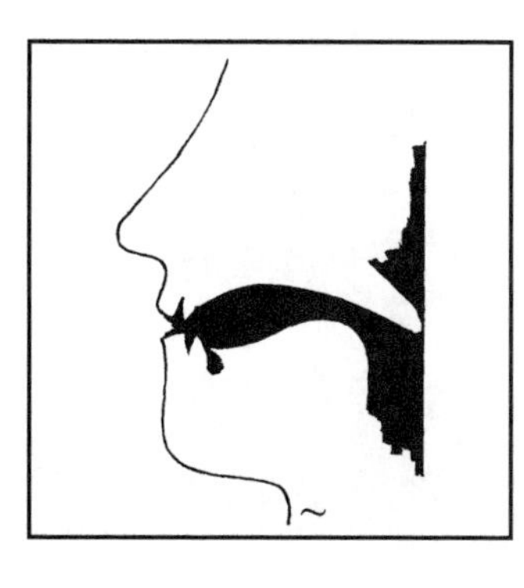
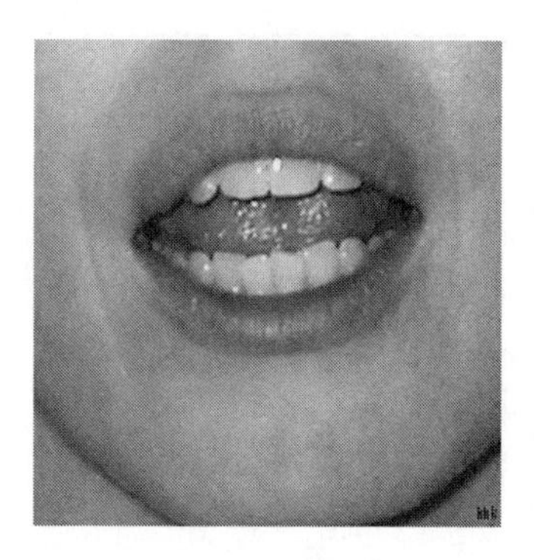
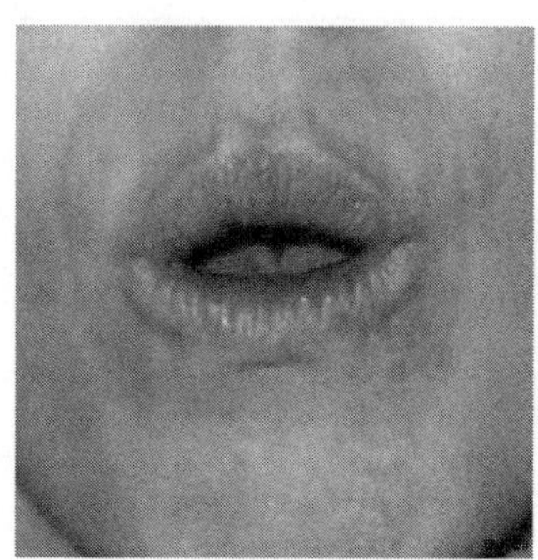

Teach this consonant blend after teaching the /k/ and /w/ sounds. The articulation positions for the sounds are assumed simultaneously. The sounds are made together. A single Lissajous pattern, paper strip movement, or meter needle movement is indicative.

Prosodic Drill

kwekwekwe kwe**kwe**kwe kwekwe**kwe**

kwekwekwekwe kwe**kwe**kwe kwekwe**kwe**kwe

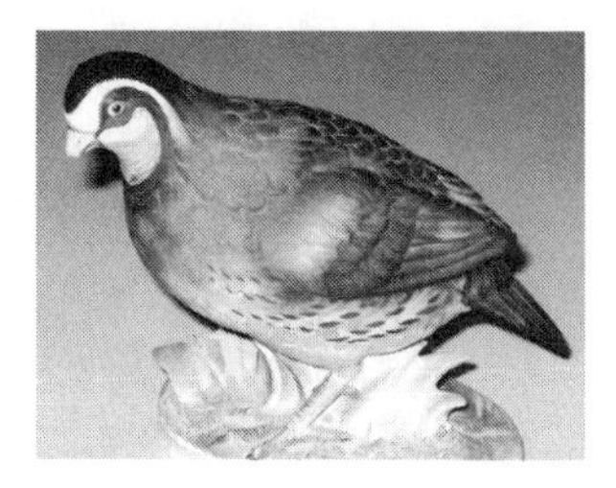

quail

That bird is a ________.

queer quill quest quake quack

quote quarrel quiet

Lesson 71 /pl-/

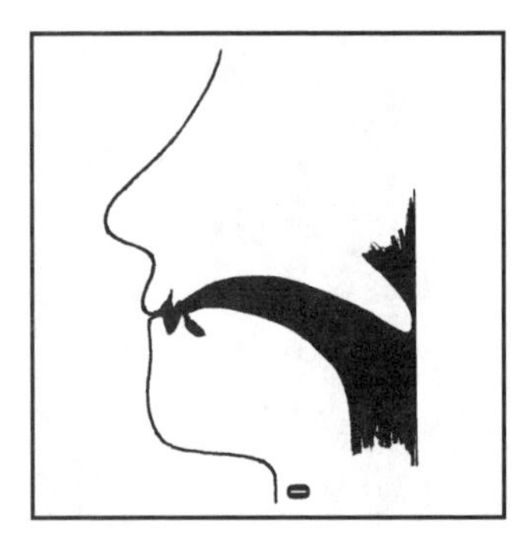
 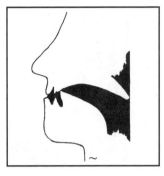
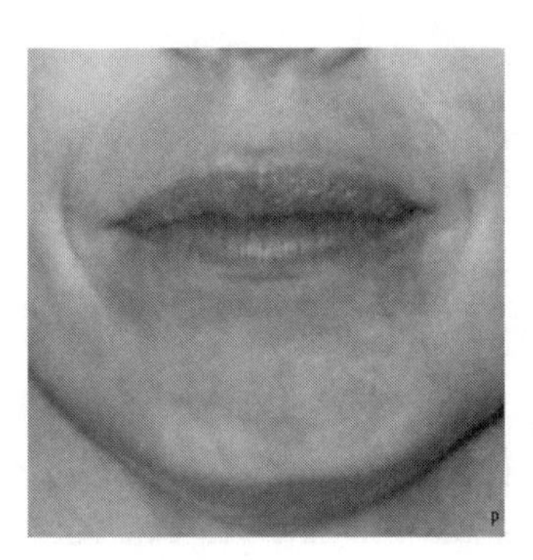
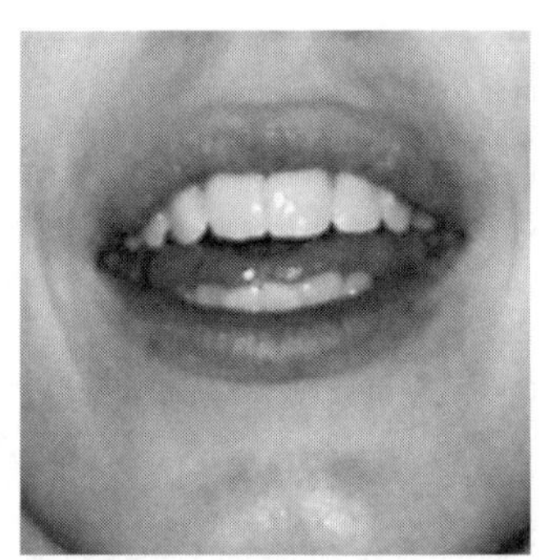

Teach this consonant blend after teaching the /p/ and /l/ sounds. The articulation positions for the sounds are assumed simultaneously. The sounds are made together. A single Lissajous pattern, paper strip movement, or meter needle movement is indicative.

Prosodic Drill

plʌpləplə plə**plʌ**plə pləplə**plʌ**

plʌpəpləplə plə**plʌ**pləplə pləplə**plʌ**plə

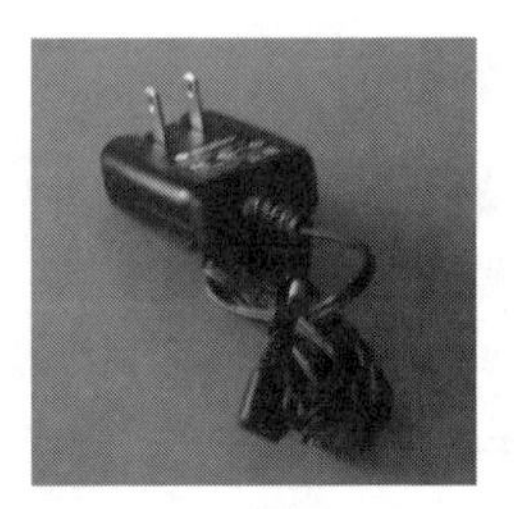

plug

Insert the ________.

please pledge play plaid plum plural

plume plot ply plow pliers

Lesson 72 /pr-/

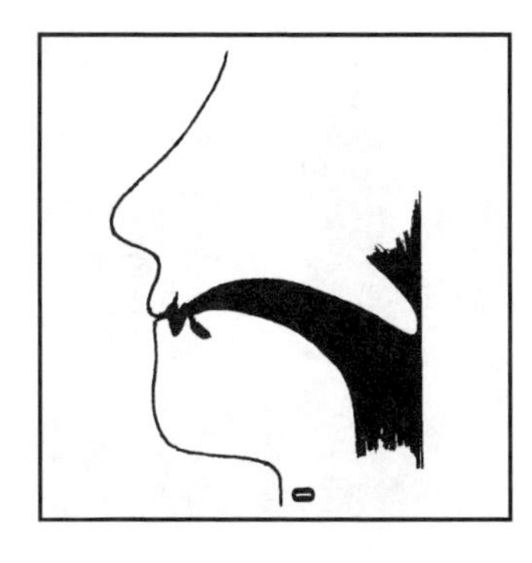
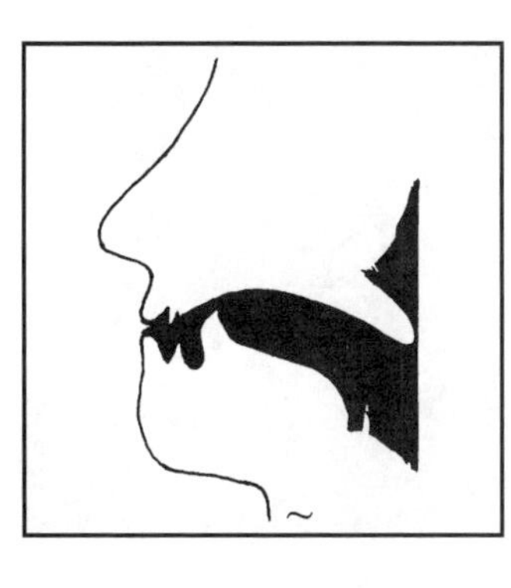
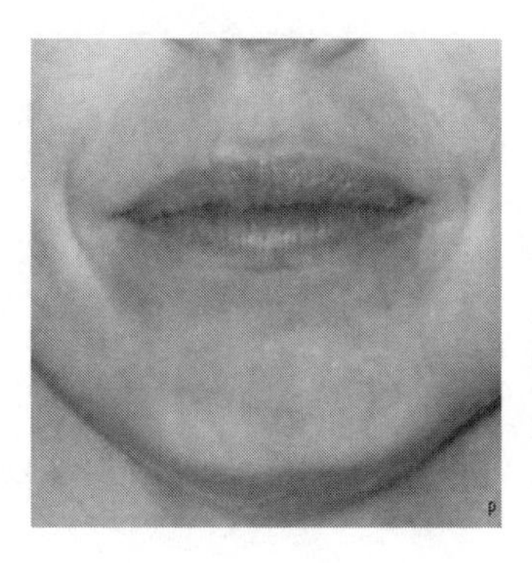
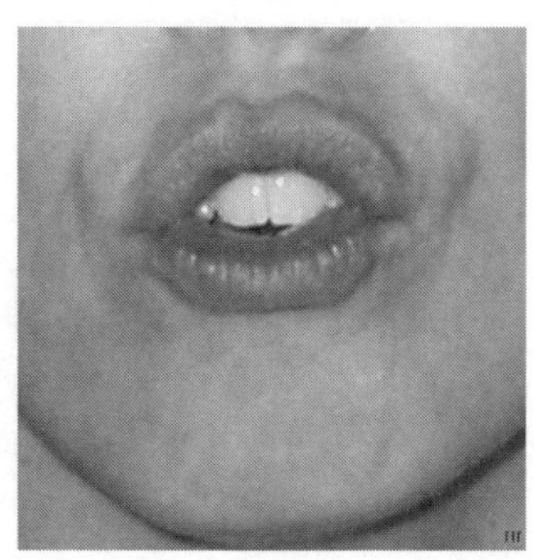

Teach this consonant blend after teaching the /p/ and /r/ sounds. The articulation positions for the sounds are assumed simultaneously. The sounds are made together. A single Lissajous pattern, paper strip movement, or meter needle movement is indicative.

Prosodic Drill

preprepre prepre**pre**pre prepre**pre**

prepreprepre pre**pre**prepre prepre**pre**pre

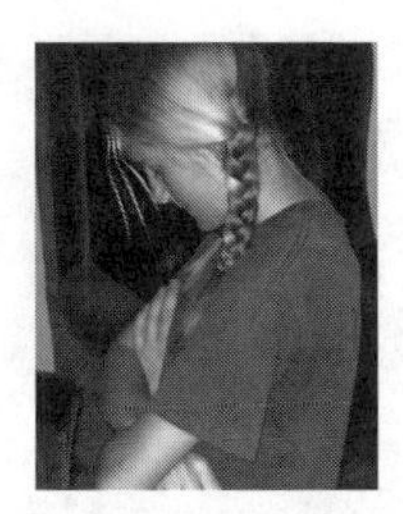

prayer

She is having a ________.

print prep praise prune

prude proud prod pry

Lesson 73 /dr-/

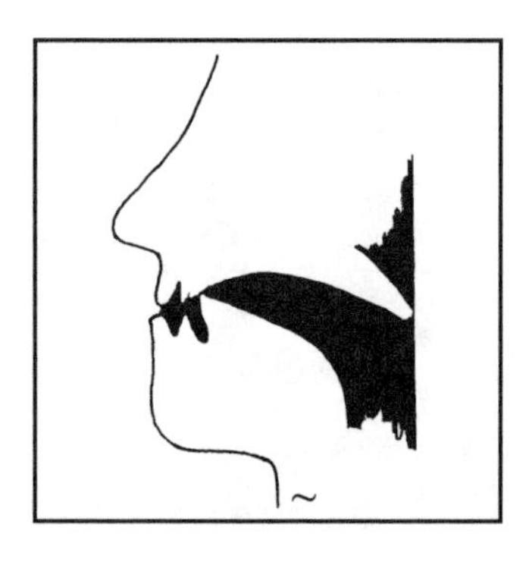
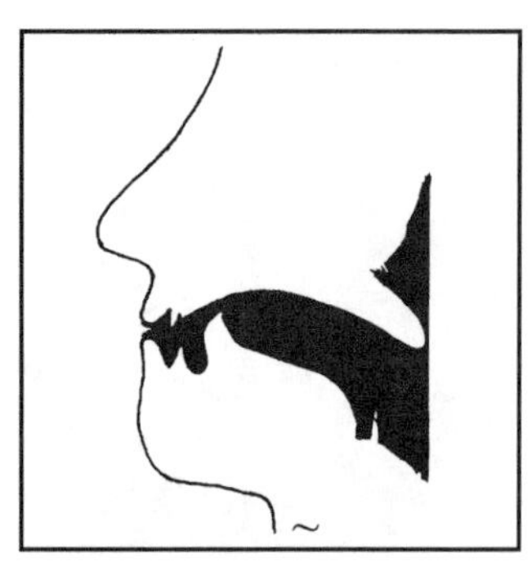
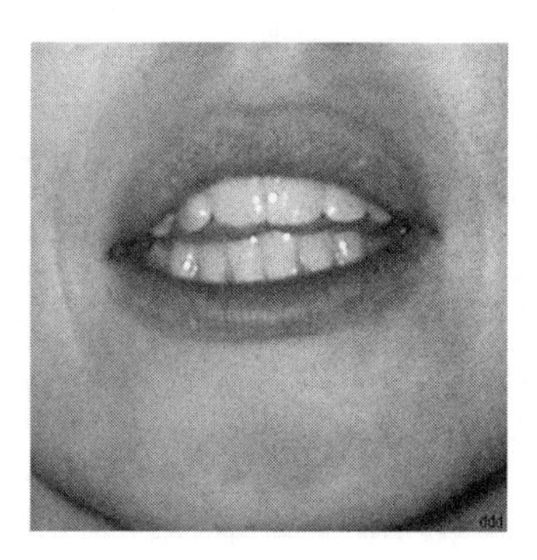
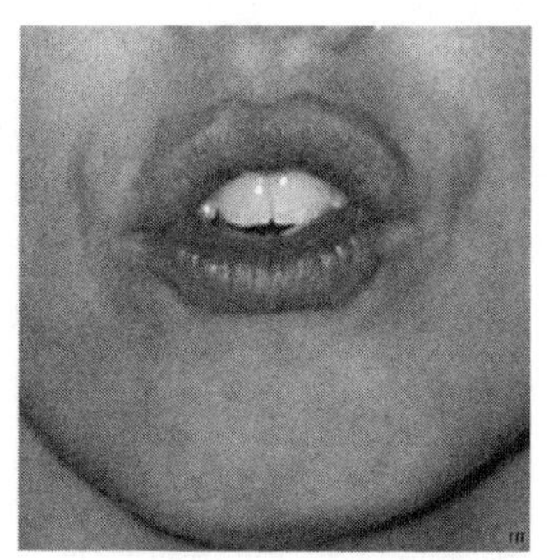

Teach this consonant blend after teaching the /d-/ and /r/ sounds. The articulation positions for the sounds are assumed simultaneously. The sounds are made together. A single Lissajous pattern, paper strip movement, or meter needle movement is indicative.

Prosodic Drill

drɛdrɛdrɛ drɛ**drɛ**drɛ drɛdrɛ**drɛ**

drɛdrɛdrɛdrɛ drɛ**drɛ**drɛdrɛ drɛdrɛ**drɛ**drɛ

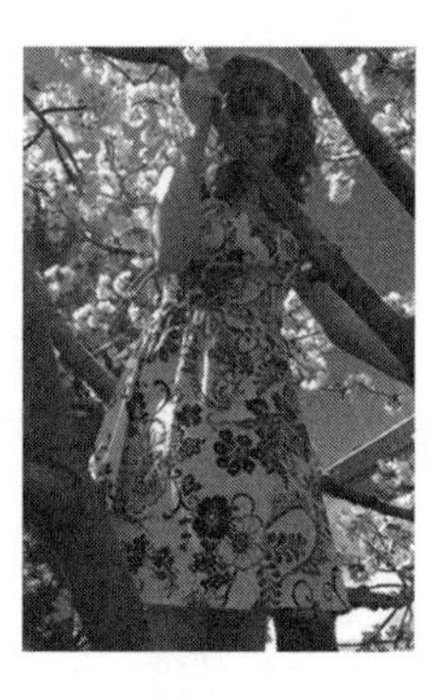

dress

She wears a ________.

dream drill dread drape drat drudge

drew droop draught dry drown

Lesson 74 /gl-/

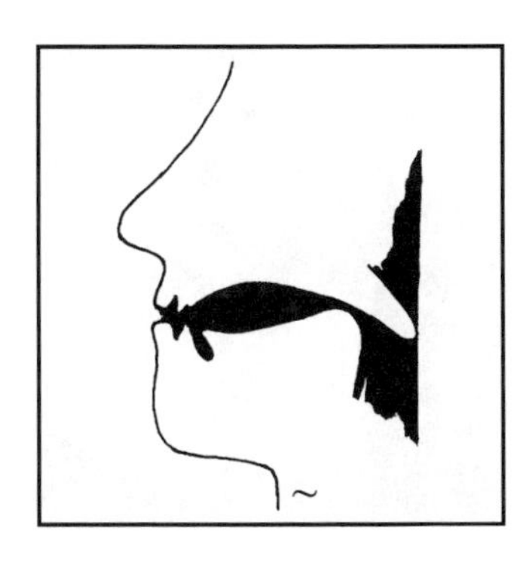

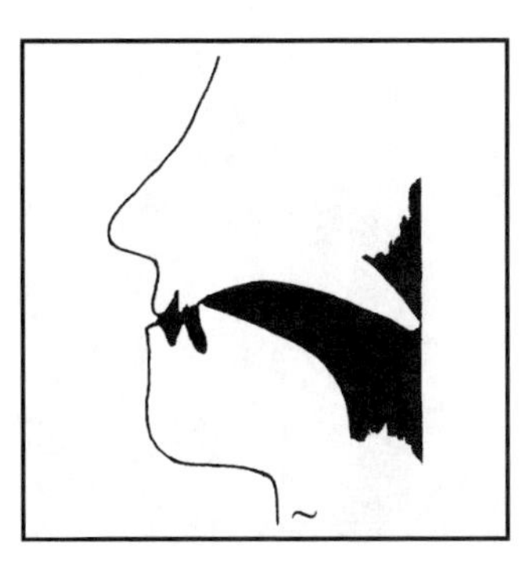

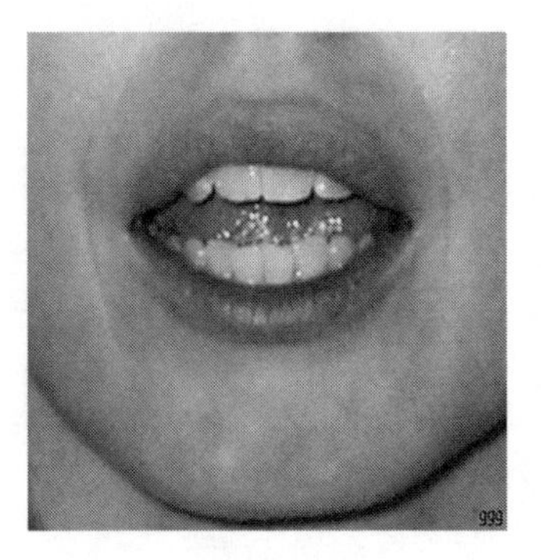

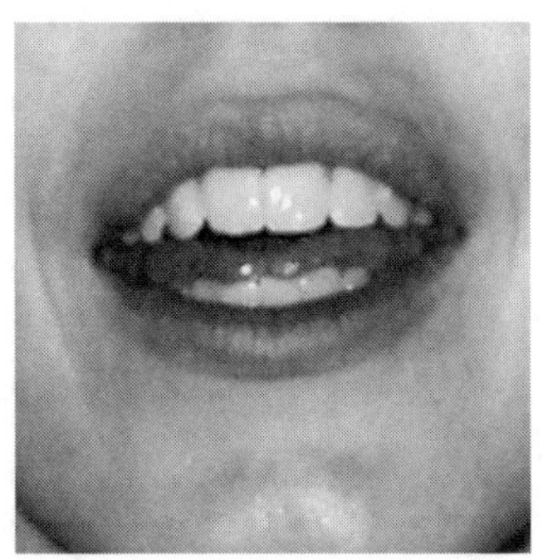

Teach this consonant blend after teaching the /g-/ and /l/ sounds. The articulation positions for the sounds are assumed simultaneously. The sounds are made together. A single Lissajous pattern, paper strip movement, or meter needle movement is indicative.

Prosodic Drill

glæglæglæ glæ**glæ**glæ glæglæ**glæ**

glæglæglæglæ glæ**glæ**glæglæ glæglæ**glæ**glæ

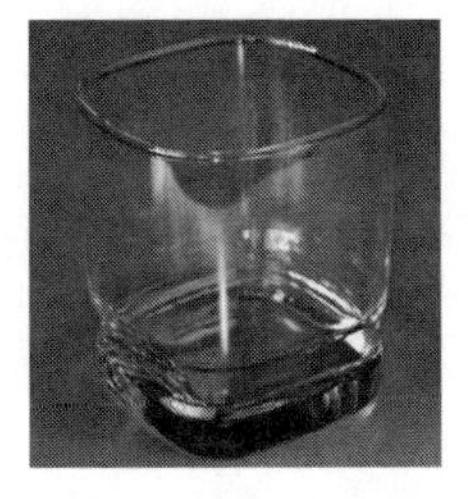

glass

Drink from the ________.

glee glimmer glade glad

gloom globe glob glide

Lesson 75 /gr-/

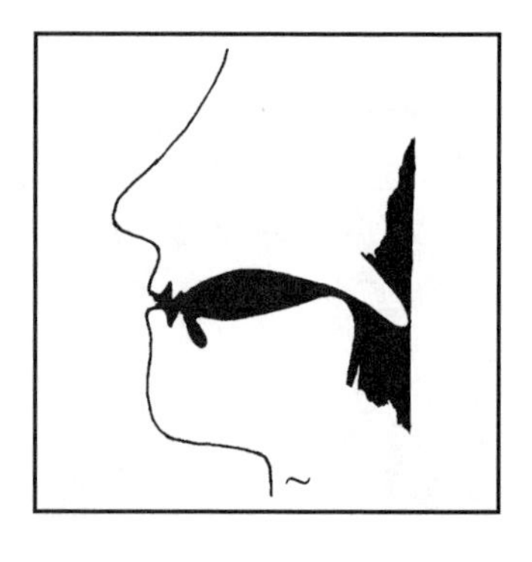 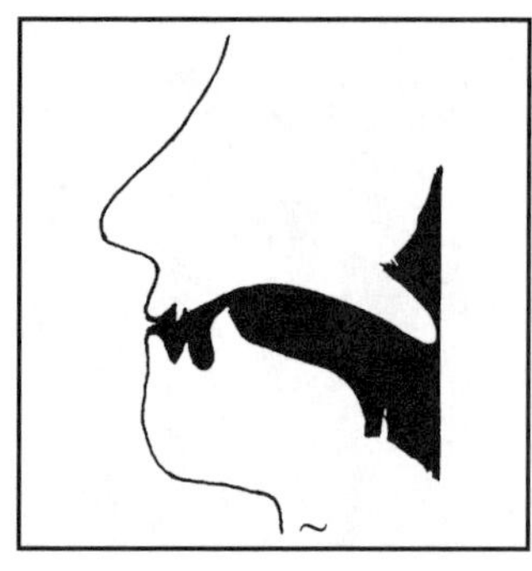 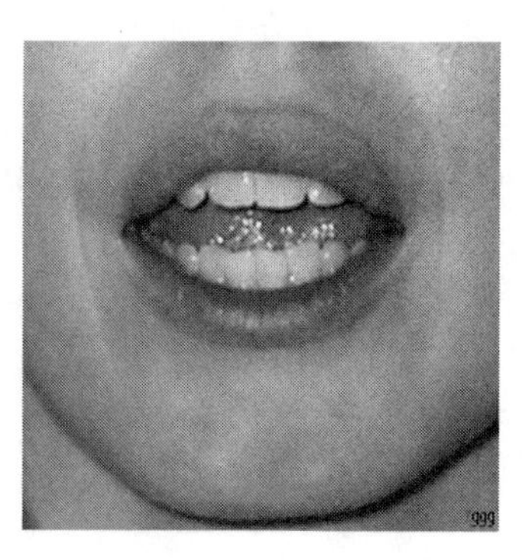 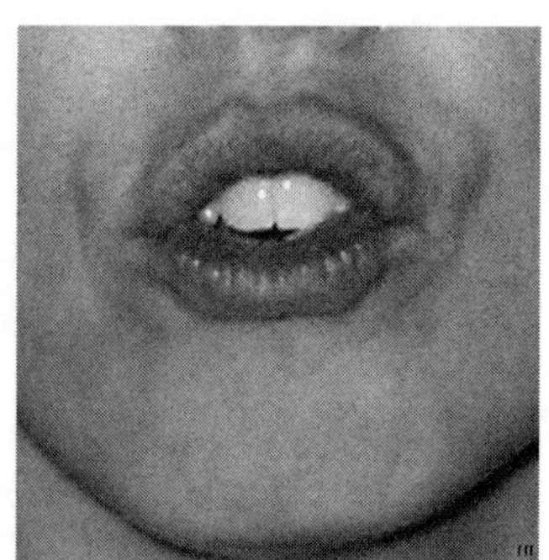

Teach this consonant blend after teaching the /g-/ and /r/ sounds. The articulation positions for the sounds are assumed simultaneously. The sounds are made together. A single Lissajous pattern, paper strip movement, or meter needle movement is indicative.

Prosodic Drill

gregregre gre**gre**gre gregre**gre**

gregregregre gre**gre**gregre gregre**gre**gre

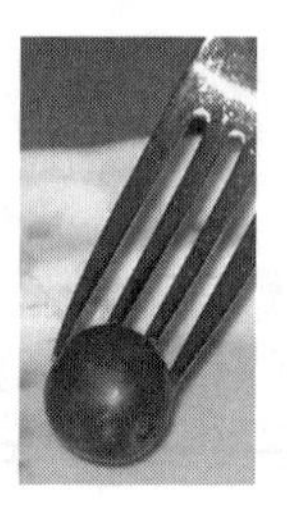

grape

Eat a ________.

grease grip great grab grub

groove grope grouse gripe

Lesson 76 /kl-/

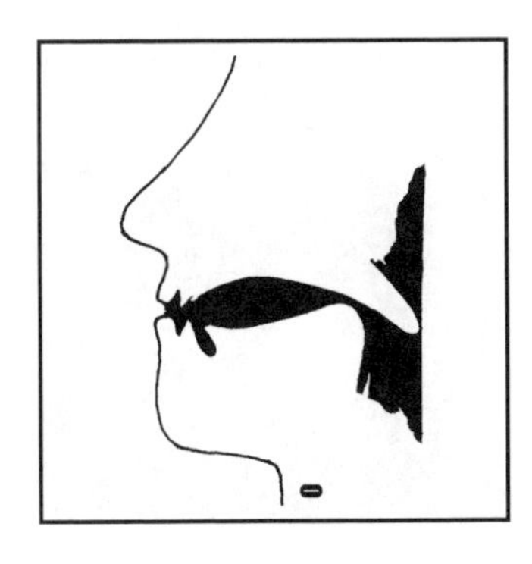
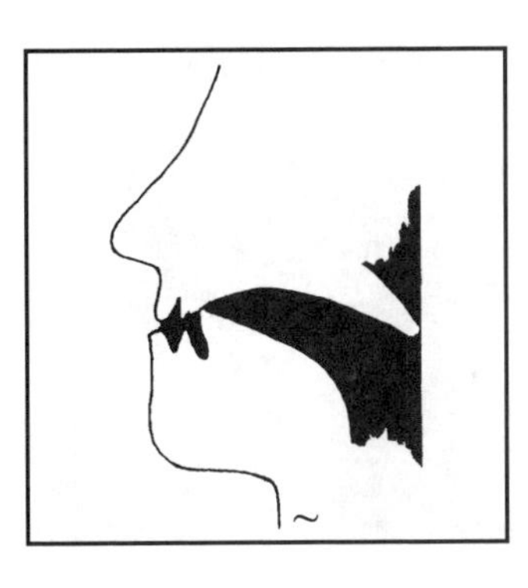
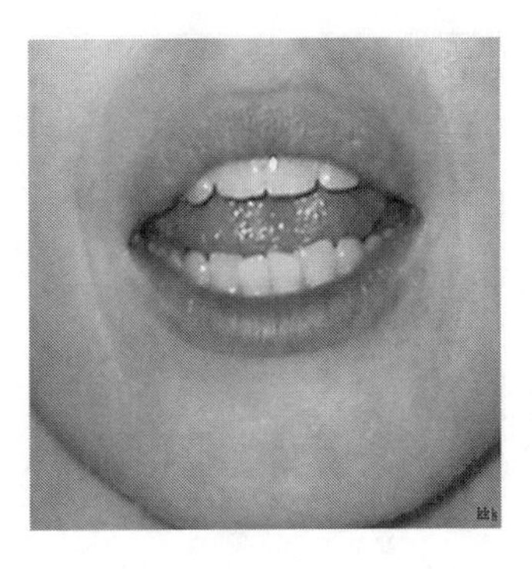
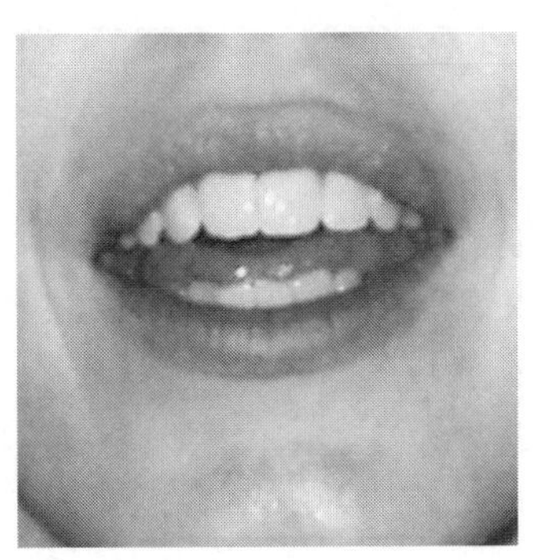

Teach this consonant blend after teaching the /k/ and /l/ sounds. The articulation positions for the sounds are assumed simultaneously. The sounds are made together. A single Lissajous pattern, paper strip movement, or meter needle movement is indicative.

Prosodic Drill

klaklakla klа**kla**kla klakla**kla**

klaklaklakla kla**kla**klakla klakla**kla**kla

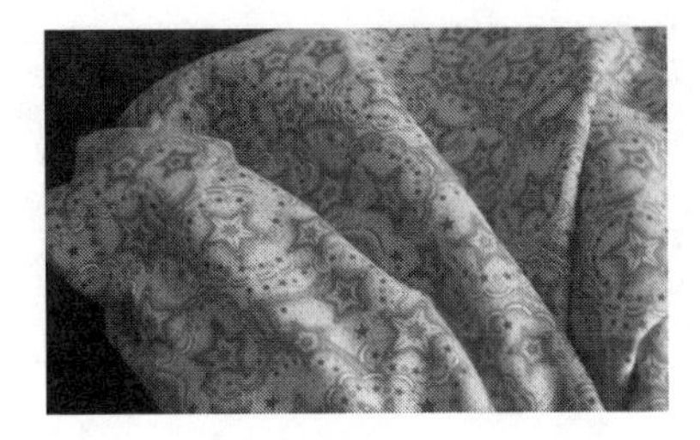

cloth

That's ________.

clean click clack cluck clerk

clue clone claw cloud climb

Lesson 77 /kr-/

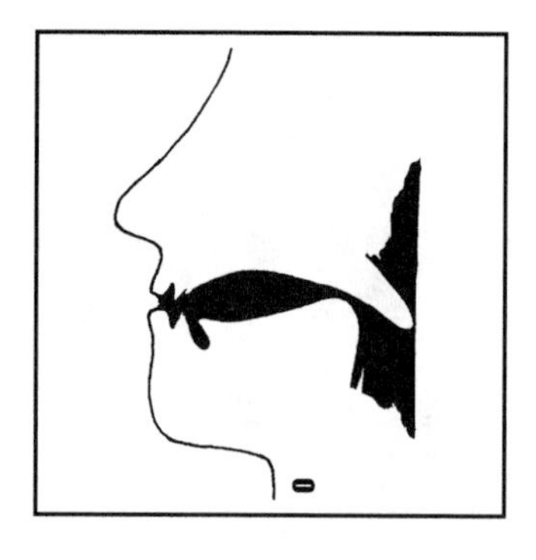
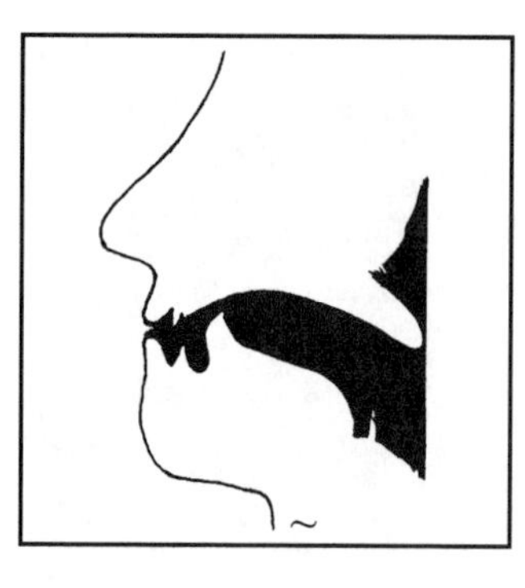
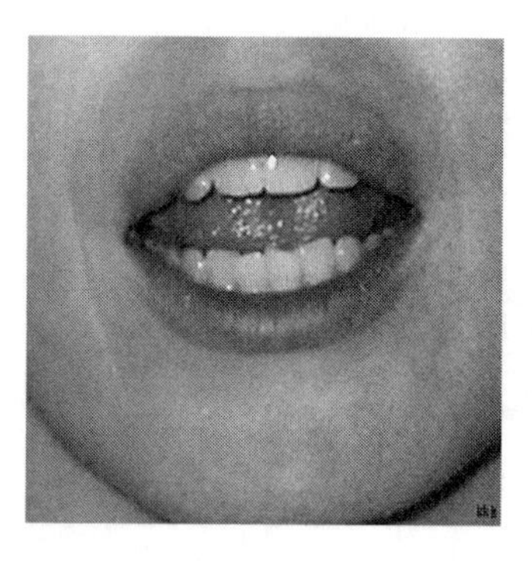
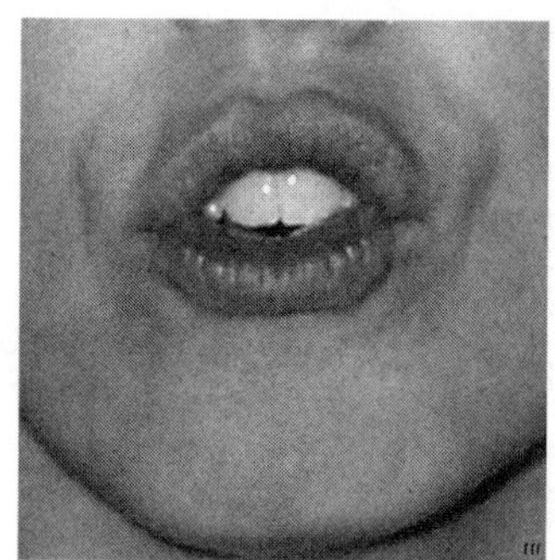

Teach this consonant blend after teaching the /k/ and /r/ sounds. The articulation positions for the sounds are assumed simultaneously. The sounds are made together. A single Lissajous pattern, paper strip movement, or meter needle movement is indicative.

Prosodic Drill

krækrækræ kræ**kræ**kræ krækræ**kræ**

krækrækrækræ kræ**kræ**krækræ krækræ**kræ**kræ

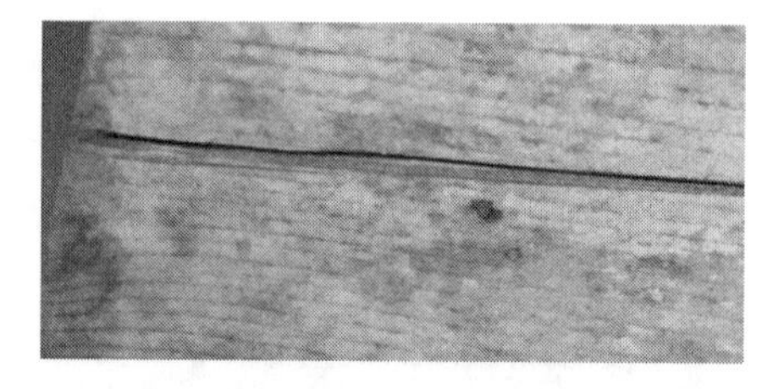

crack

The board has a ________.

creek critter cress cram crumb

cruel crow craw crowd cry

Lesson 78 /tr-/

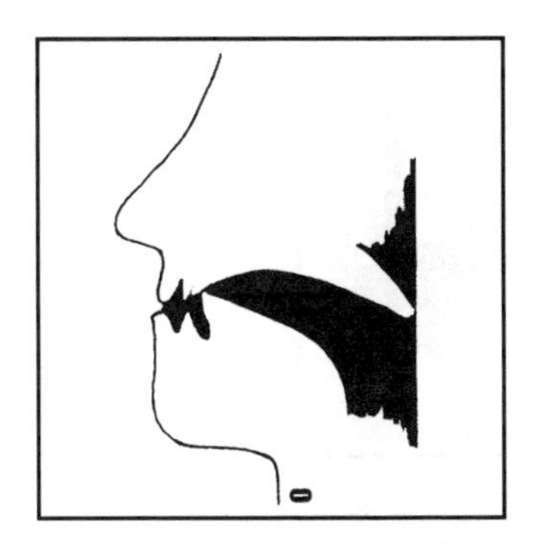
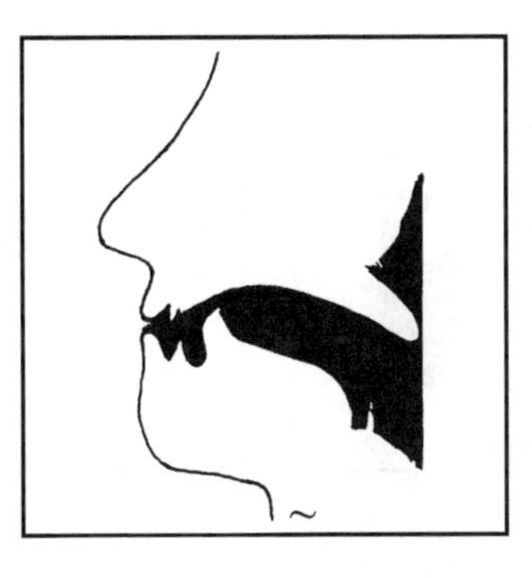
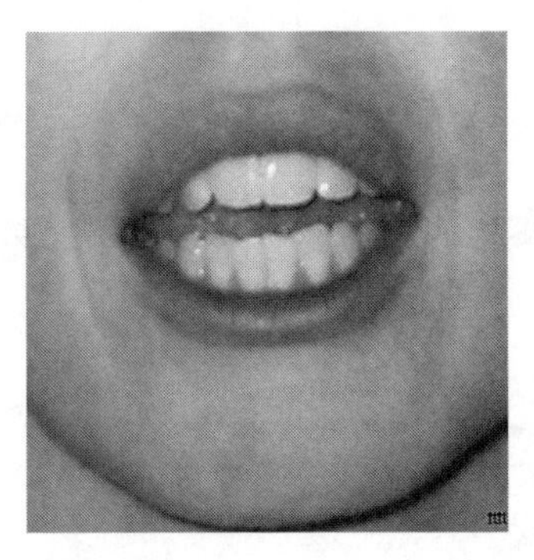
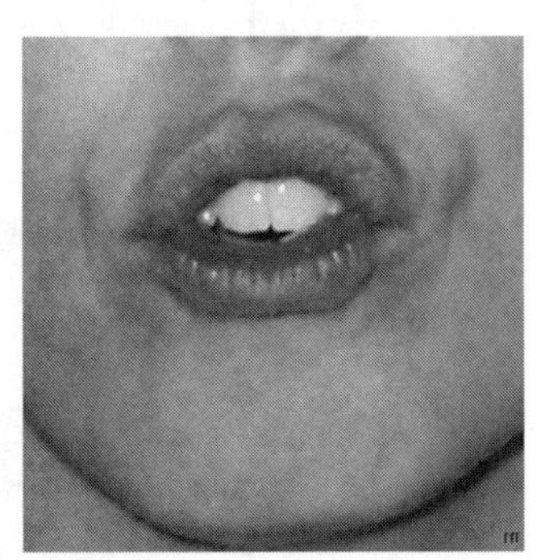

Teach this consonant blend after teaching the /t/ and /r/ sounds. The articulation positions for the sounds are assumed simultaneously. The sounds are made together. A single Lissajous pattern, paper strip movement, or meter needle movement is indicative.

Prosodic Drill

tritritri tri**tri**tri tri**tri**tri

tritritritri tri**tri**tritri tritri**tri**tri

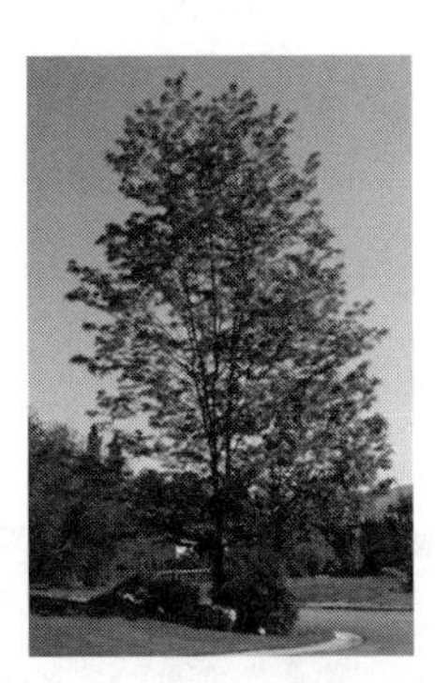

tree

That is a ________.

treat trip train trap truck

true troll trot trout try

Lesson 79 /spl-/

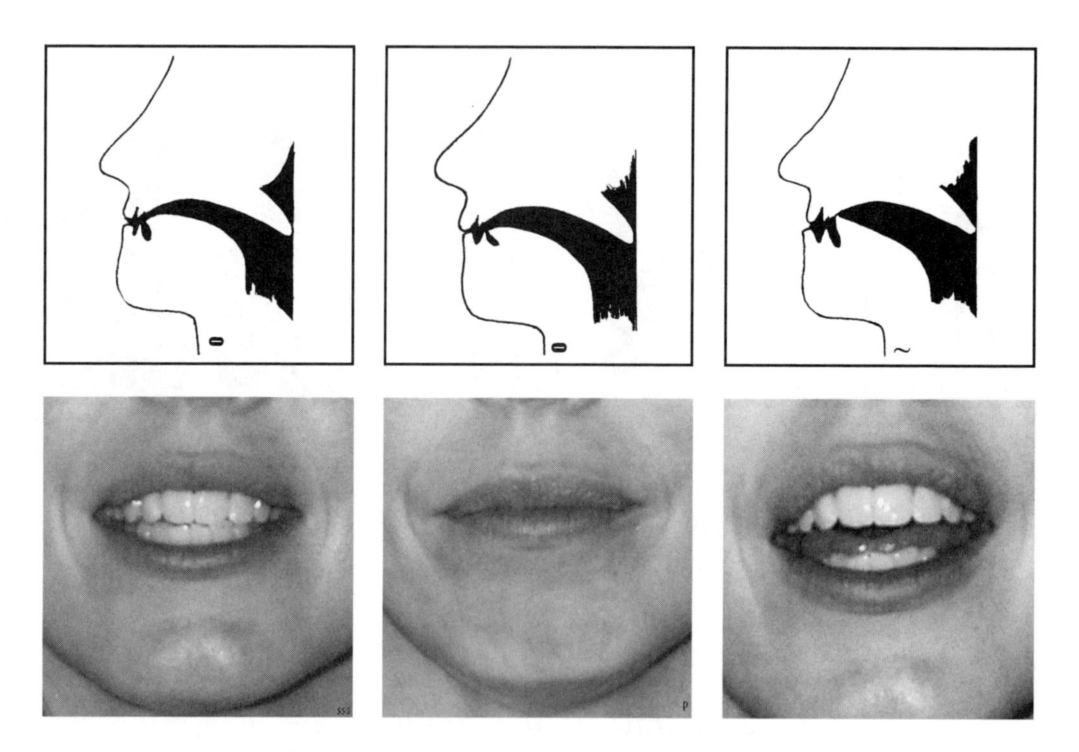

Teach this consonant blend after teaching the /s/, /p/, and /l/ sounds. Say the first sound, then the second and third sounds together, faster and faster, until the /spl-/ blend occurs. The successive parts of this blend are indicated by Lissajous patterns and paper strip and meter needle movements.

Prosodic Drill

splæsplæsplæ splæ**splæ**splæ splæsplæ**splæ**

splæsplæsplæ splæ**splæ**splæsplæ splæsplæ**splæ**splæ

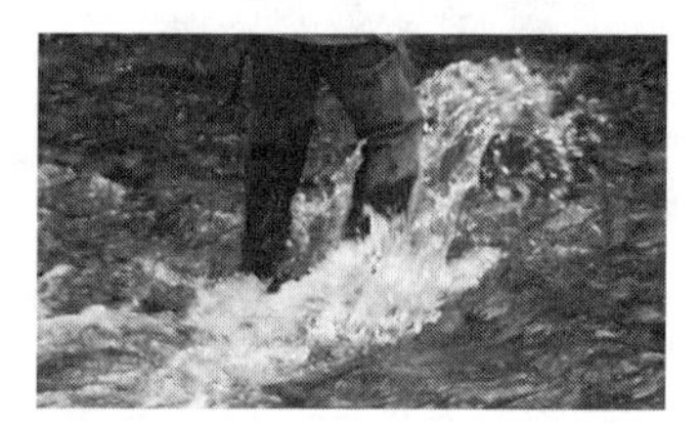

splash

See the water ________.

spleen split splendid splat

splurge splice

Lesson 80 /spr-/

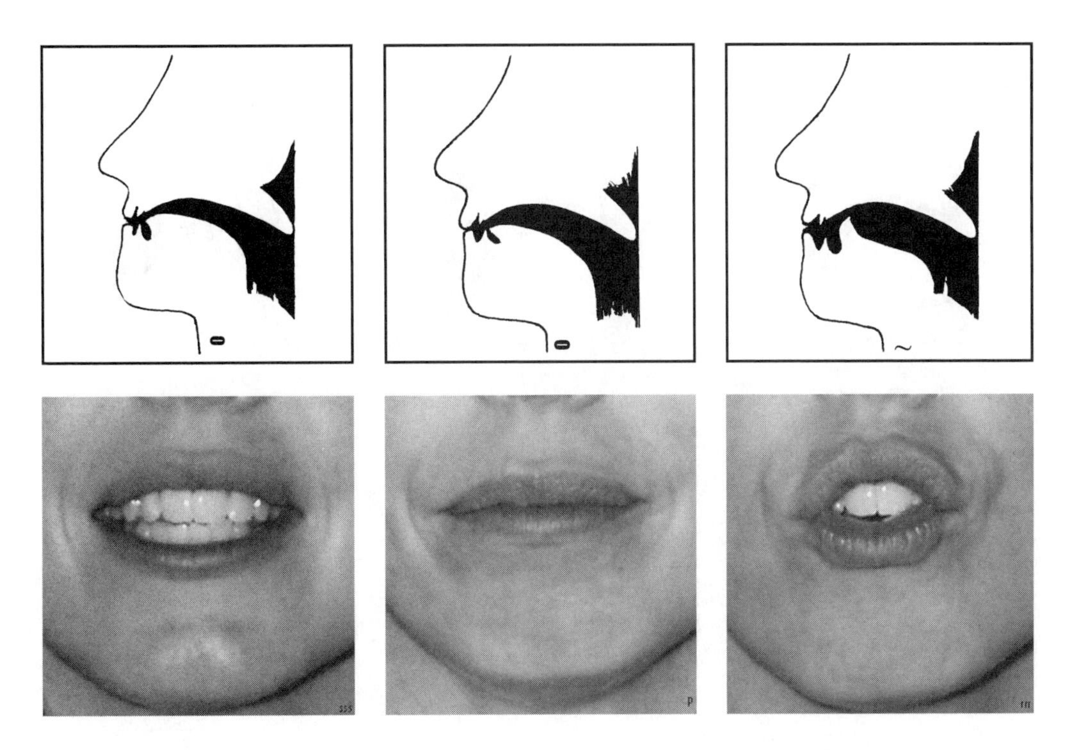

Teach this consonant blend after teaching the /s/, /p/, and /r/ sounds. Say the first sound, then the second and third sounds together, faster and faster, until the /spr-/ blend occurs. The successive parts of this blend are indicated by Lissajous patterns and paper strip and meter needle movements.

Prosodic Drill

spresprespre spre**spre**spre sprespre**spre**

sprespresprespre spre**spre**sprespre sprespre**spre**spre

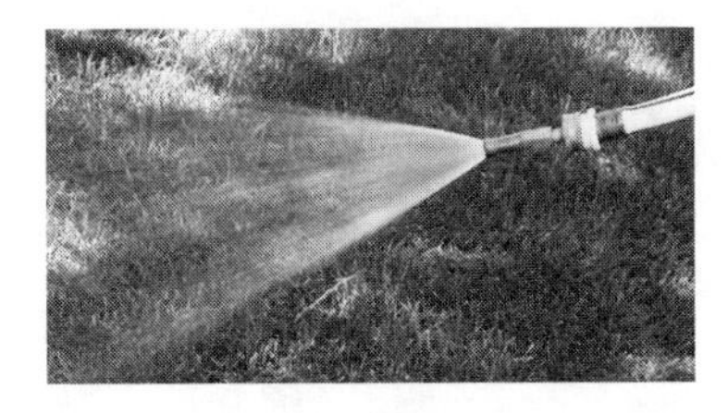

spray

See the water ________.

spree spring spread sprat

spruce sprawl sprout

Lesson 81 /str-/

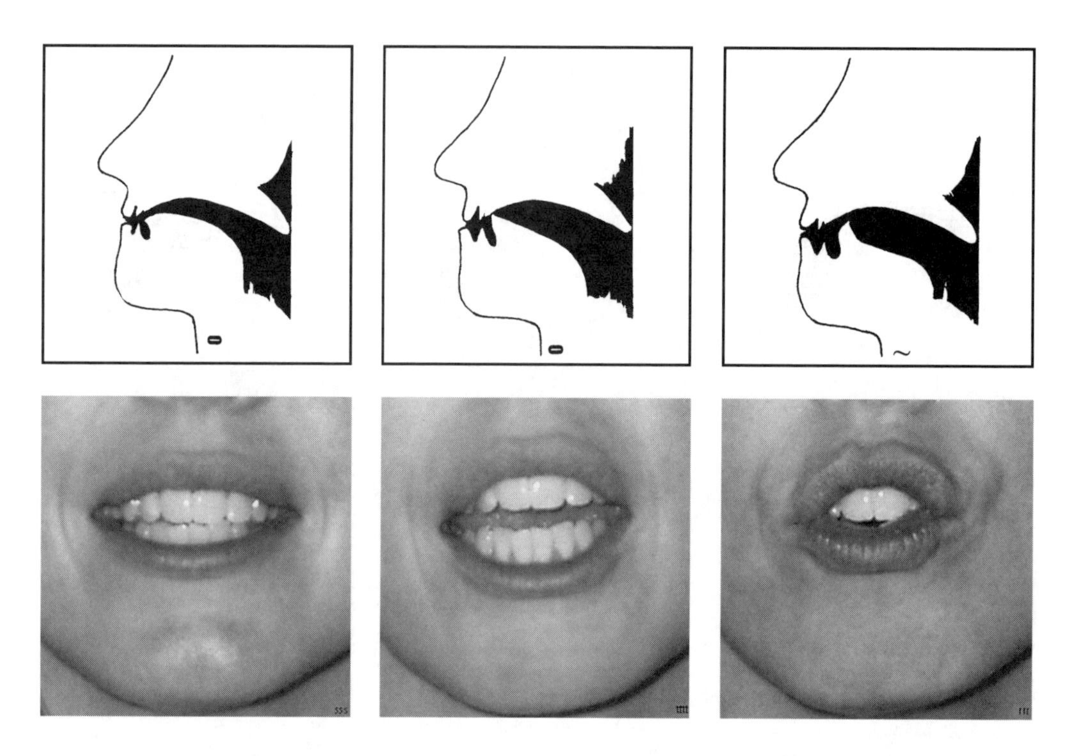

Teach this consonant blend after teaching the /s/, /t/, and /r/ sounds. Say the first sound, then the second and third sounds together, faster and faster, until the /str-/ blend occurs. The successive parts of this blend are indicated by Lissajous patterns and paper strip and meter needle movements.

Prosodic Drill

stristristri stri**stri**stri stristri**stri**

stristristristri stri**stri**stristri stristri**stri**stri

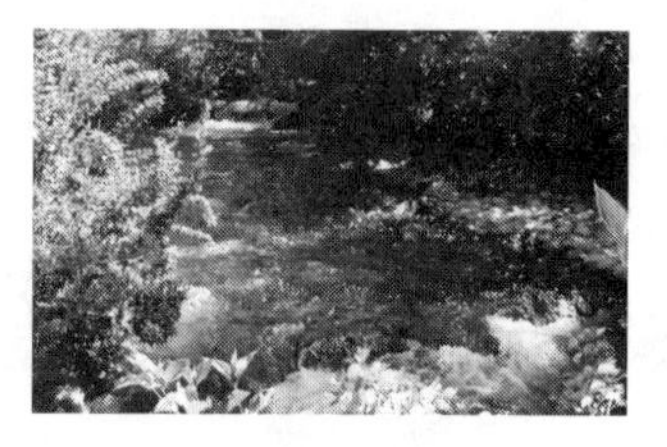

stream

That is a ________.

streak strip stretch strange strap strut

strove straw stride

Lesson 82 /-fs/

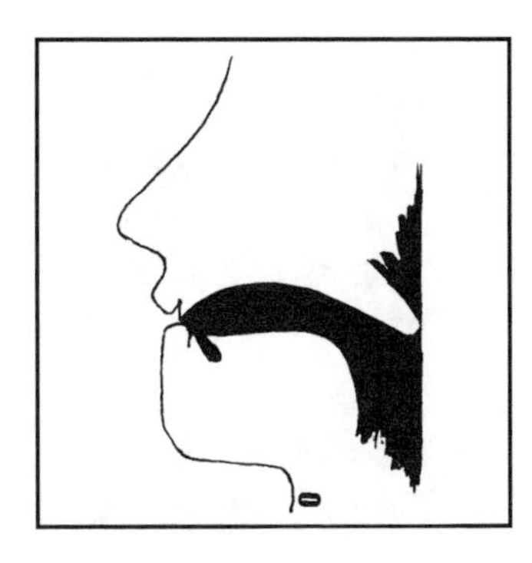
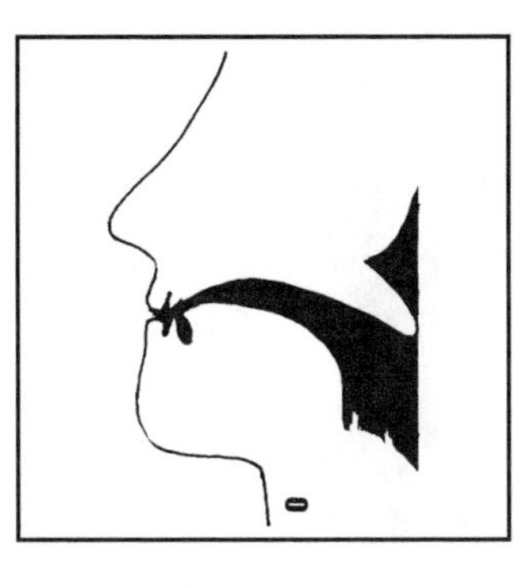
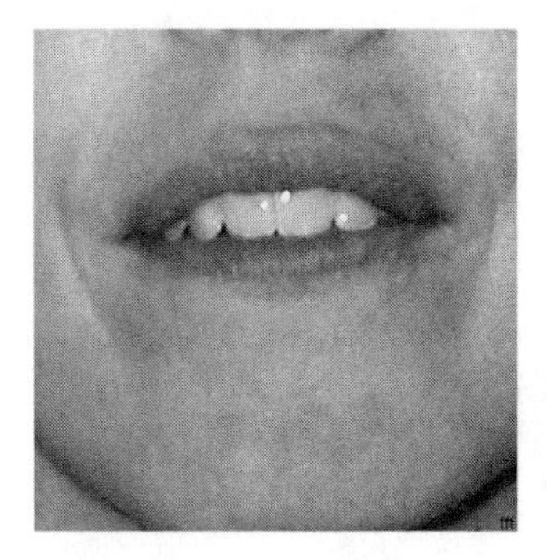
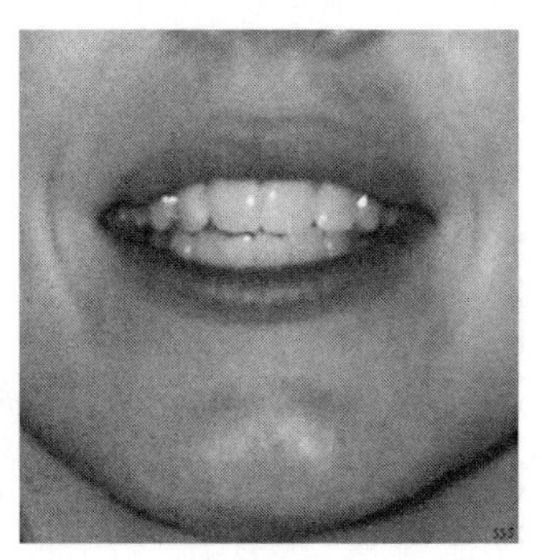

Teach this consonant blend after teaching the /f/ and /s/ sounds. Say the two sounds in succession, faster and faster, until /-fs/ occurs. Both sounds are voiceless and high frequency. The successive parts of this blend are indicated by Lissajous patterns, paper strip movements, and meter needle movements.

Prosodic Drill

ʌfsəfsəfs əfs**ʌfs**əfs əfsəfs**ʌfs**

ʌfsəfsəfsəfs əfs**ʌfs**əfsəfs əfsəfs**ʌfs**əfs

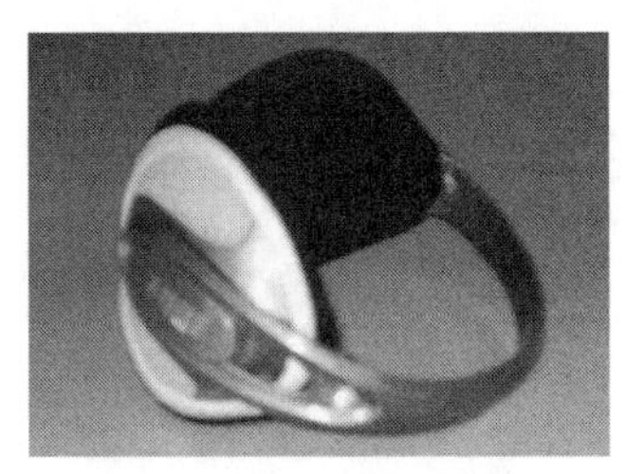

muffs

Those are ear ________.

reefs riffs chefs safes puffs

laughs surfs roofs loafs coughs

Lesson 83 /-lz/

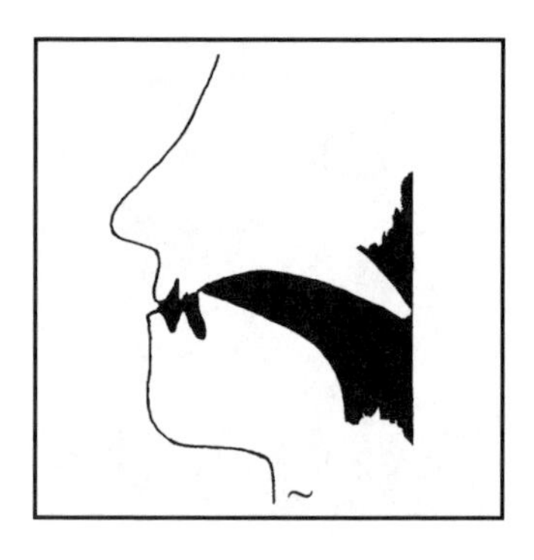
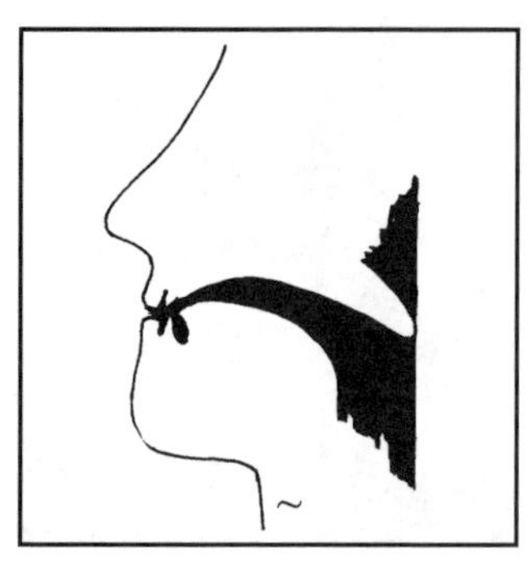
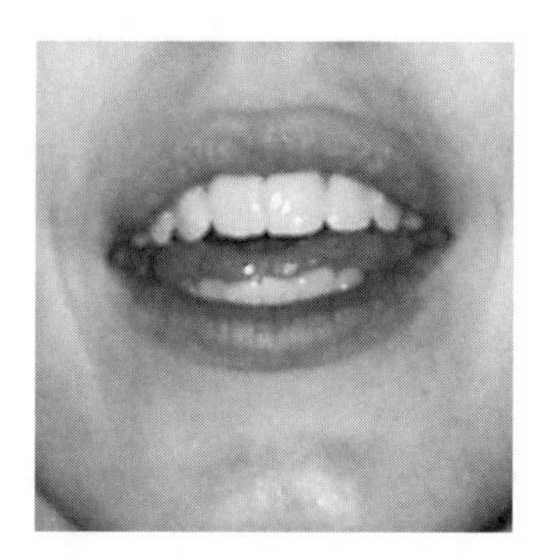
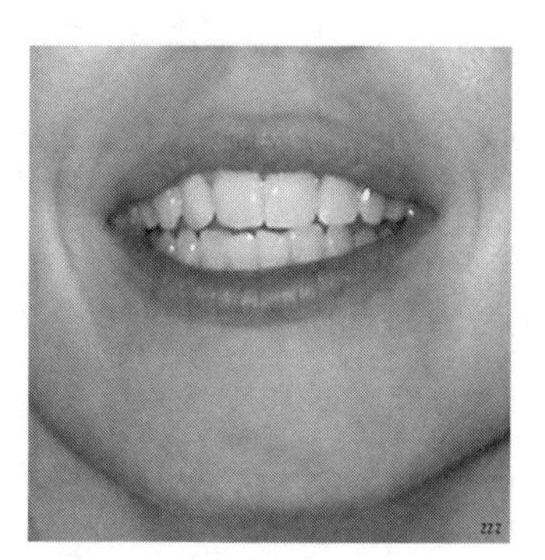

Teach this consonant blend after teaching the /l/ and /z/ sounds. Say the two sounds in succession, faster and faster, until /-lz/ occurs. Both sounds are voiced. The first is low frequency, the second low and high frequency. The successive parts of this blend are indicated by Lissajous patterns and meter needle movements.

Prosodic Drill

ɔlzɔlzɔlz ɔlz**ɔlz**ɔlz ɔlzɔlz**ɔlz**

ɔlzɔlzɔlzɔlz ɔlz**ɔlz**ɔlzɔlz ɔlzɔlz**ɔlz**ɔlz

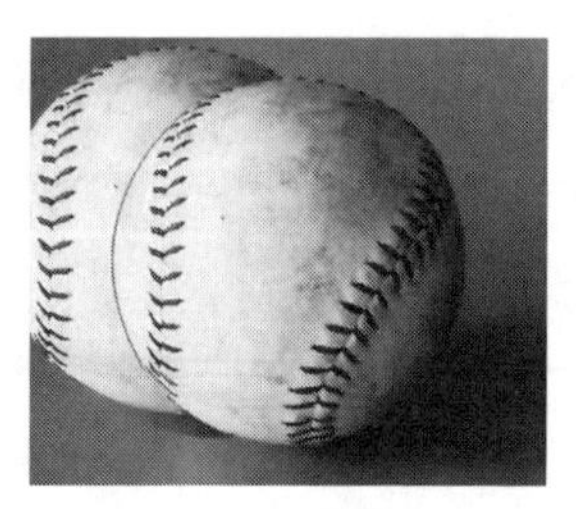

balls

Give me the ________.

peels bills sells pails pals pulls

pearls pools poles towels piles

Lesson 84 /-mz/

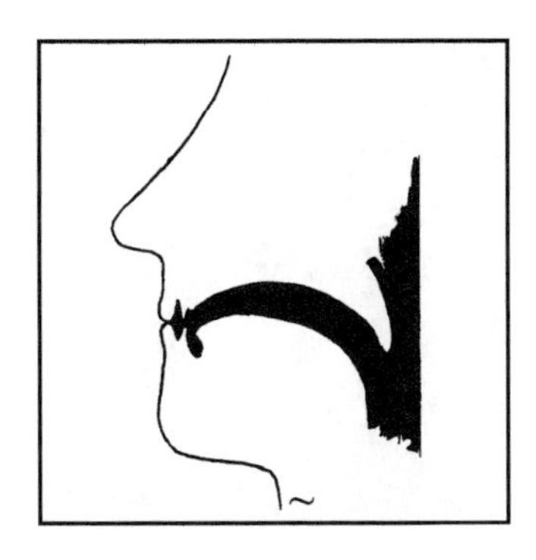
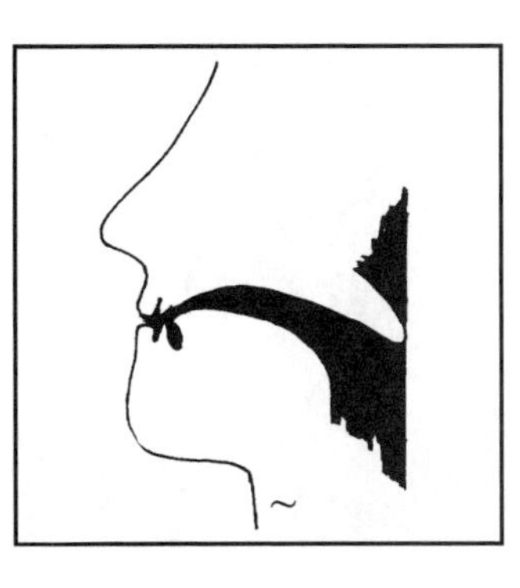
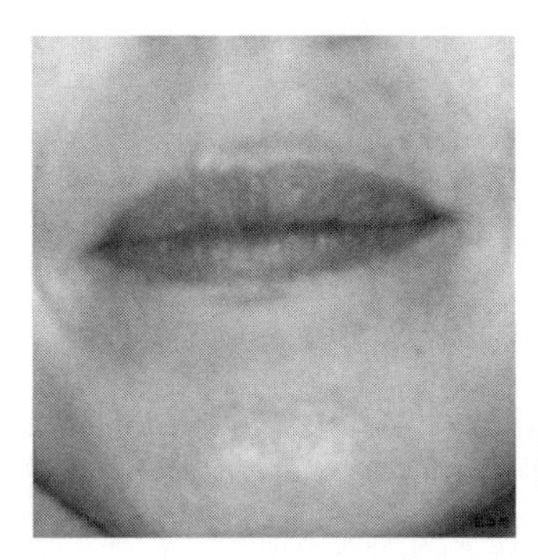
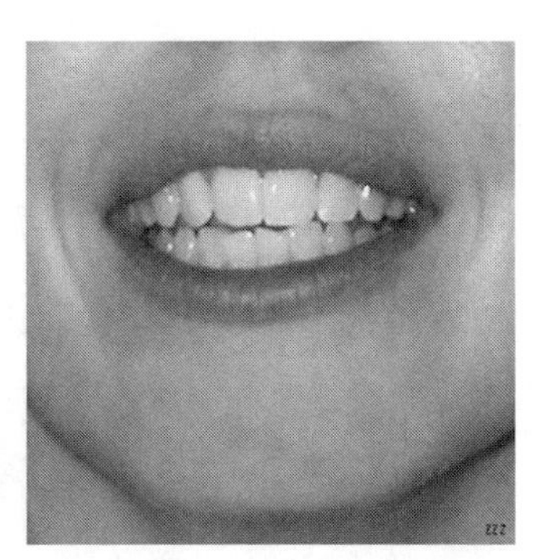

Teach this consonant blend after teaching the /m/ and /z/ sounds. Say the two sounds in succession, faster and faster, until /-mz/ occurs. The first sound is nasal and low frequency, the second oral and low and high frequency. The successive parts of this blend are indicated by Lissajous patterns, paper strip movements, and meter needle movements.

Prosodic Drill

ʌmzəmzəmz əmz**ʌmz**əmz əmzəmz**ʌmz**

ʌmzəmzəmzəmz əmz**ʌmz**əmzəmz əmzəmz**ʌmz**əmz

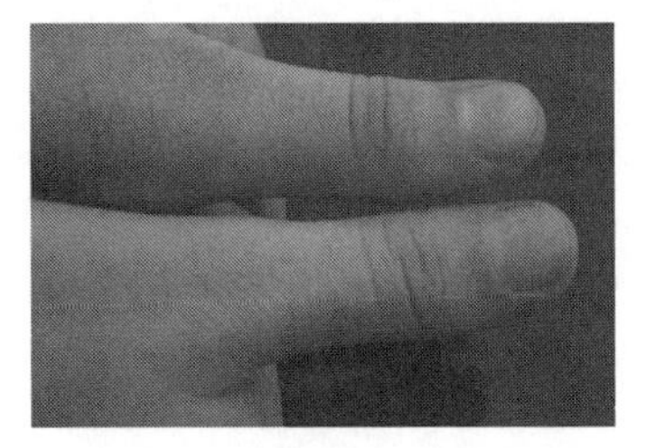

thumbs

We have two ________.

beams limbs tames comes worms

booms foams bombs times

Lesson 85 /-nz/

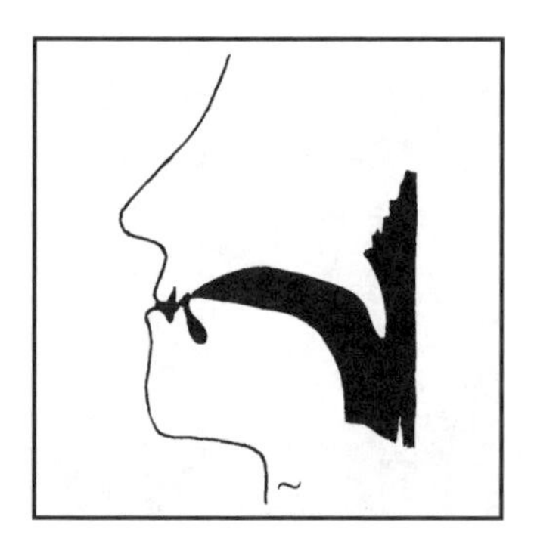
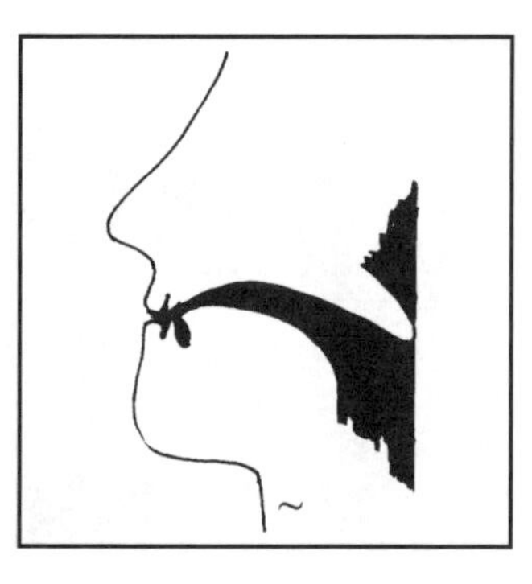
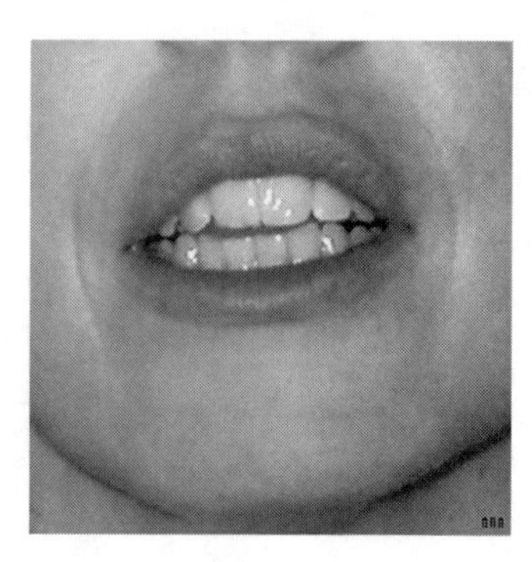
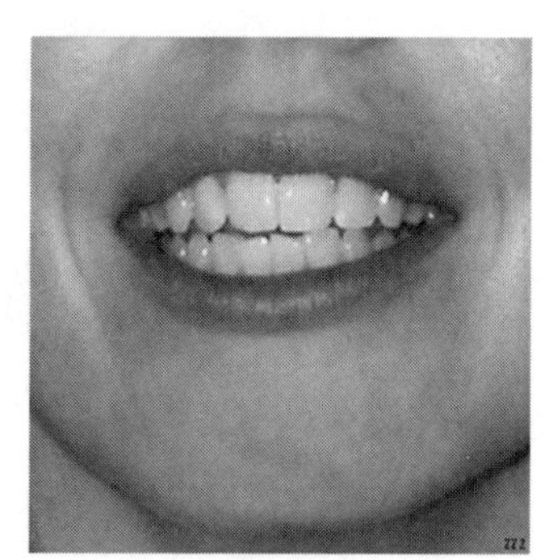

Teach this consonant blend after teaching the /n/ and /z/ sounds. Say the two sounds in succession, faster and faster, until /-nz/ occurs. The first sound is nasal and low frequency, the second oral and low and high frequency. The successive parts of this blend are indicated by Lissajous patterns, paper strip movements, and meter needle movements.

Prosodic Drill

ɔɪnzɔɪnzɔɪnz ɔɪnz**ɔɪnz**ɔɪnz ɔɪnzɔɪnz**ɔɪnz**

ɔɪnzɔɪnzɔɪnzɔɪnz ɔɪnz**ɔɪnz**ɔɪnzɔɪnz ɔɪnzɔɪnz**ɔɪnz**ɔɪnz

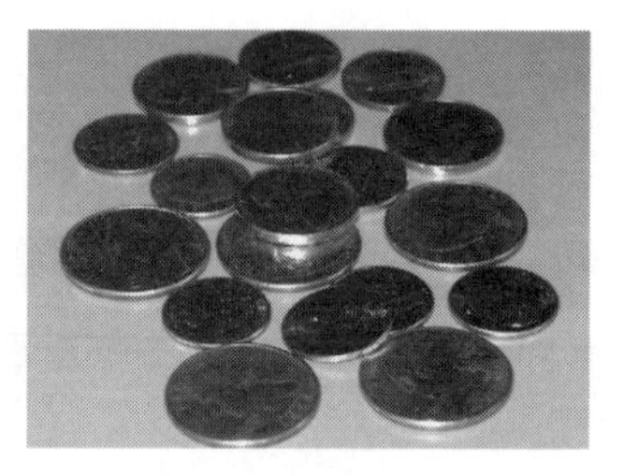

coins

These are ________.

beans pins hens panes pans turns

spoons tones lawns towns signs

Lesson 86 /-sn/

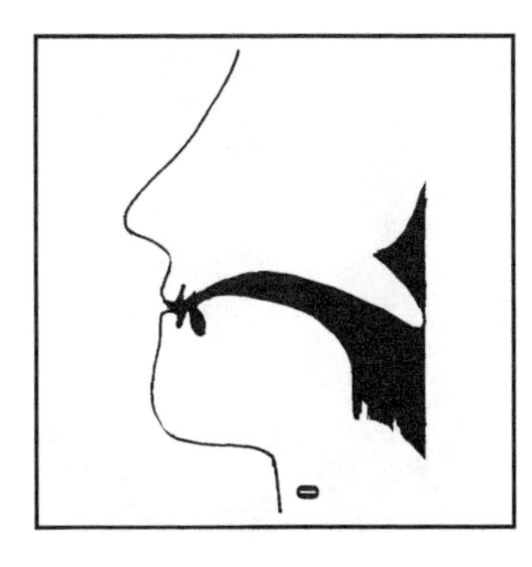
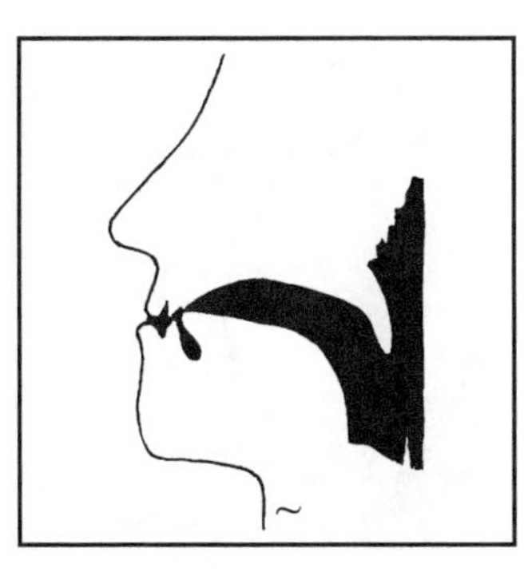
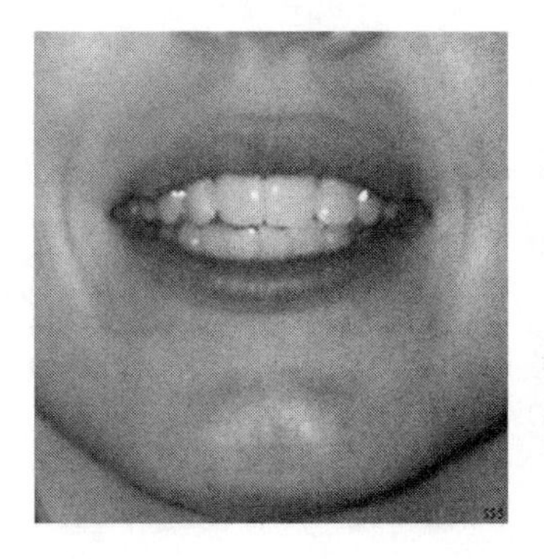
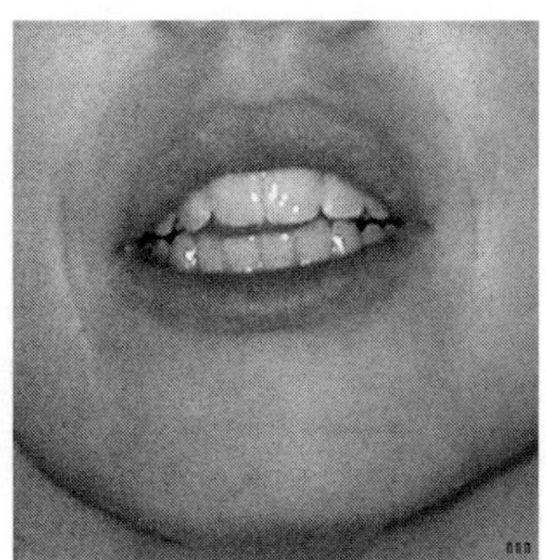

Teach this consonant blend after teaching the /s/ and /n/ sounds. Say the two sounds in succession, faster and faster, until /-sn/ occurs. The first sound is voiceless and high frequency, the second voiced and low frequency. The successive parts of this blend are indicated by Lissajous patterns, paper strip movements, and meter needle movements.

Prosodic Drill

ɪsnɪsnɪsn ɪsn**ɪsn**ɪsn ɪsnɪsn**ɪsn**

ɪsnɪsnɪsnɪsn ɪsn**ɪsn**ɪsnɪsn ɪsnɪsn**ɪsn**ɪsn

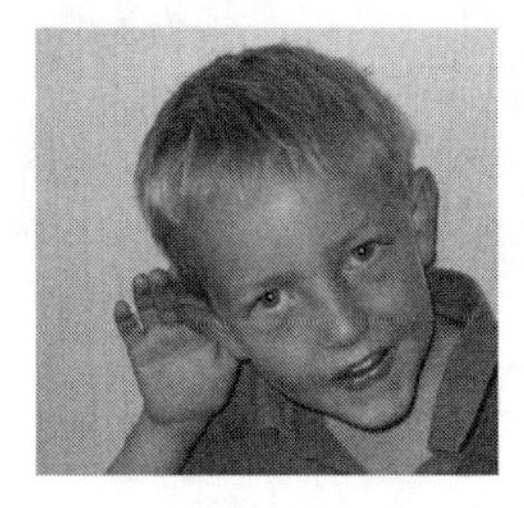

listen

Try to ________.

glisten hasten chasten mason

boatswain moisten

Lesson 87 /vz/

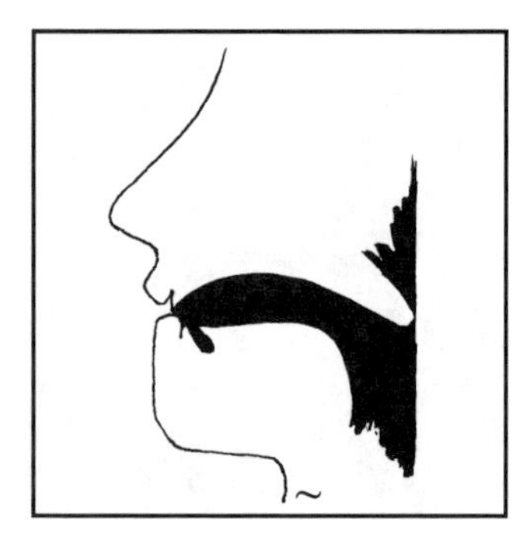
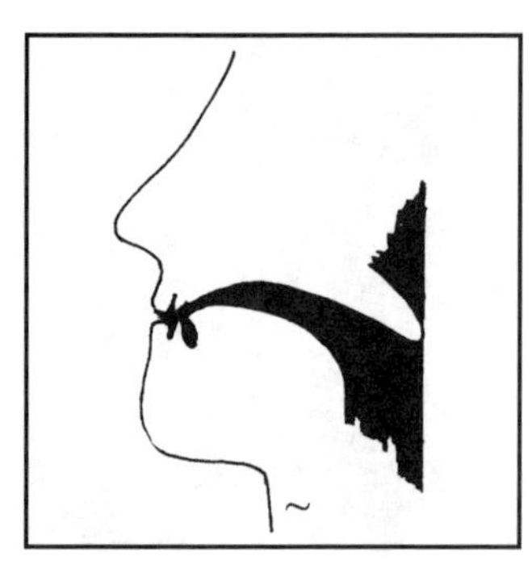
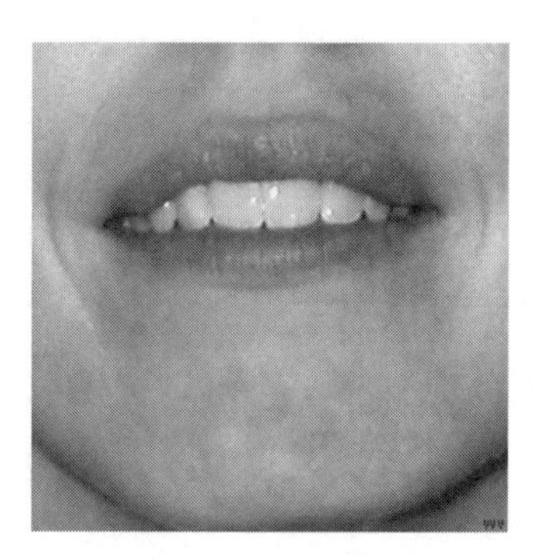
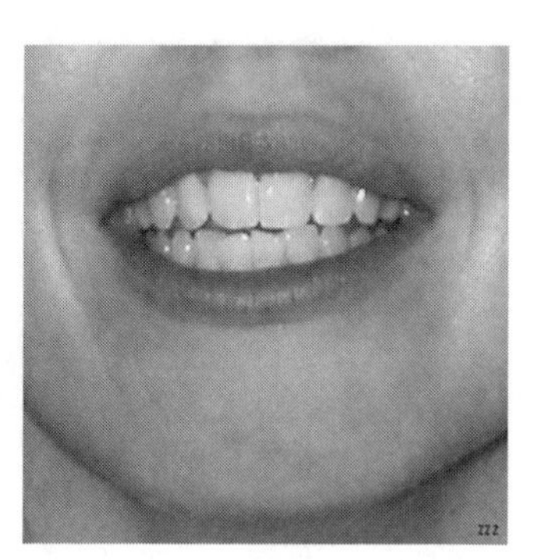

Teach this consonant blend after teaching the /v/ and /z/ sounds. Say the two sounds in succession, faster and faster, until /-vz/ occurs. They each have low and high frequency buzz energies. The successive parts of this blend are indicated by Lissajous patterns, paper strip movements, and meter needle movements.

Prosodic Drill

aɪvzaɪvzaɪvz aɪvz**aɪvz**aɪvz aɪvzaɪvz**aɪvz**

aɪvzaɪvzaɪvzaɪvz aɪvz**aɪvz**aɪvzaɪvz aɪvzaɪvz**aɪvz**aɪvz

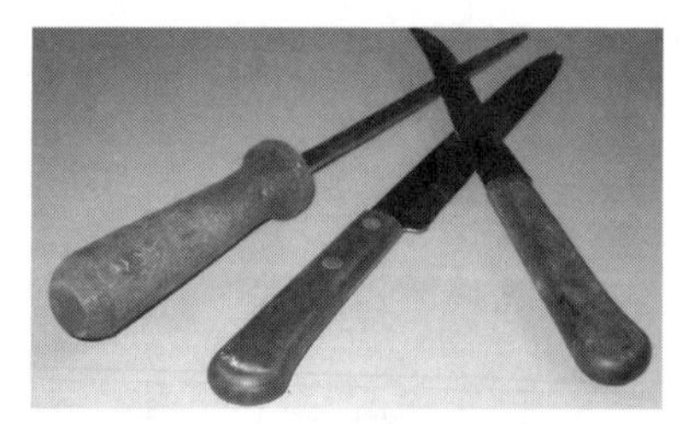

knives

Sharpen the ________.

leaves lives saves calves

loves moves coves lives

Lesson 88 /-rn/

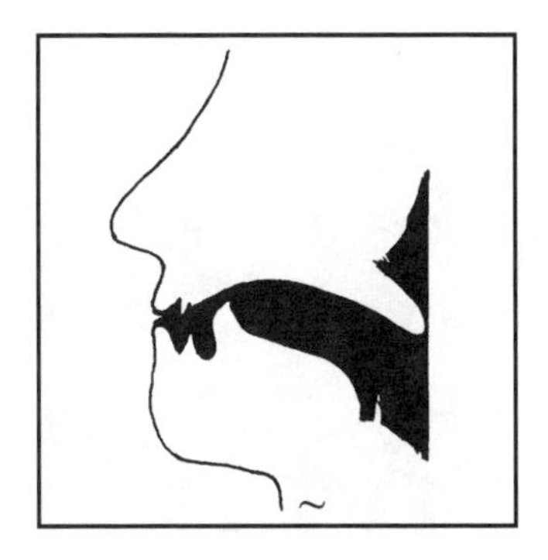
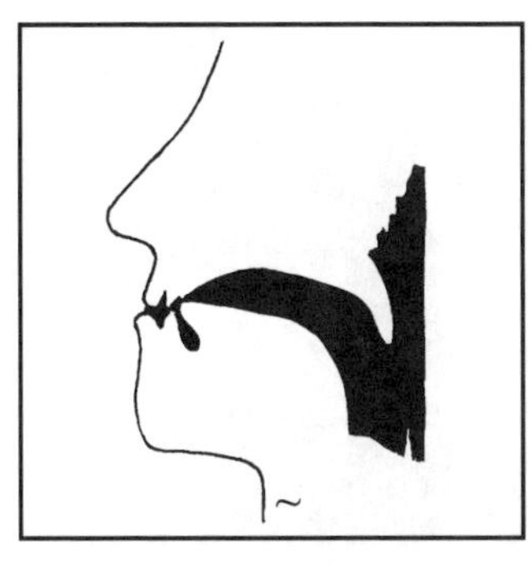
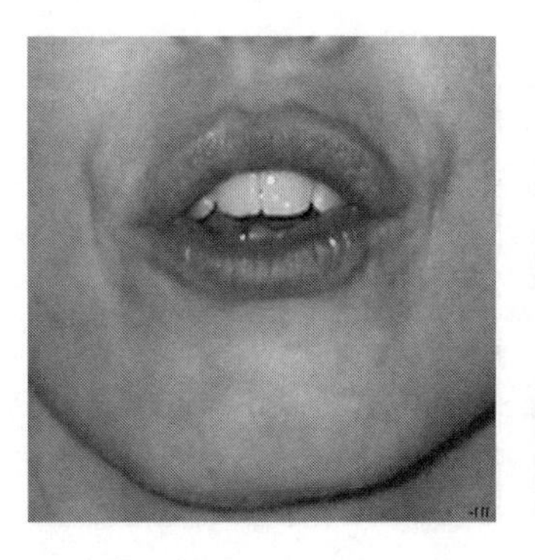
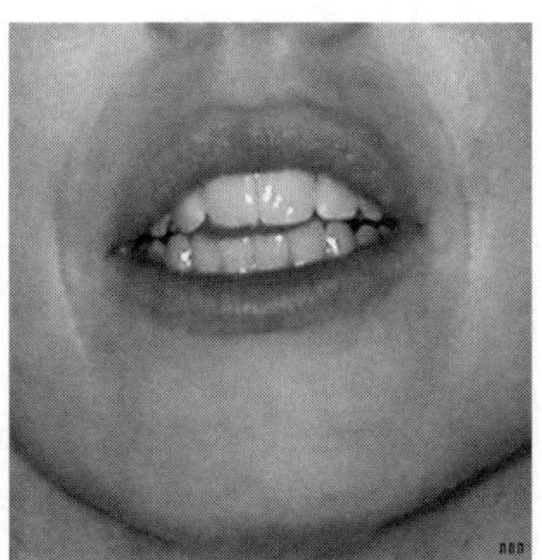

Teach this consonant blend after teaching the /-r/ and /n/ sounds. Say the two sounds in succession, faster and faster, until /-rn/ occurs. The first sound is oral and low and mid frequency, the second nasal and low frequency. The successive parts of this blend are indicated by Lissajous patterns and meter needle movements.

Prosodic Drills

arnarnarn   arn**arn**arn   arnarn**arn**

arnarnarnarn   arn**arn**arnarn   arnarn**arn**arn

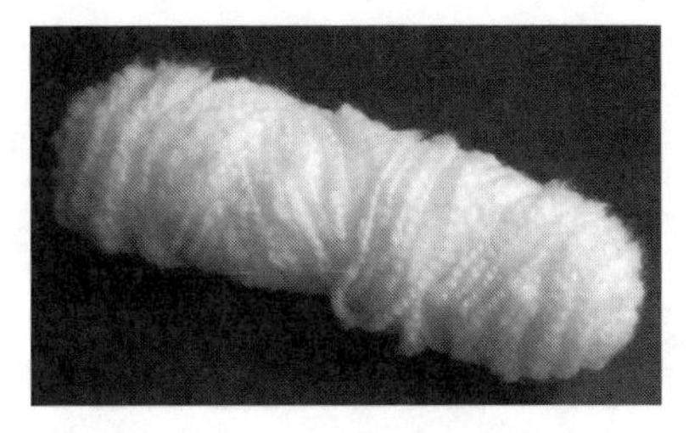

yarn

A piece of ________.

burn   fern   learn   turn

corn   torn   worn   barn

Lesson 89 /-ft/

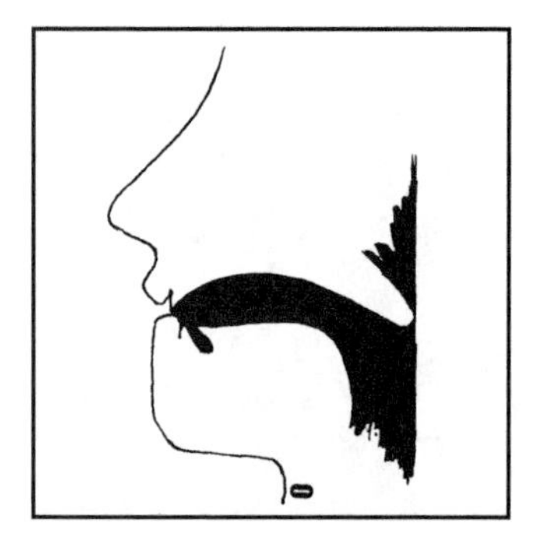
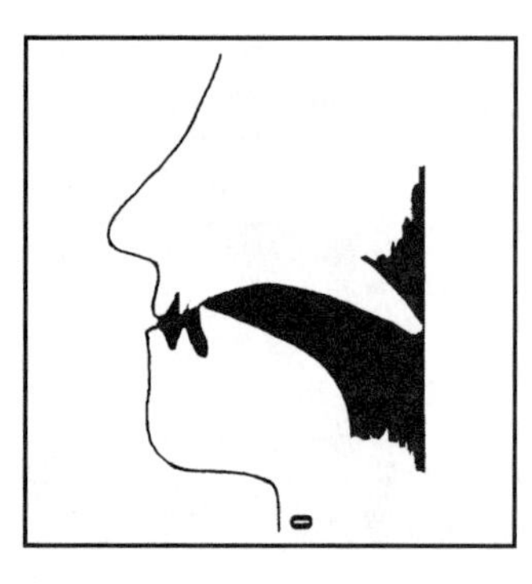
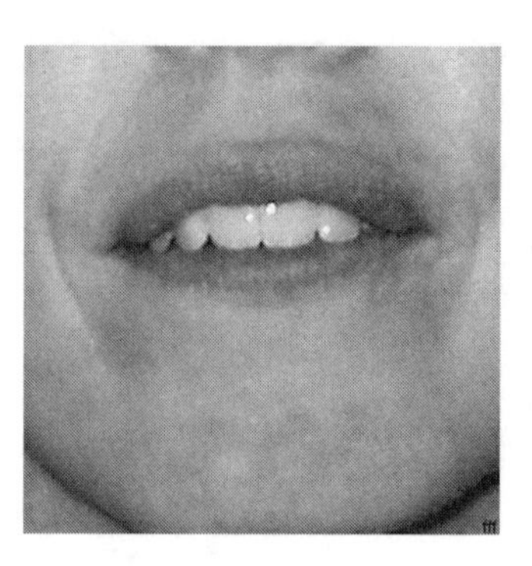
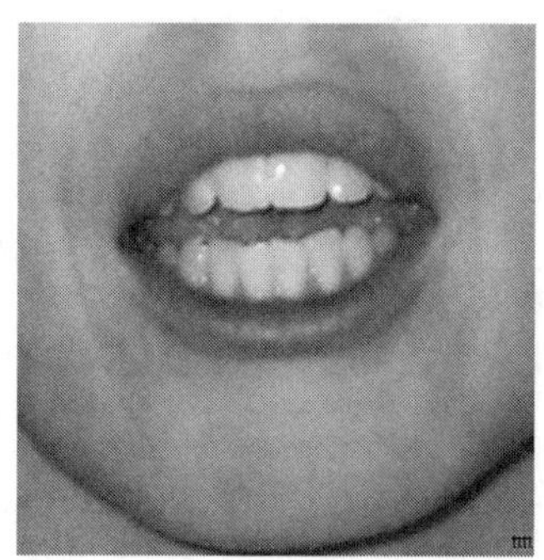

Teach this consonant blend after teaching the /f/ and /t/ sounds. Say the two sounds in succession, faster and faster, until /-ft/ occurs. The two sounds are voiceless, the first a high frequency fricative, the second a low-mid-high frequency stop-plosive. The successive parts of this blend are indicated by Lissajous patterns, paper strip movements, and meter needle movements.

Prosodic Drill

ɪftɪftɪft   ɪft**ɪft**ɪft   ɪftɪft**ɪft**

ɪftɪftɪftɪft   ɪft**ɪft**ɪftɪft   ɪftɪft**ɪft**ɪft

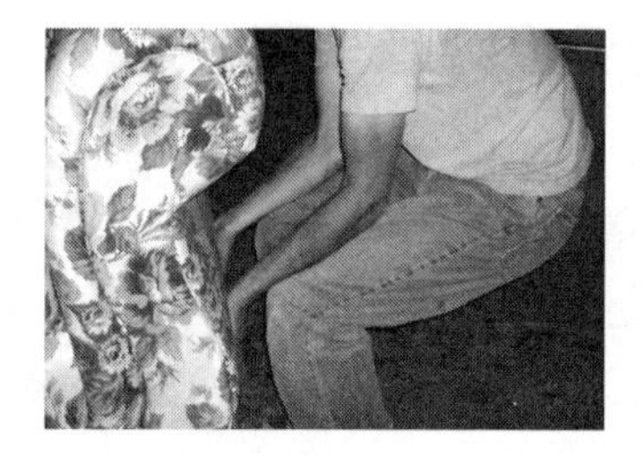

lift

Try to ________.

leafed   gift   left   raft   puffed

goofed   loafed   soft   knifed

Lesson 90 /-ld/

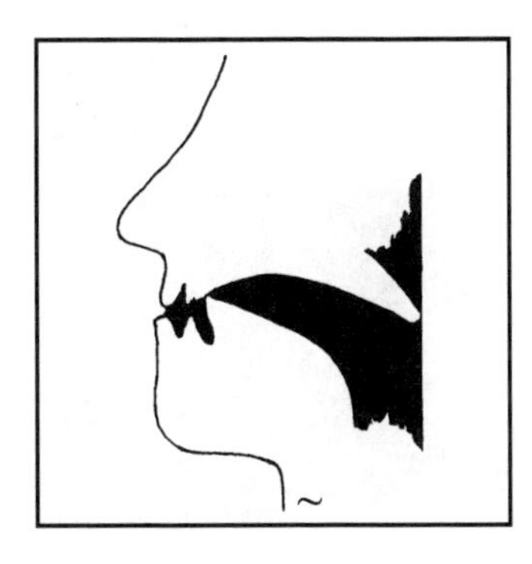
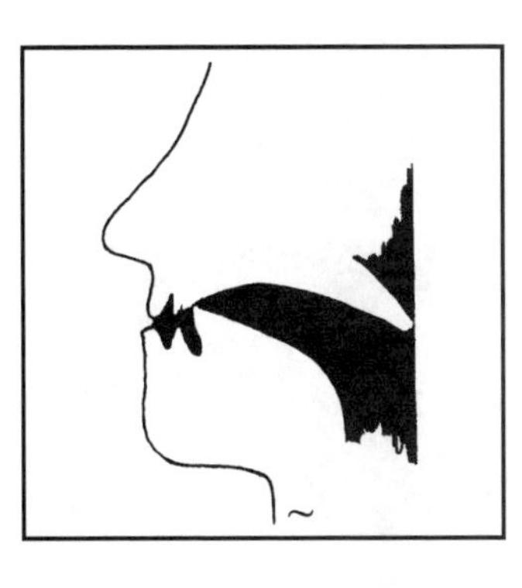
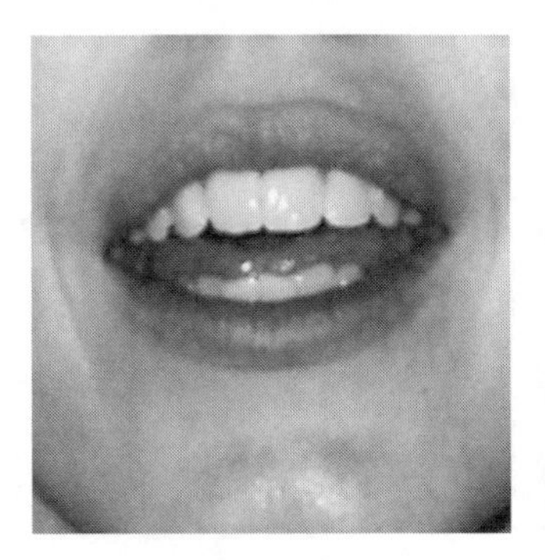
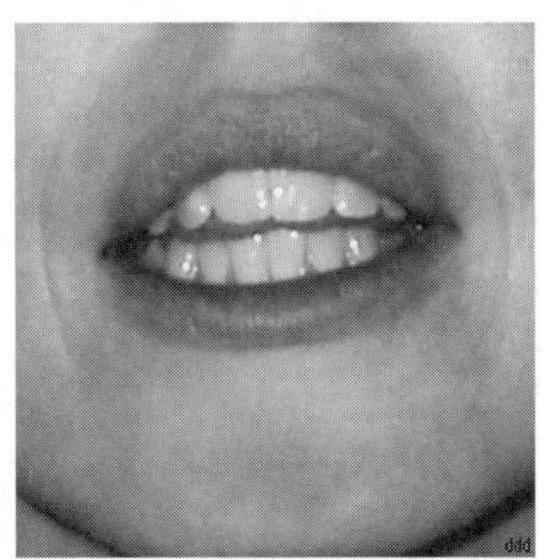

Teach this consonant blend after teaching the /l/ and /d/ sounds. Say the two sounds in succession, faster and faster, until /-ld/ occurs. The two sound are voiced and oral, the first a glide, the second a stop. The first is lower frequency than the second. The successive parts of this blend are indicated by Lissajous patterns and meter needle movements.

Prosodic Drill

ɪldɪldɪld ɪld**ɪld**ɪld ɪldɪld**ɪld**

ɪldɪldɪldɪld ɪld**ɪld**ɪldɪld ɪldɪld**ɪld**ɪld

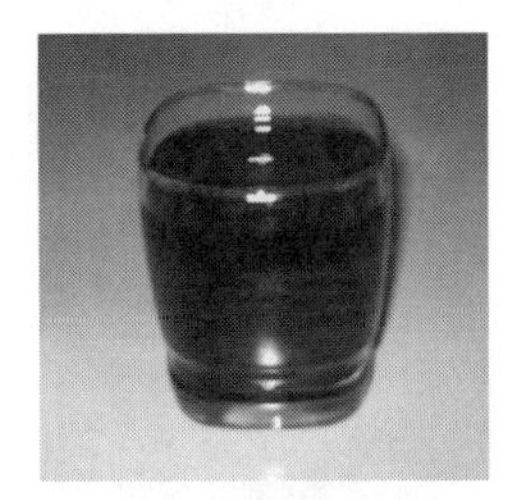

filled

The glass is ________.

heeled killed felled mailed curled

pooled sold mauled howled piled

Lesson 91 /-lp/

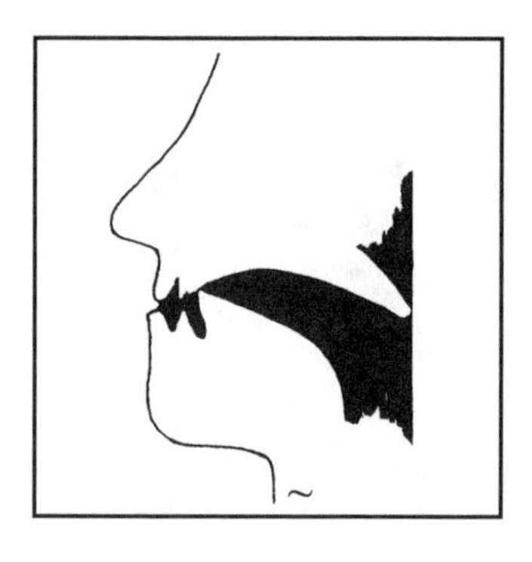
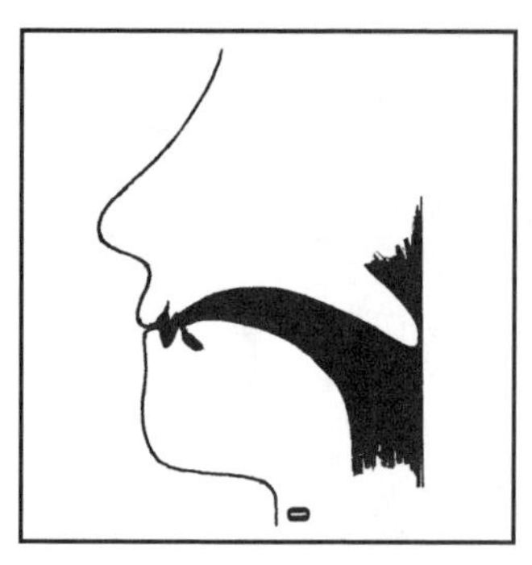
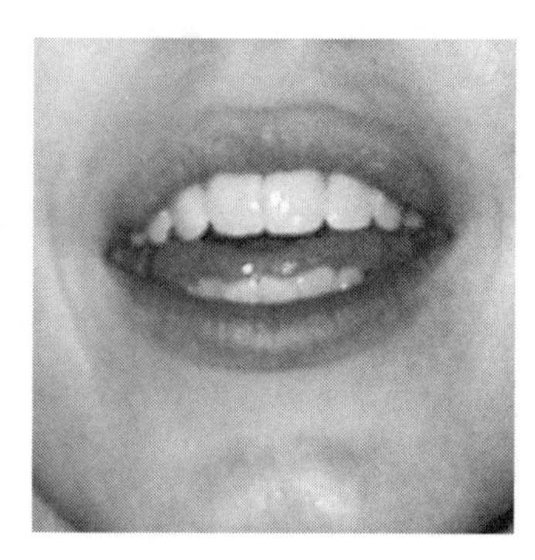
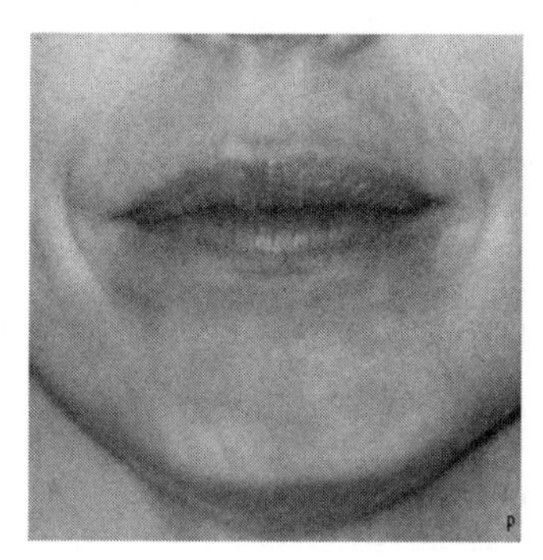

Teach this consonant blend after teaching the /l/ and /p/ sounds. Say the two sounds in succession, faster and faster, until the /-lp/ occurs. The first sound is a glide, the second a stop plosive. Both are low frequency. The successive parts of this blend are indicated by Lissajous patterns and meter needle movements.

Prosodic Drill

ɛlpɛlpɛlp ɛlp**ɛlp**ɛlp ɛlpɛlp**ɛlp**

ɛlpɛlpɛlpɛlp ɛlp**ɛlp**ɛlpɛlp ɛlpɛlp**ɛlp**ɛlip

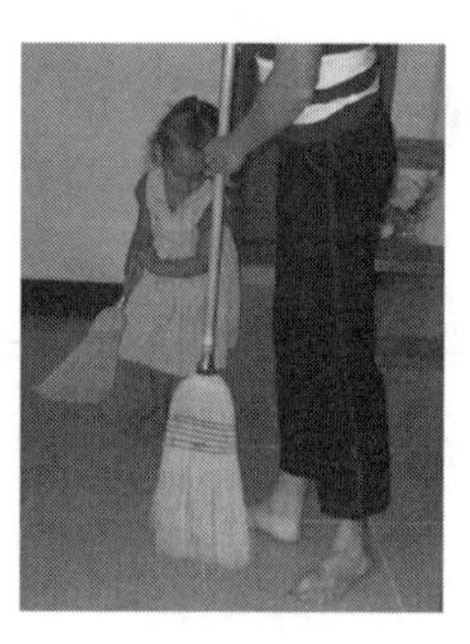

whelp

The little girl is a ________.

help kelp pulp gulp

Lesson 92 /-mp/

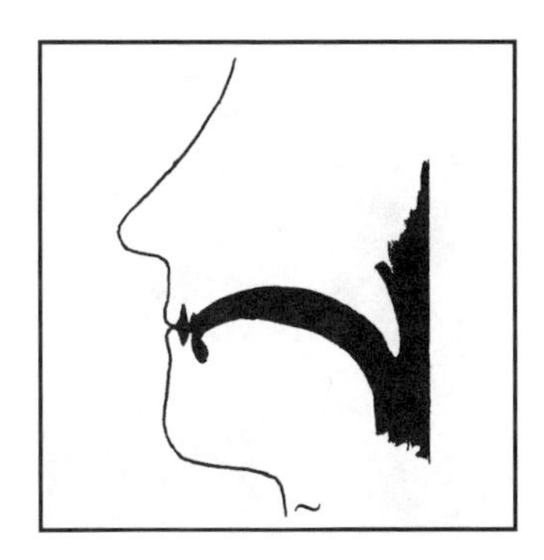
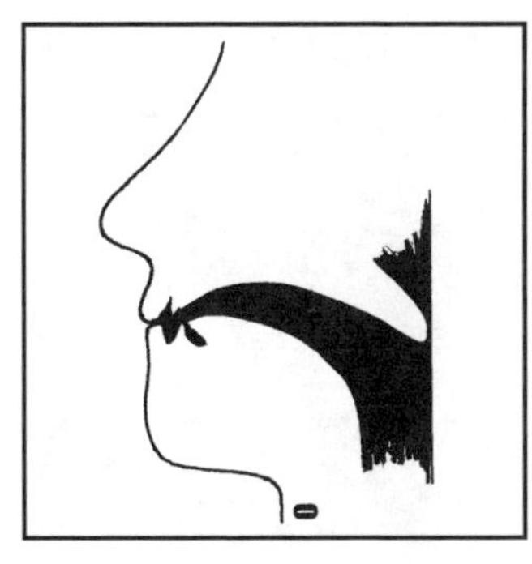
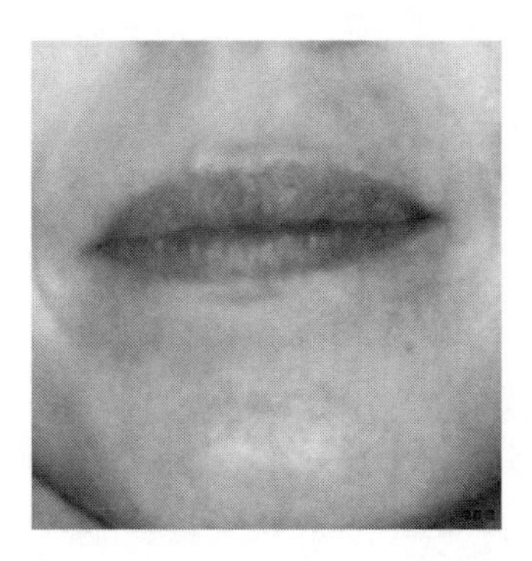
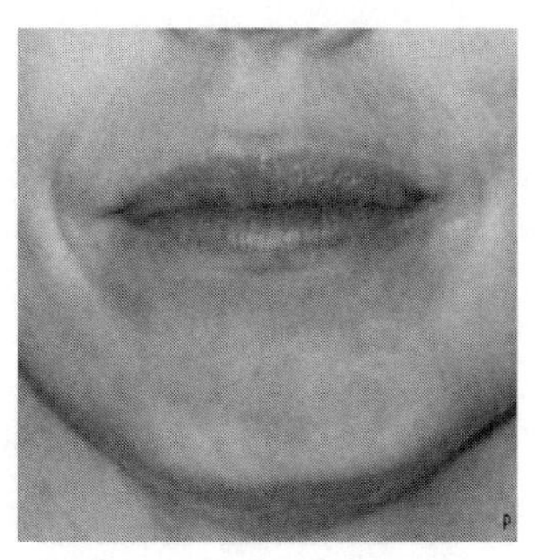

Teach this consonant blend after teaching the /m/ and /p/ sounds. Release the first sound, a lip shut nasal, with the second sound, a lip shut stop plosive. Both are low frequency voiced sounds. The successive parts of this blend are indicated by Lissajous patterns and meter needle movements.

Prosodic Drill

æmpæmpæmp æmp**æmp**æmp æmpæmp**æmp**

æmpæmpæmp æmp**æmp**æmp æmpæmp**æmp**æmp

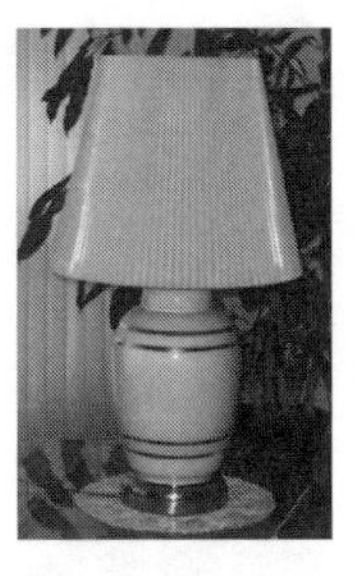

lamp

Turn off the ________.

limp hemp camp

hump pump chump pomp

Lesson 93 /-nd/

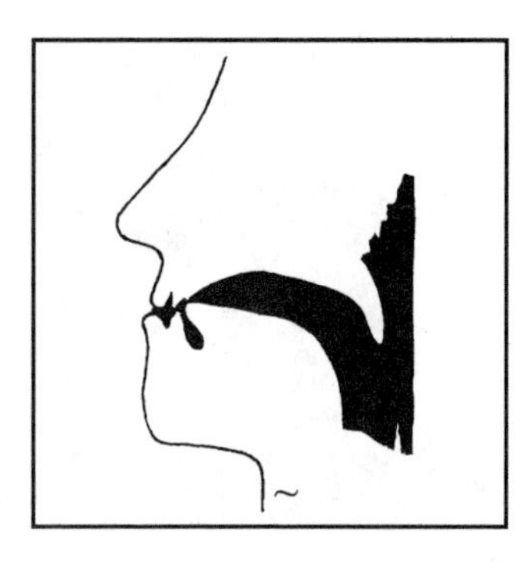 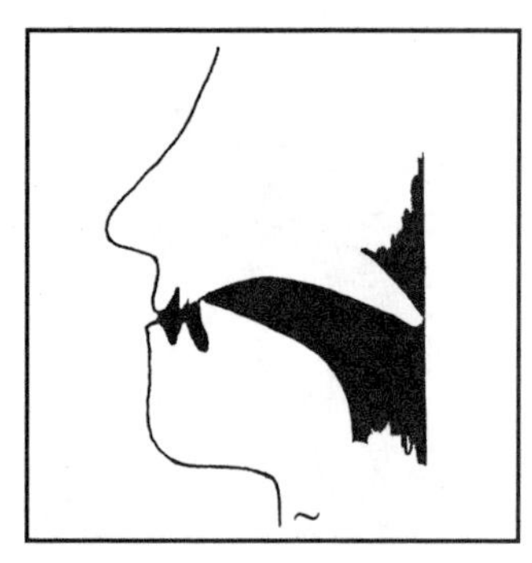 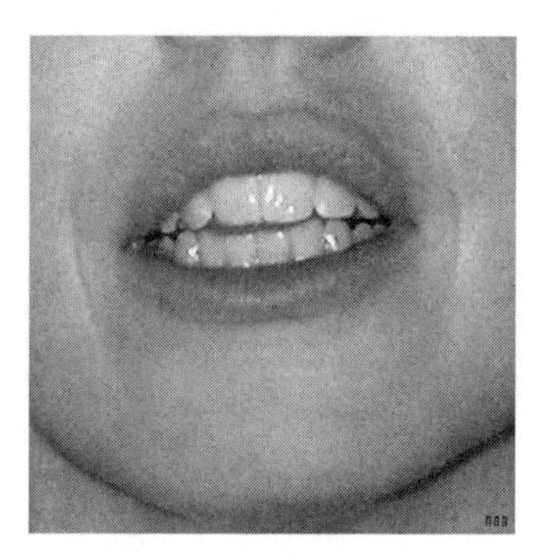 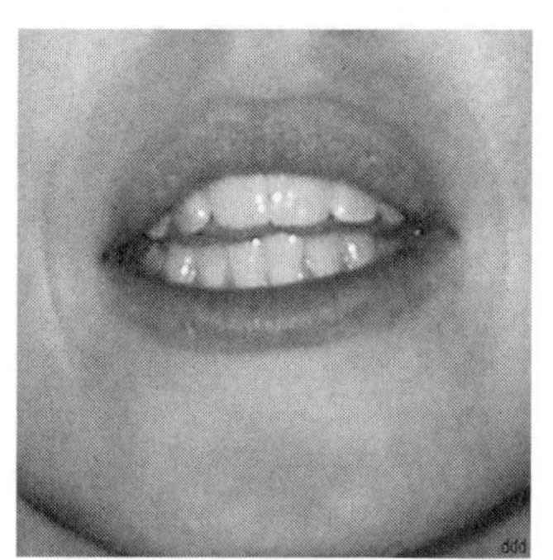

Teach this consonant blend after teaching the /n/ and /-d/ sounds. Release the first sound, a lingua-alveolar nasal, with the second sound, a lingua-alveolar stop. The first sound is low frequency, the second mid-high frequency. The successive parts of this blend are indicated by Lissajous patterns and meter needle movements.

Prosodic Drill

ændændænd ænd**ænd**ænd ændænd**ænd**

ændændændænd ænd**ænd**ændænd ændænd**ænd**ænd

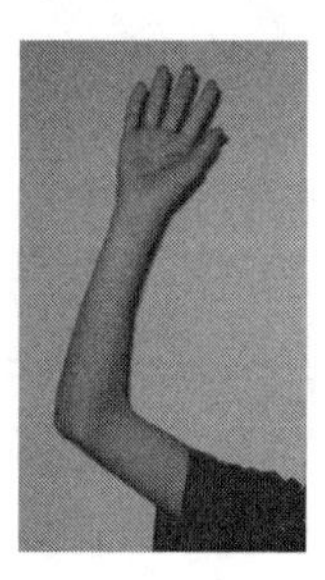

hand

Raise your ________.

leaned wind send band fund

tuned phoned bond sound shined

Lesson 94 /-nt/

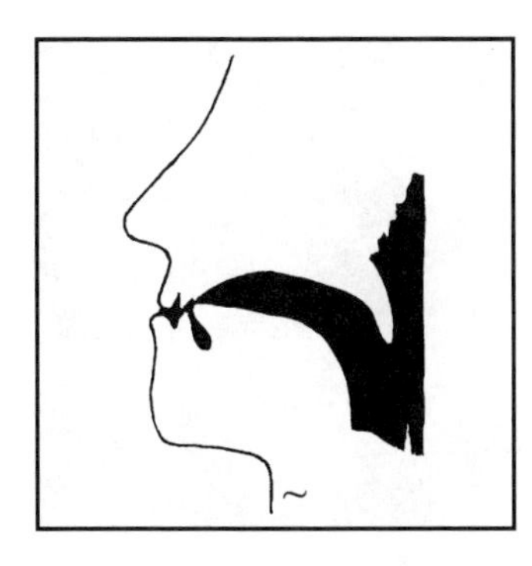 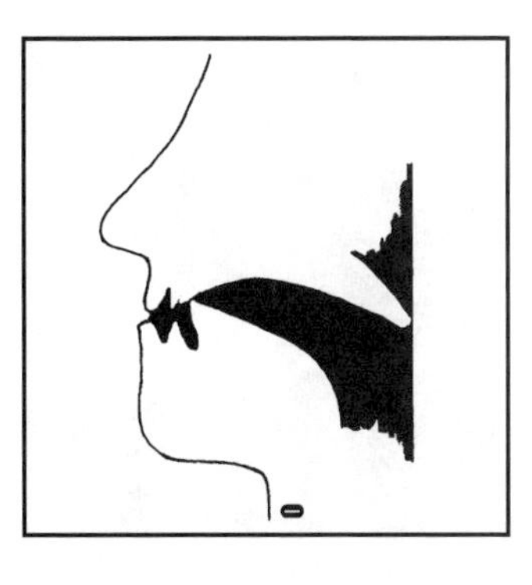 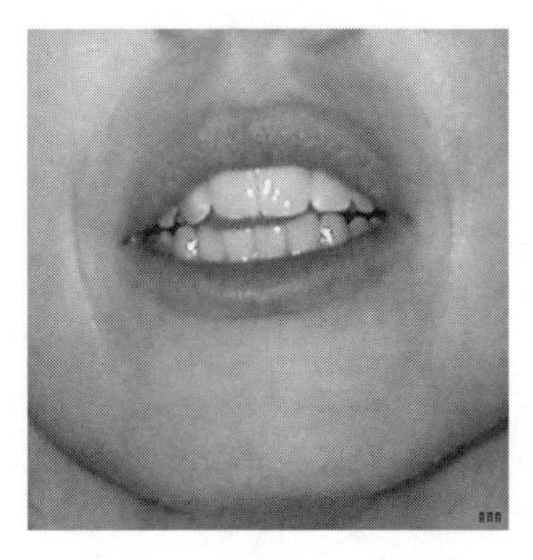 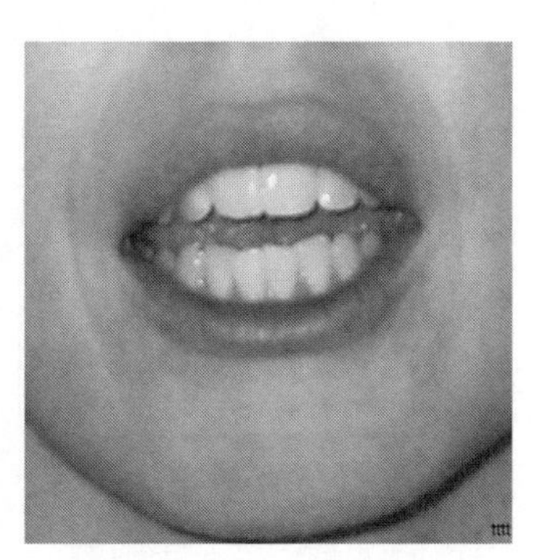

Teach this consonant blend after teaching the /n/ and /t/ sounds. Release the first sound, a lingua-alveolar nasal, with the second sound, a voiceless lingua-alveolar stop. The first is low frequency, the second mid-high frequency. The successive parts of this blend are indicated by Lissajous patterns and meter needle movements.

Prosodic Drill

ententent enn**ent**ent entent**ent**

entententent ent**ent**entent entent**ent**ent

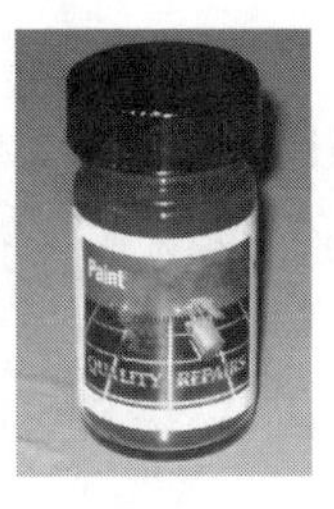

paint

A can of ________.

lint tint taint chant punt

don't gaunt mount pint

Lesson 95 /-ntʃ/

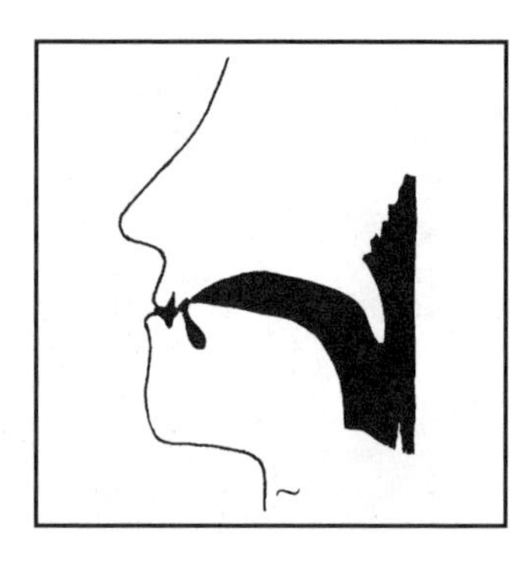
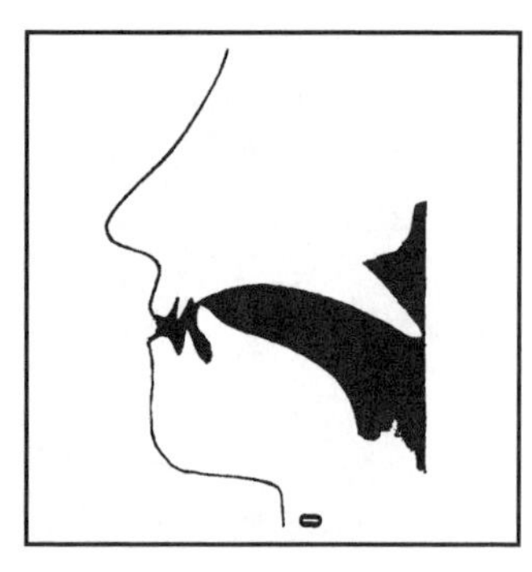
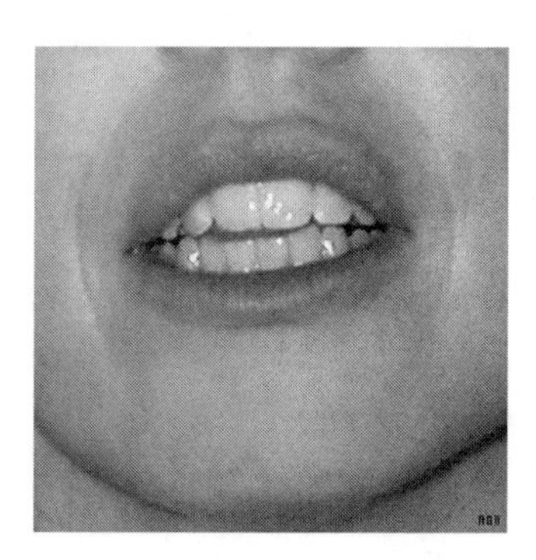
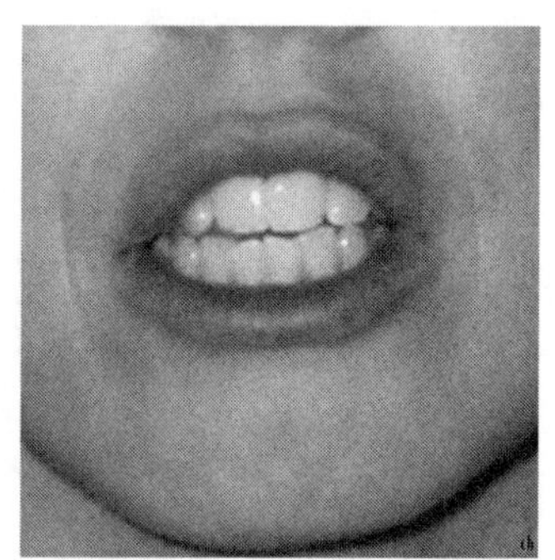

Teach this consonant blend after teaching the /n/ and /tʃ/ sounds. Say the two sounds in succession, faster and faster, until the /-ntʃ/ blend occurs. The first is nasal and low frequency, the second fricative stop and mid-high frequency. The successive parts of this blend are indicated by Lissajous patterns and meter needle movements.

Prosodic Drill

ɛntʃɛntʃɛntʃ   ɛntʃ**ɛntʃ**ɛntʃ   ɛntʃɛntʃ**ɛntʃ**

ɛntʃɛntʃɛntʃɛntʃ   ɛntʃ**ɛntʃ**ɛntʃɛntʃ   ɛntʃɛntʃ**ɛntʃ**ɛntʃ

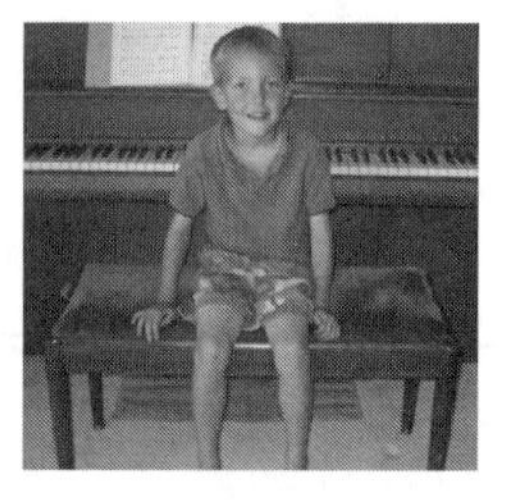

bench

Sit on a ________.

pinch   wrench   ranch   lunch

brunch   haunch   launch

Lesson 96 /-ŋk/

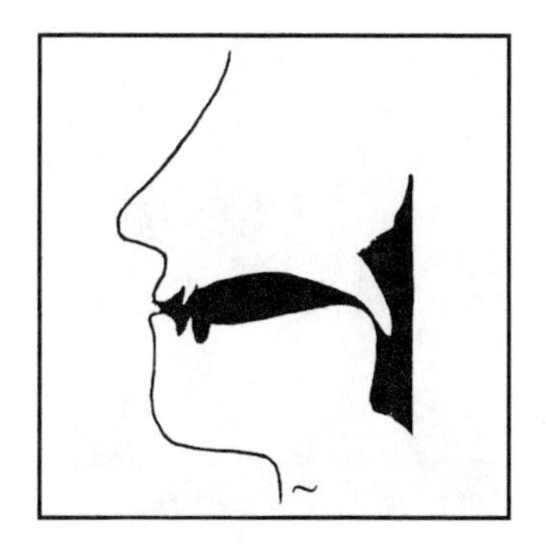

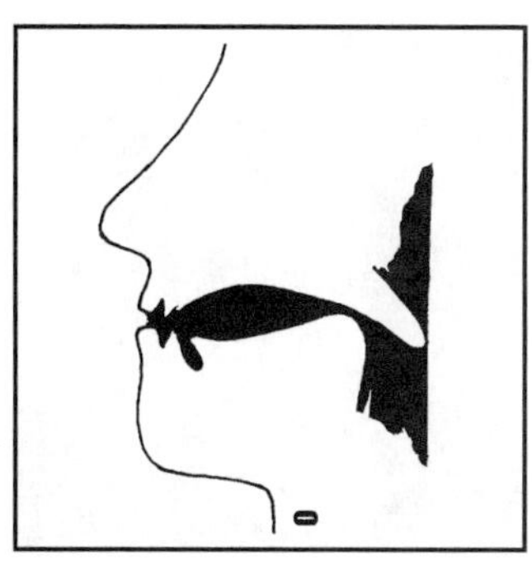

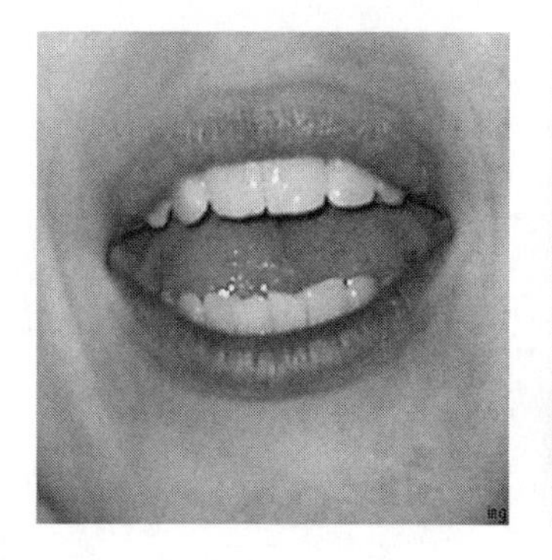

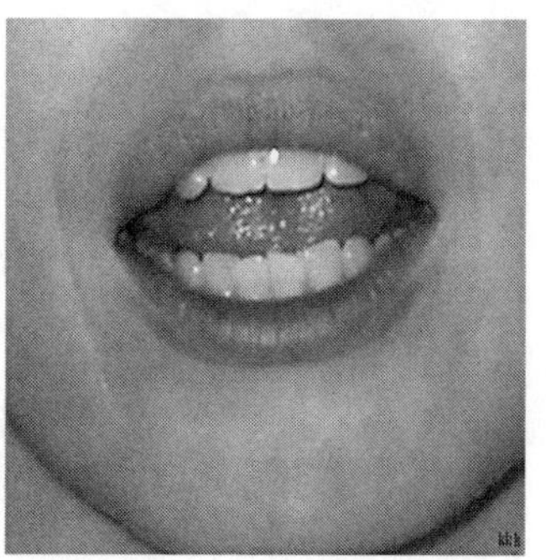

Teach this consonant blend after teaching the /ŋ/ and /k/ sounds. Release the first sound, a lingua-velar nasal, with the second sound, a lingua-velar stop. The first is low frequency, the second mid-high frequency. The successive parts of this blend are indicated by Lissajous, meter needle, and paper strip movements.

Prosodic Drill

ɪŋkɪŋkɪŋk ɪŋk**ɪŋk**ɪŋk ɪŋkɪŋk**ɪŋk**

ɪŋkɪŋkɪŋkɪŋk ɪŋk**ɪŋk**ɪŋkɪŋk ɪŋkɪŋk**ɪŋk**ɪŋk

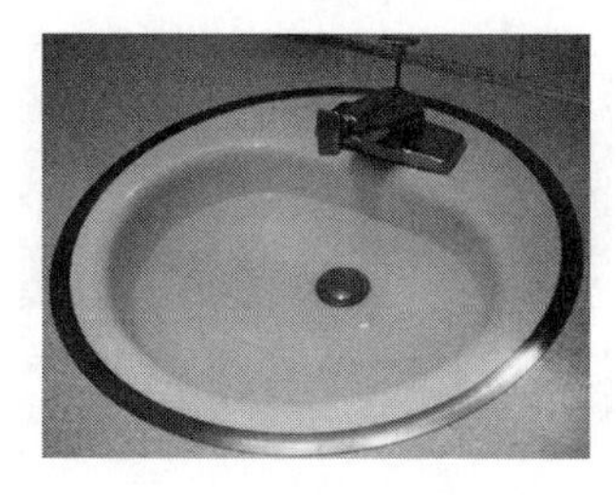

sink

Fill the ________.

pink thank bank

dunk punk sunk tank

Lesson 97 /-sp/

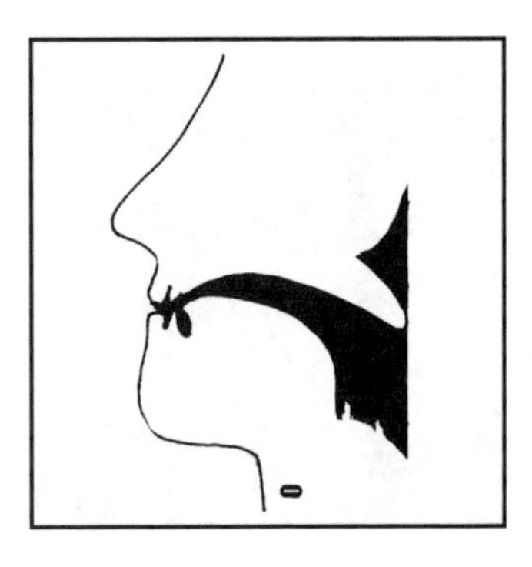
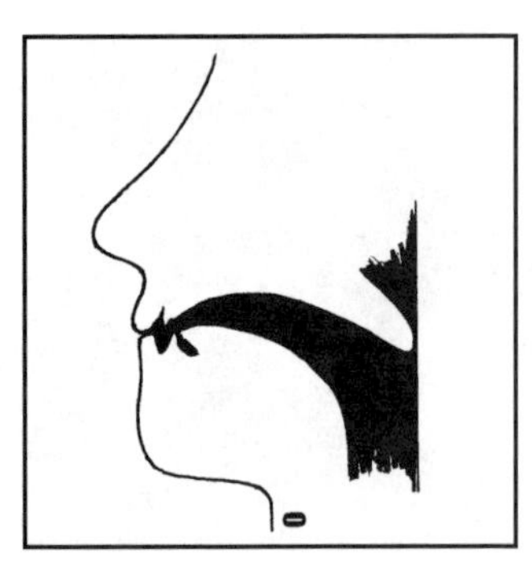
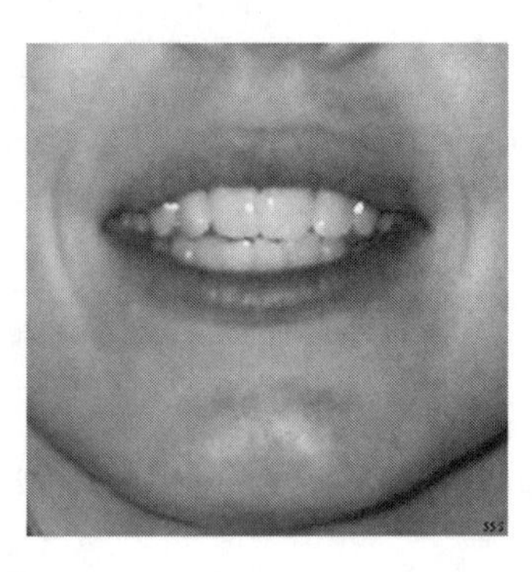
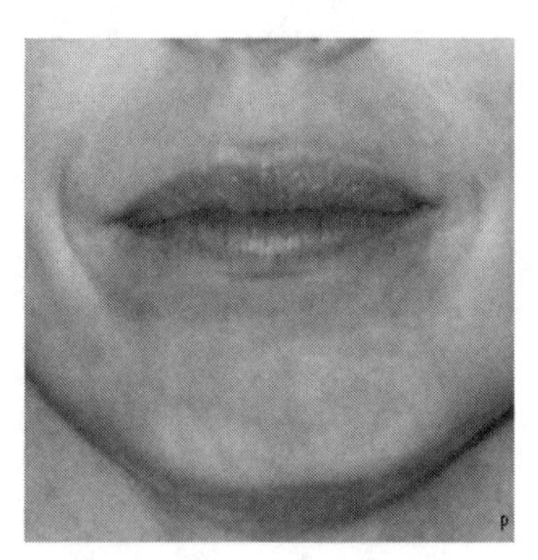

Teach this consonant blend after teaching the /s/ and /p/ sounds. Say the two sounds in succession, faster and faster, until /-sp/ occurs. The first is a voiceless high frequency fricative, the second a voiceless low frequency stop plosive. The successive parts of this blend are indicated by Lissajous patterns and paper strip and meter needle movements.

Prosodic Drill

æspæspæsp æsp**æsp**æsp æspæsp**æsp**

æspæspspæsp æsp**æsp**æspæsp æspæsp**æsp**æsp

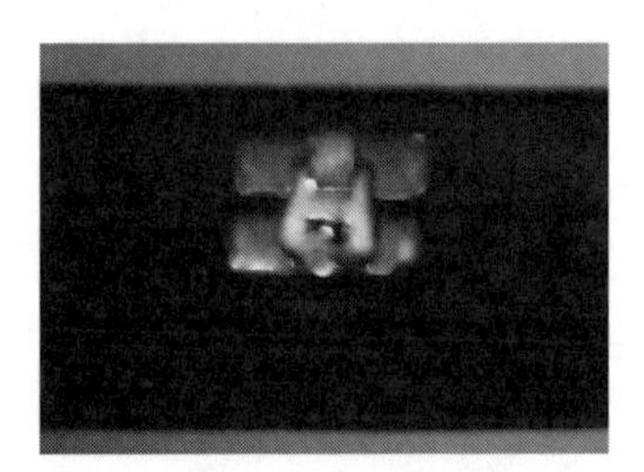

clasp

That's a ________.

lisp crisp gasp asp cusp

Lesson 98 /-st/

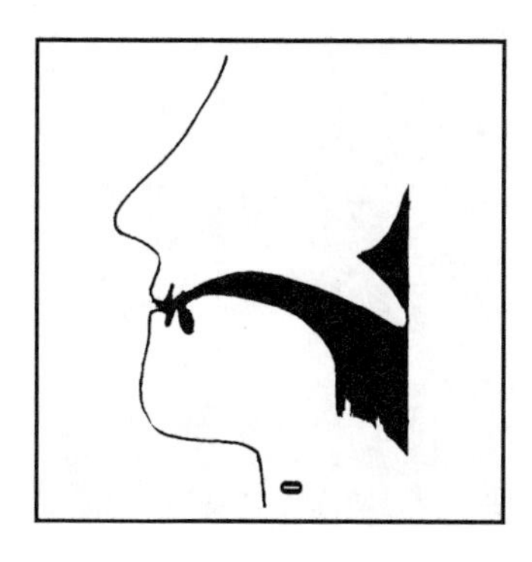
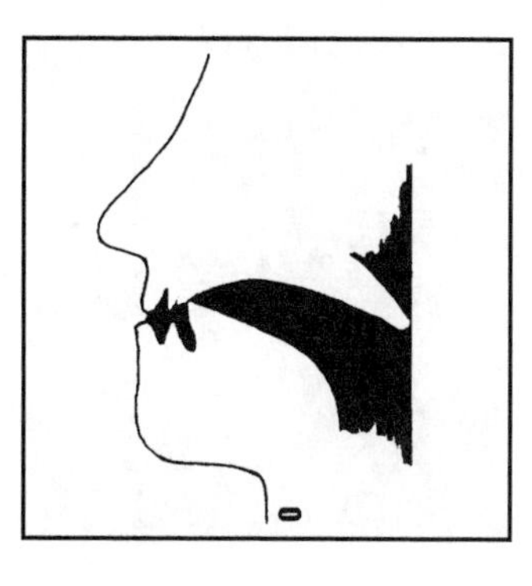
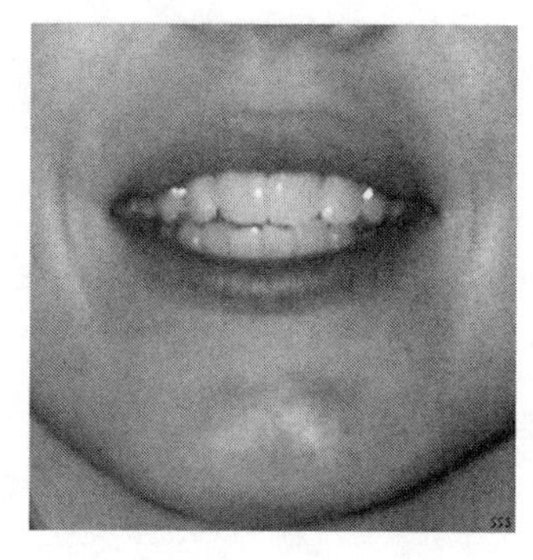
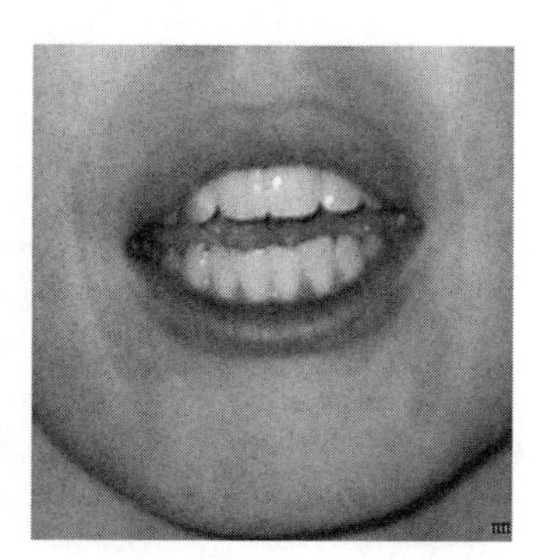

Teach this consonant blend after teaching the /s/ and /t/ sounds. Say the two sounds in succession, faster and faster, until the /-st/ occurs. The first is a voiceless high frequency fricative, the second a voiceless mid-high frequency stop plosive. The successive parts of this blend are indicated by Lissajous patterns and paper strip and meter needle movements.

Prosodic Drill

ɪstɪstɪst ɪst**ɪst**ɪst ɪstɪst**ɪst**

ɪstɪstɪstɪst ɪst**ɪst**ɪstɪst ɪstɪst**ɪst**ɪst

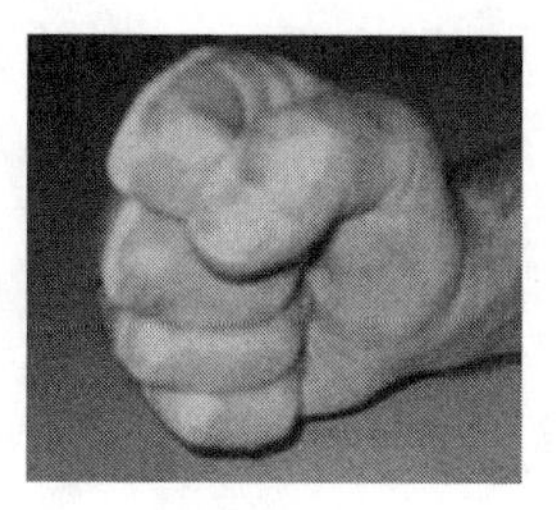

fist

Clench your ________.

feast list messed faced past cursed

boost roast cost doused heist

Lesson 99 /-sk/

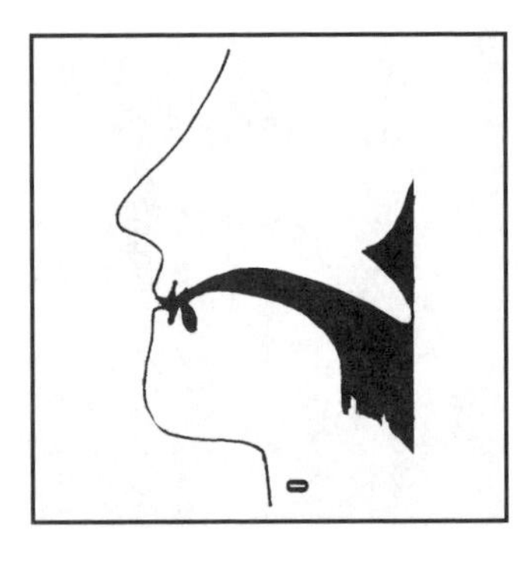
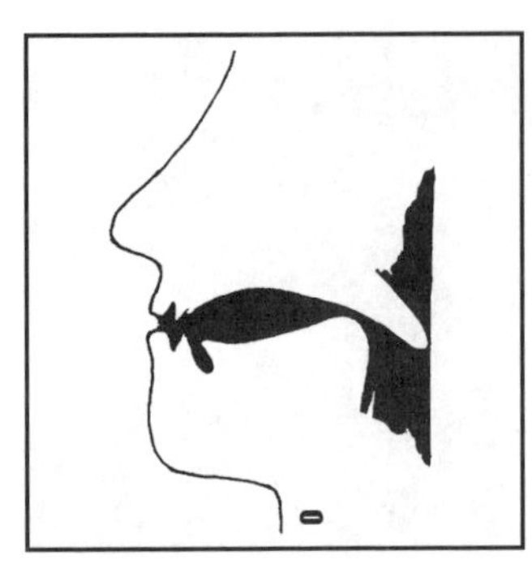
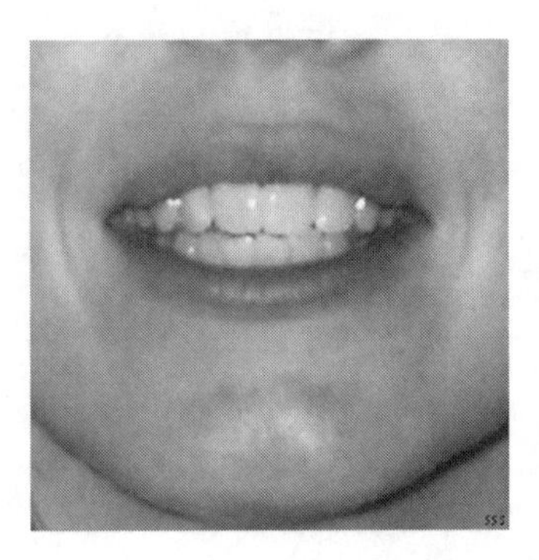
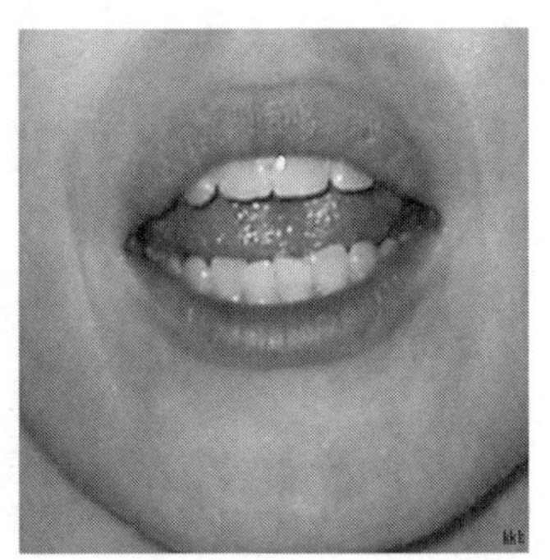

Teach this consonant blend after teaching the /s/ and /k/ sounds. Say the two sounds in succession, faster and faster, until the /-sk/ occurs. The first is a voiceless high frequency fricative, the second a voiceless mid-high frequency stop-plosive. The successive parts of this blend are indicated by Lissajous patterns and paper strip and meter needle movements.

Prosodic Drill

ɛskɛskɛsk ɛsk**ɛsk**ɛsk ɛskɛsk**ɛsk**

ɛskɛskɛskɛsk ɛsk**ɛsk**ɛsɛsk ɛskɛsk**ɛsk**ɛsk

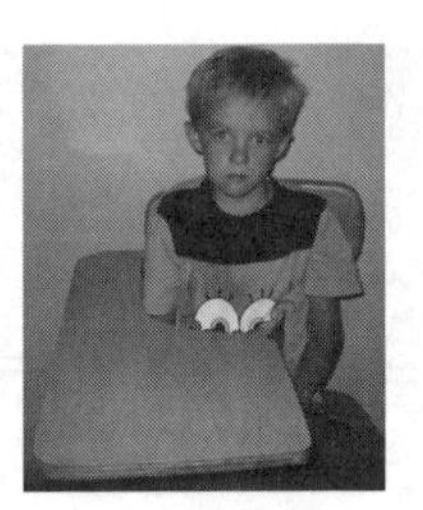

desk

Sit at the ________.

disc risk brisk frisk

bask dusk mosque

Lesson 100 /-vd/

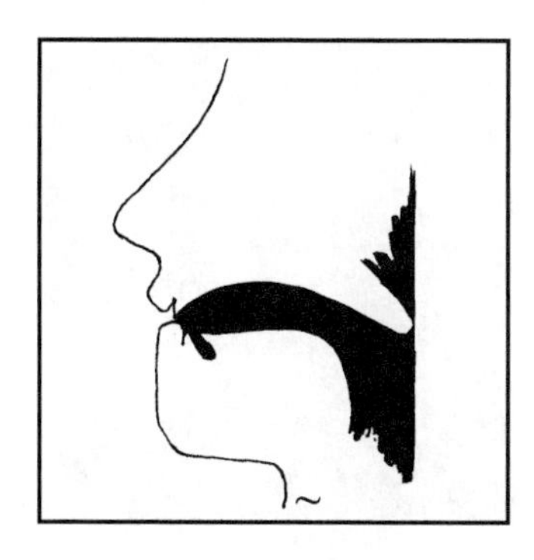
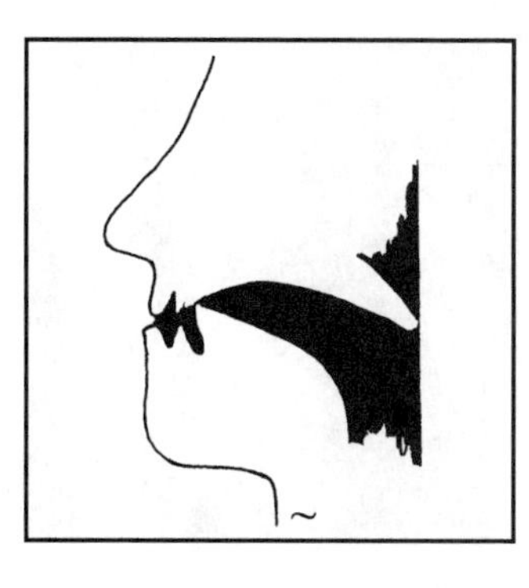
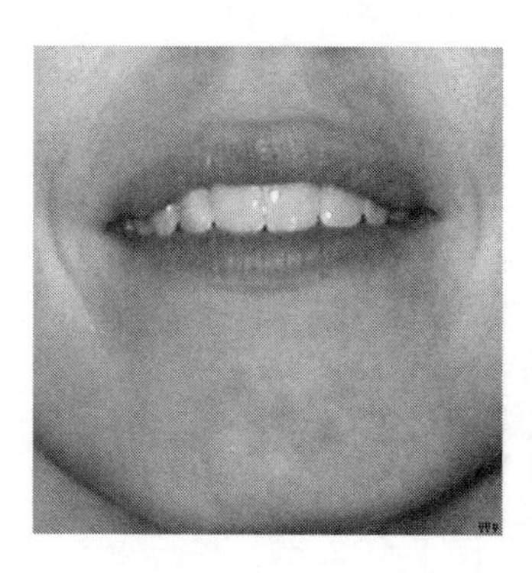
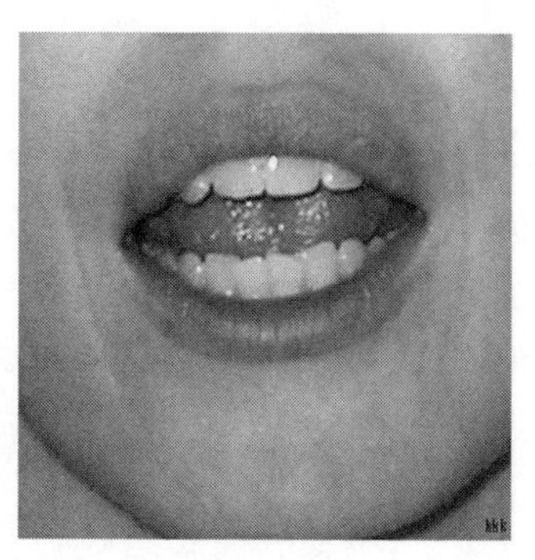

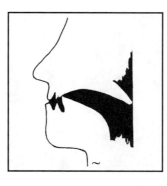

Teach this consonant after teaching the /v/ and /-d/ sounds. Say these two voiced sounds in succession, faster and faster, until the /-vd/ occurs. The first is a fricative, the second a stop. The successive parts of this blend are indicated by Lissajous patterns and meter needle movements.

Prosodic Drill

ʌvdəvdəvd   əvd**ʌvd**əvd   əvdəvd**ʌvd**

ʌvdəvdəvdəvd   əvd**ʌvd**əvdəvd   əvdəvd**ʌvd**əvd

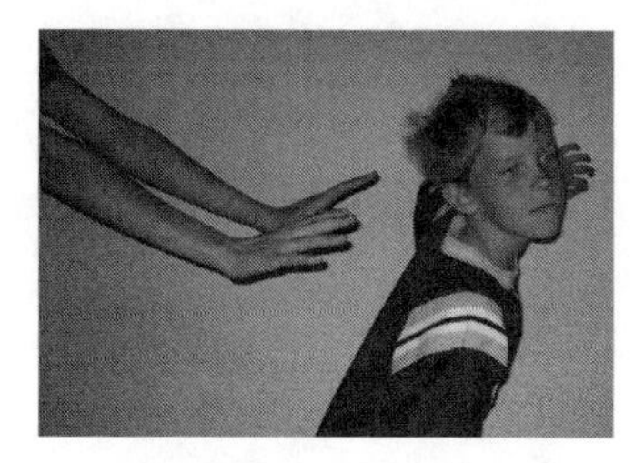

shoved

He was ________.

peeved   lived   paved   calved   gloved   served

moved   roved   dived

Lesson 101 /-rk/

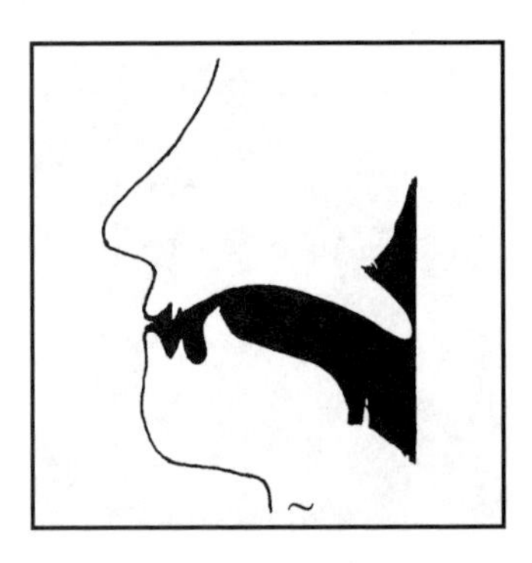
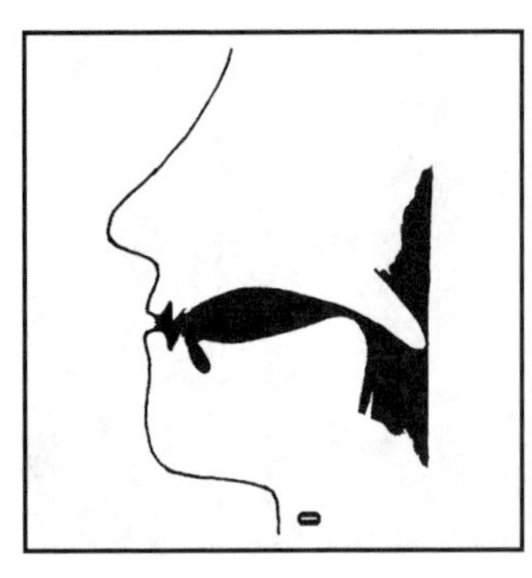
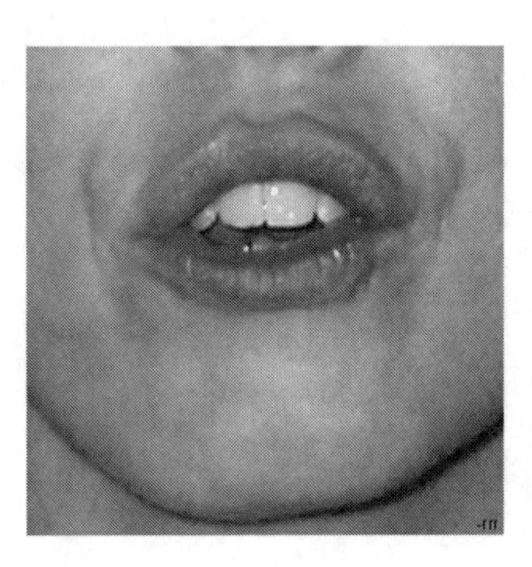
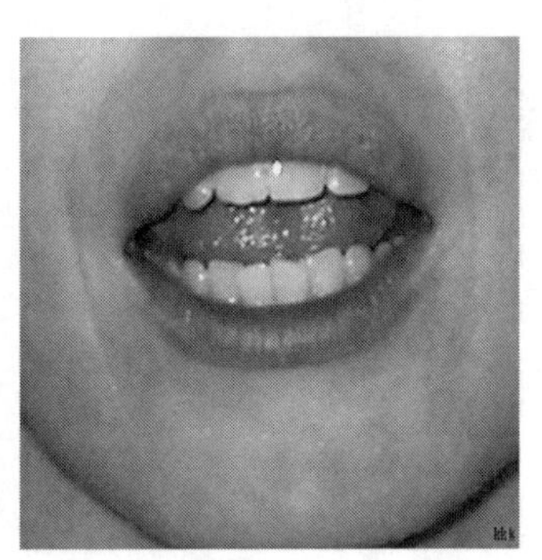

Teach this consonant blend after teaching /ʊr/, /or/, /ɑr/, and /k/. Then, say each of /ʊr/, /or/, and /ɑr/ before saying /k/ repeatedly, faster and faster, until /ʊrk/, /ork/, and /ɑrk/ are said. The successive parts of the /-rk/ blend are indicated by Lissajous pattern, paper strip, and meter needle movements.

Prosodic Drill

orkorkork orkor**ork**ork orkork**ork**

orkorkorkork ork**ork**orkork orkork**ork**ork

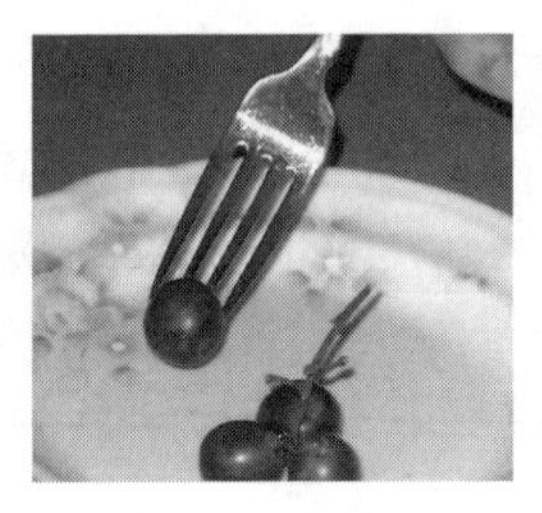

fork

Eat with a ________.

perk jerk work torque cork

hark bark dark lark mark

Lesson 102 /-bl/

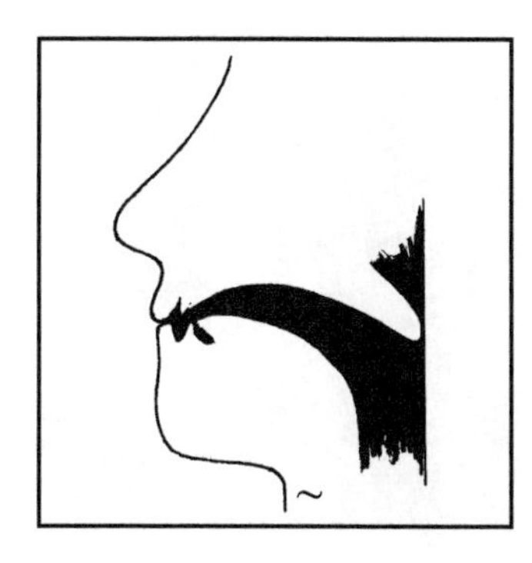

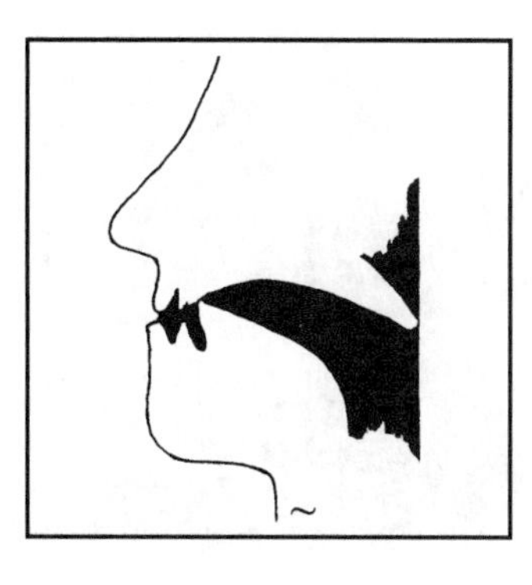

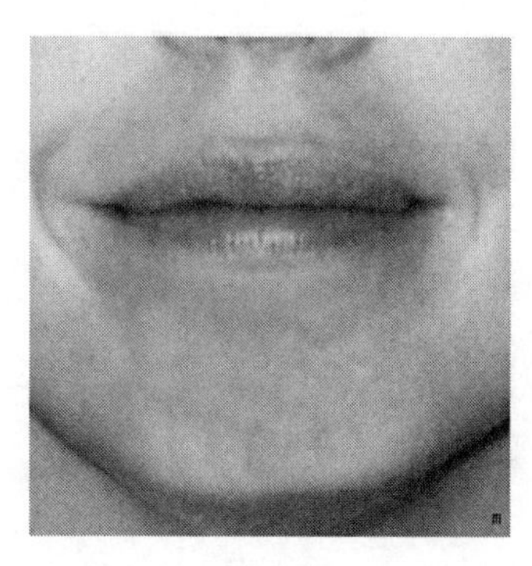

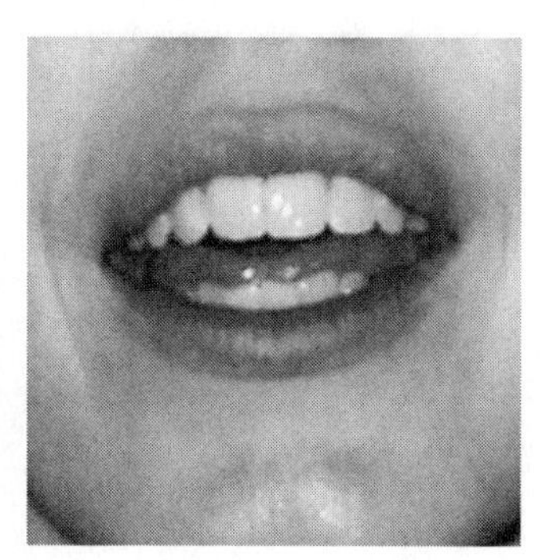

Teach this consonant blend after teaching the /b-/ and /l/ sounds. Begin saying this blend as a syllable, with the /ə/ vowel (unstressed /ʌ/ vowel) between the /b-/ and /l/. Say /bəl/ faster and faster, until it becomes /bl/. This blend is indicated by a single Lissajous pattern, paper strip movement, or meter needle movement.

Prosodic Drill

ebleblebl ebl**ebl**ebl ebleb l**ebl**

eblebleblebl ebl**ebl**eblebl ebleb**ebl**ebl

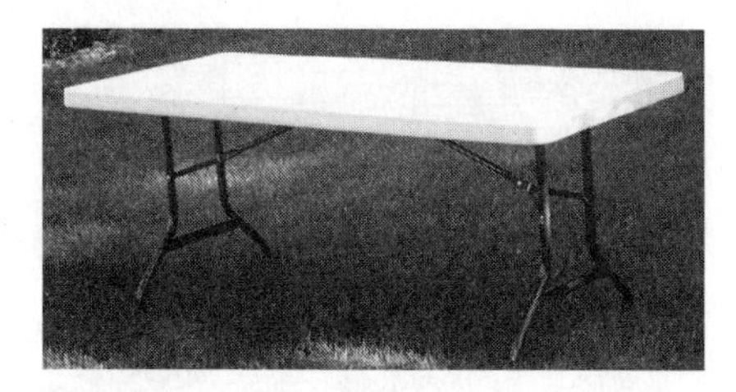

table

Sit at the ________.

feeble nibble pebble babble double

herbal mobile hobble bible

Lesson 103 /-dl/

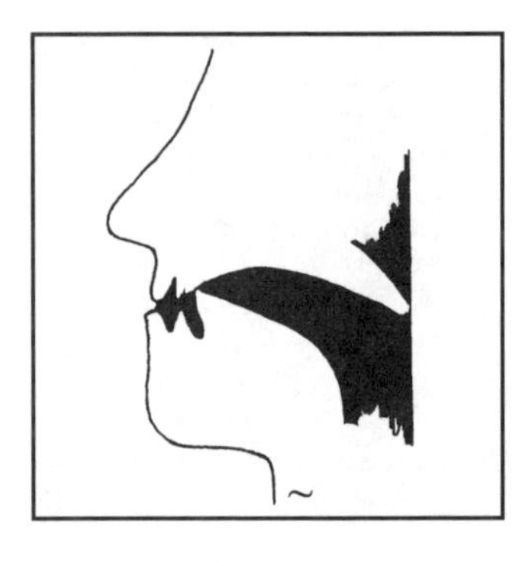
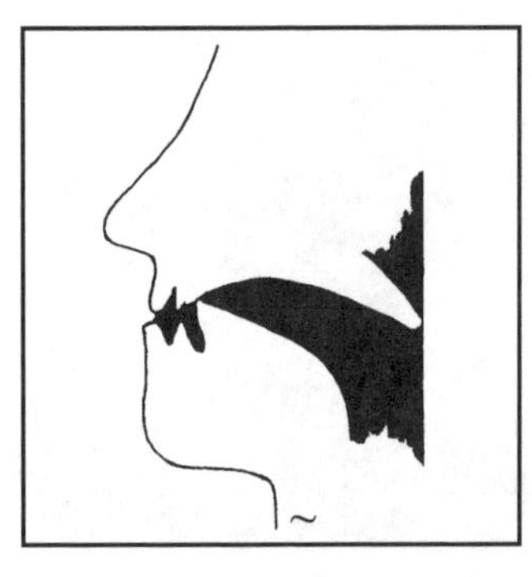
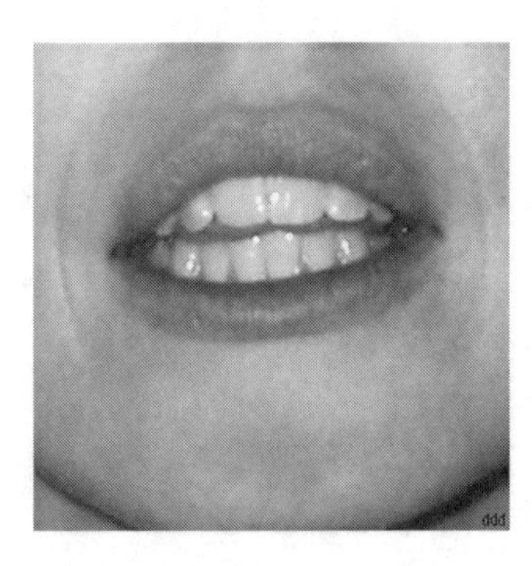
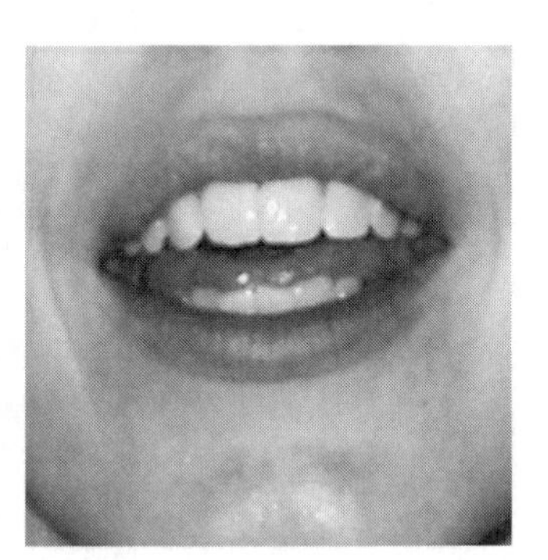

Teach this consonant blend after teaching the /d-/ and /l/ sounds. Begin saying this blend as a syllable, with the /ə/ vowel (unstressed /ʌ/ vowel) between the /d-/ and /l/. Say /dəl/ faster and faster, until it becomes /dl/. This blend is indicated by a single Lissajous pattern, paper strip movement, or meter needle movement.

Prosodic Drill

idlidlidl idl**idl**idl idlidl**idl**

idlidlidlidl idl**idl**idlidl idlidl**idl**idl

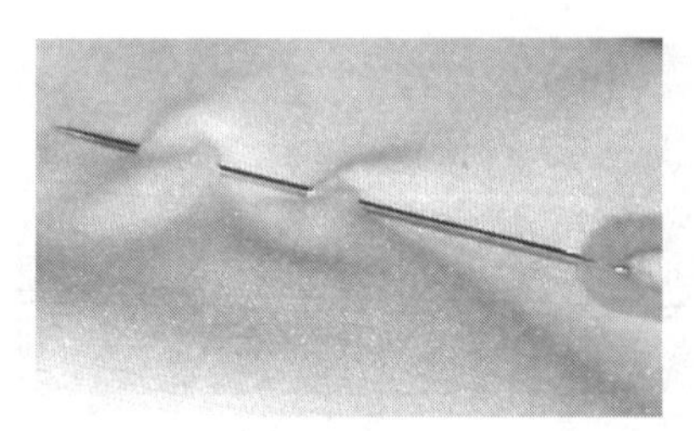

needle

Sew with a ________.

piddle pedal saddle puddle

poodle modal waddle tidal

Lesson 104 /-dz/

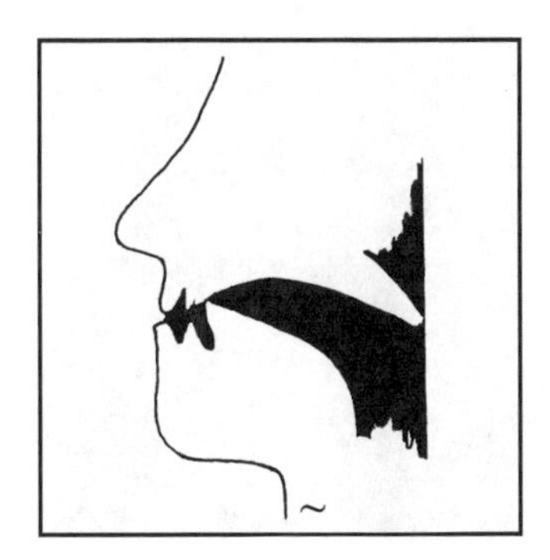
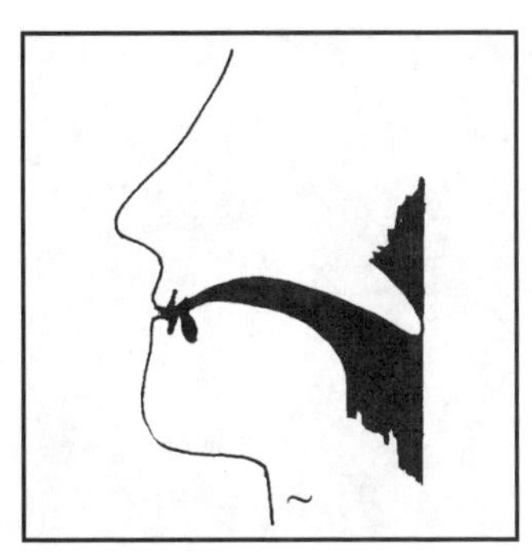
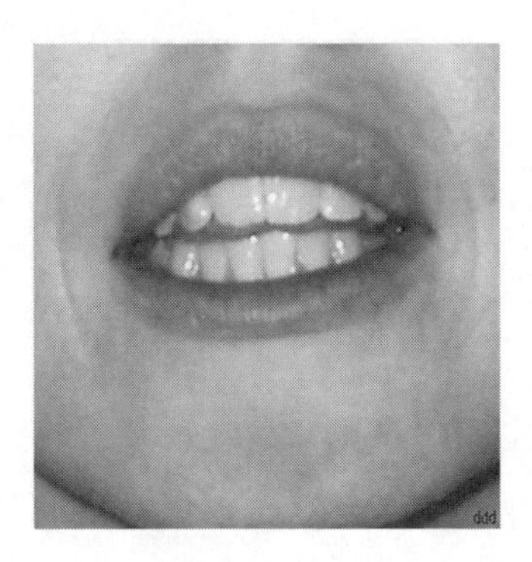
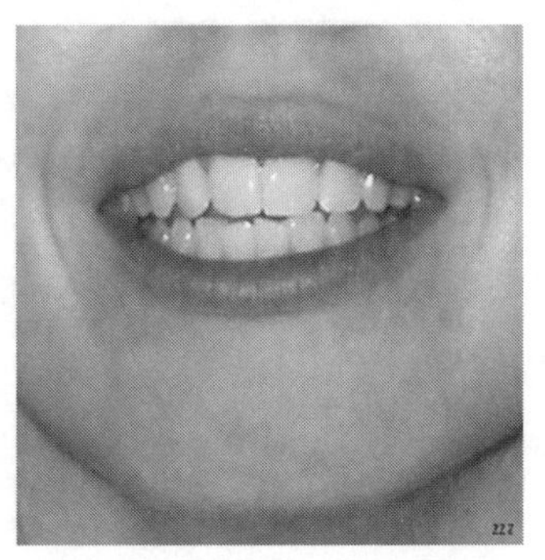

Teach this consonant blend after teaching the /-d/ and /z/ sounds. Momentarily dam up air behind the tongue tip raised to the alveolar ridge. Then, say the /z/. Repeat this procedure until the /-dz/ occurs. This voiced stop-fricative blend is indicated by a single Lissajous pattern, paper strip movement, or meter needle movement.

Prosodic Drill

idzidzidz idz**idz**idz idzidz**idz**

idzidzidzidz idz**idz**idzidz idzidz**idz**idz

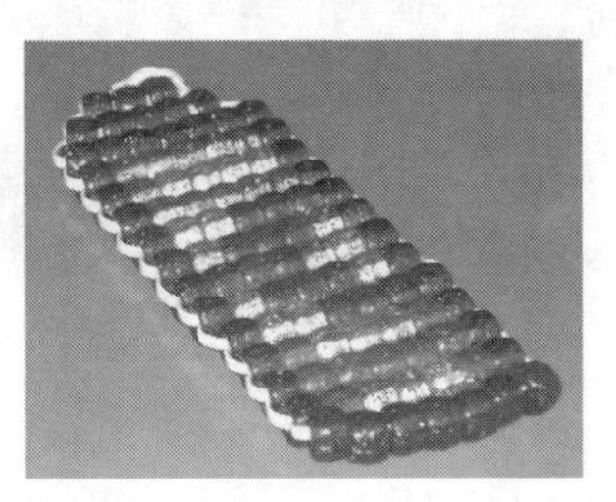

beads

String the ________.

seeds lids heads maids pads buds birds

moods toads suds hides

Lesson 105 /-ps/

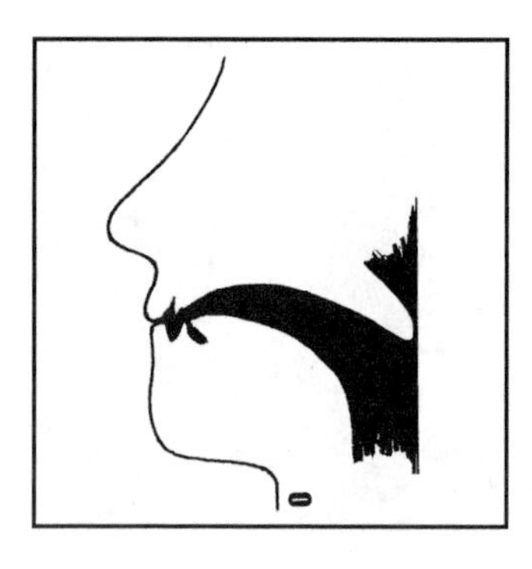
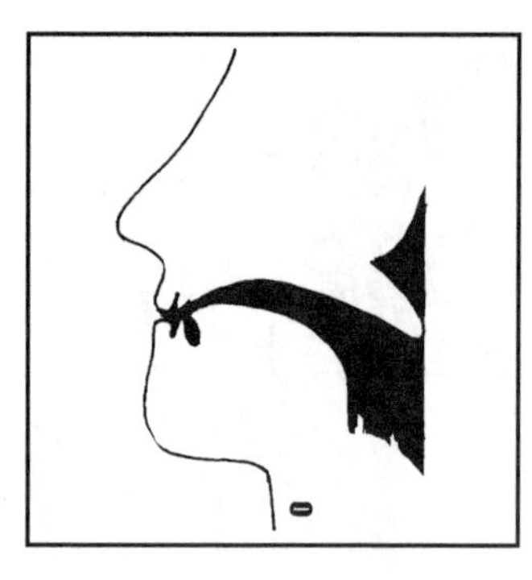
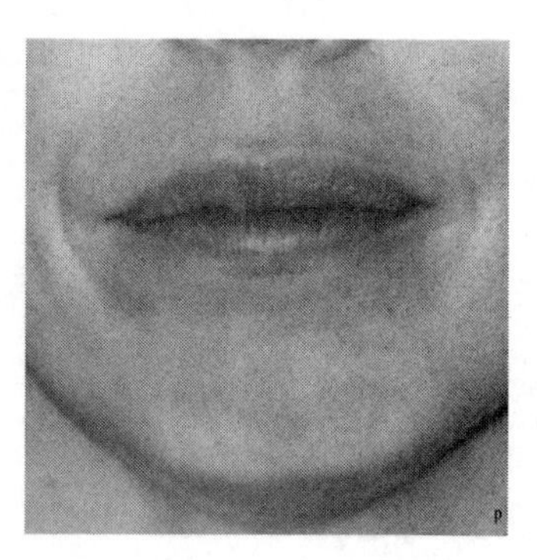
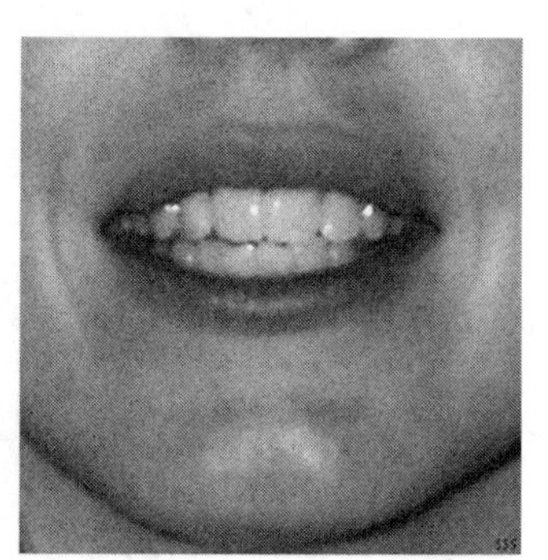

Teach this consonant blend after teaching the /p-/ and /s/ sounds. Momentarily dam air behind the shut lips. Then, say the /s/. Repeat this procedure until the /-ps/ occurs. This voiceless stop-fricative blend is indicated by a single Lissajous pattern, paper strip movement, or meter needle movement.

Prosodic Drill

opsopsops ops**ops**ops opsops**ops**

opsopsopsops ops**ops**opsops opsops**ops**ops

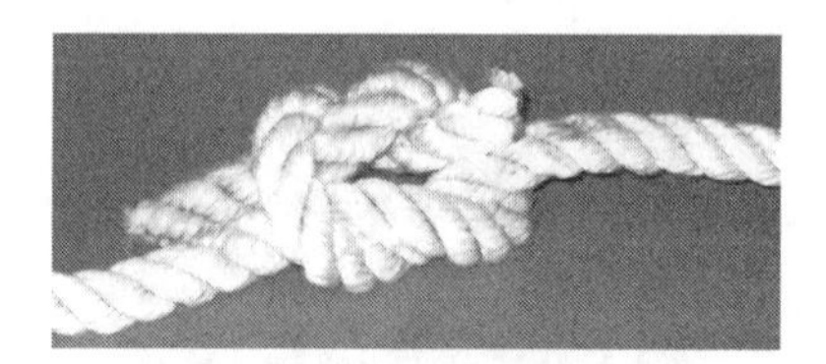

ropes

Tie the ________.

peeps hips reps shapes chaps cups

burps loops lopes mops pipes

Lesson 106 /-tl/

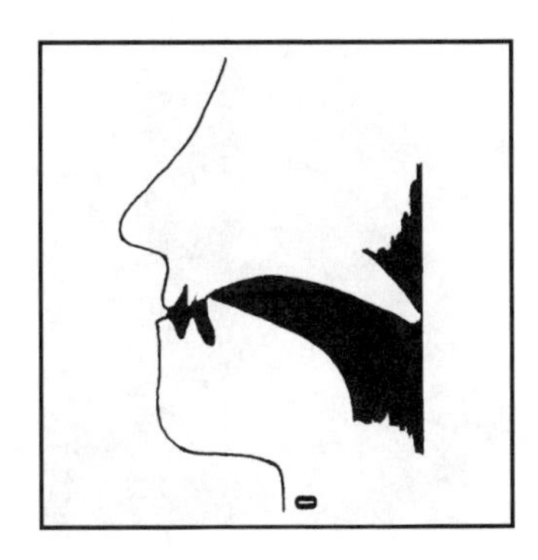

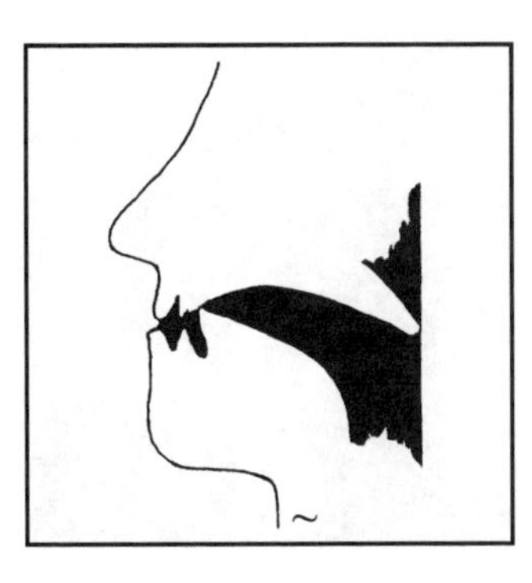

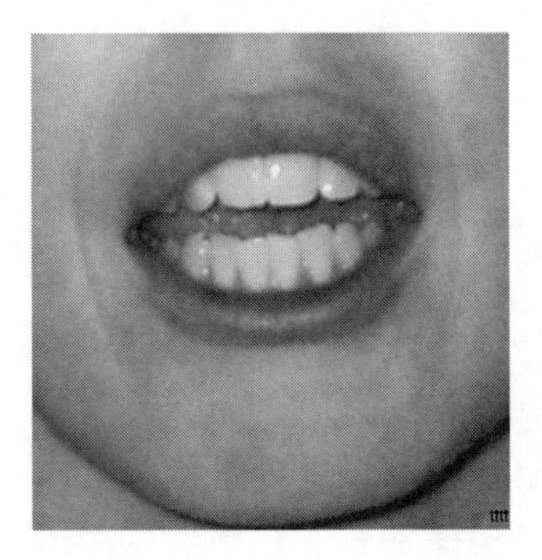

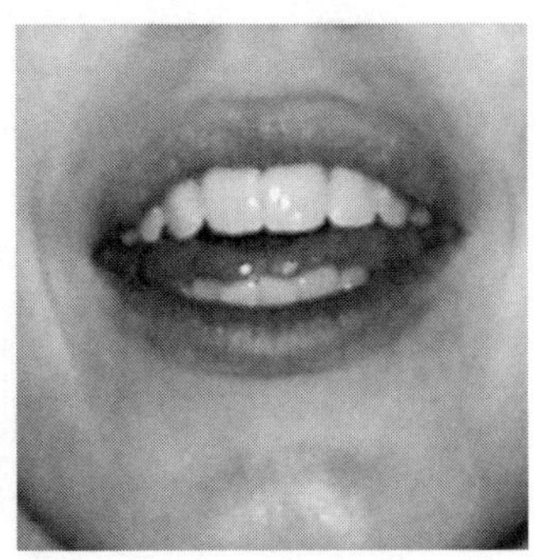

Teach this consonant blend after teaching the /t/ and /l/. Momentarily dam air behind the tongue tip raised to the alveolar ridge. Then, say the /l/. Repeat this procedure until /-tl/ occurs. This voiceless-voiced, stop-lateral glide blend is indicated by a single Lissajous pattern, paper strip movement, or meter needle movement.

Prosodic Drill

atlatlatl atl**atl**atl atlatl**atl**

atlatlatlatl atl**atl**atlatl atlatl**atl**atl

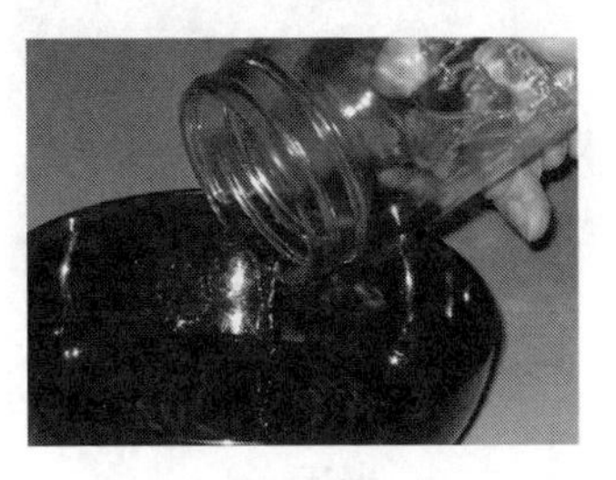

bottle

Empty the ________.

beetle petal rattle

turtle total title

Lesson 107 /-tn/

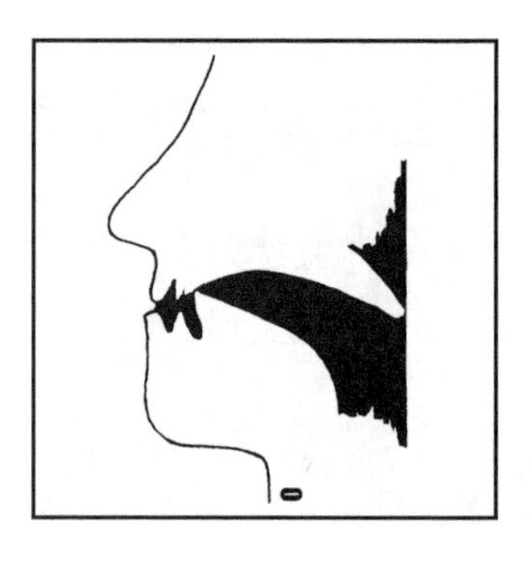
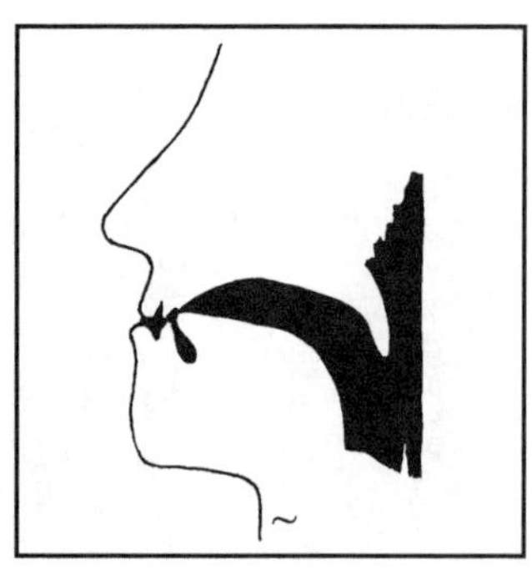
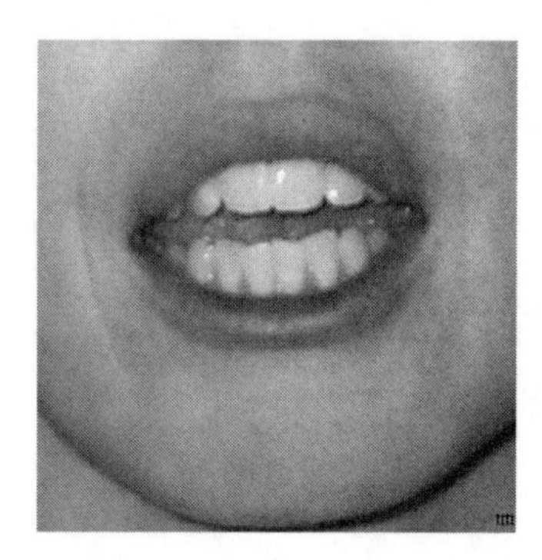
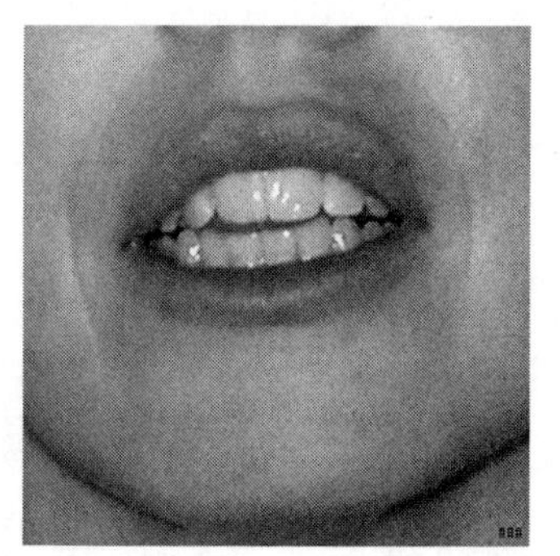

Teach this consonant blend after teaching the /t-/ and /n/. Begin saying this blend as a syllable, with the /ə/ between the /t-/ and /n/. Say /tən/ faster and faster, until it becomes /tn/. This blend is indicated by a single Lissajous pattern, paper strip movement, or meter needle movement.

Prosodic Drill

ɪtnɪtnɪtn ɪtn**ɪtn**ɪtn ɪtnɪtn**ɪtn**

ɪtnɪtnɪtnɪtn ɪtn**ɪtn**ɪtnɪtn ɪtnɪtn**ɪtn**ɪtn

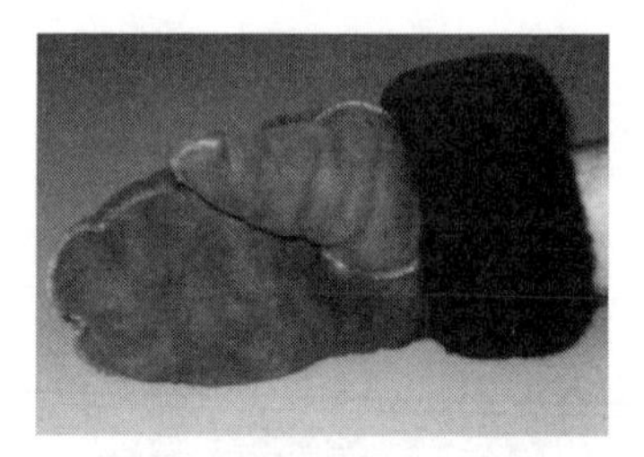

mitten

Slip on the ________.

beaten bitten batten curtain

lighten cotton brighten

Lesson 108 /-ts/

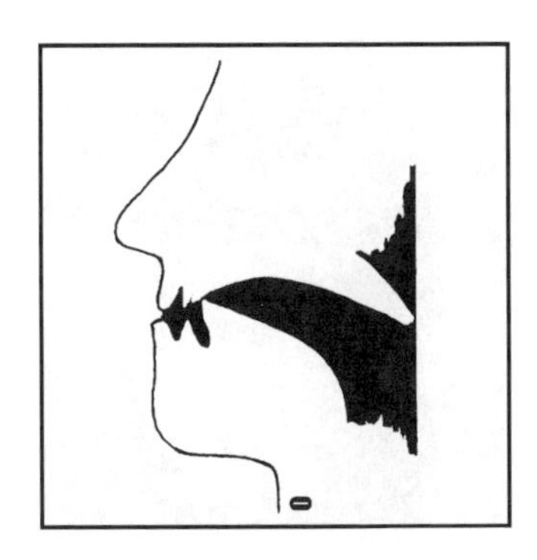

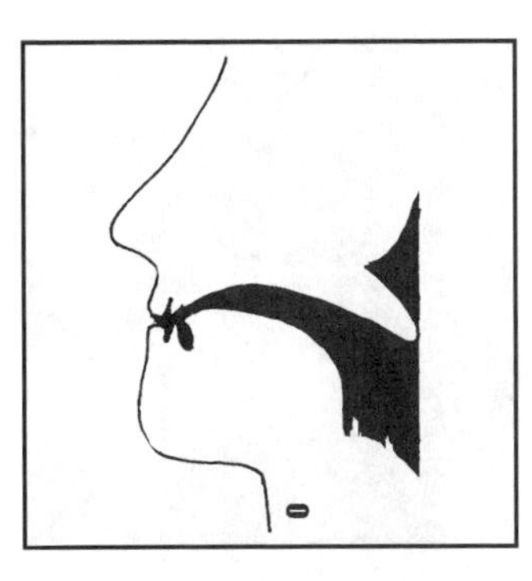

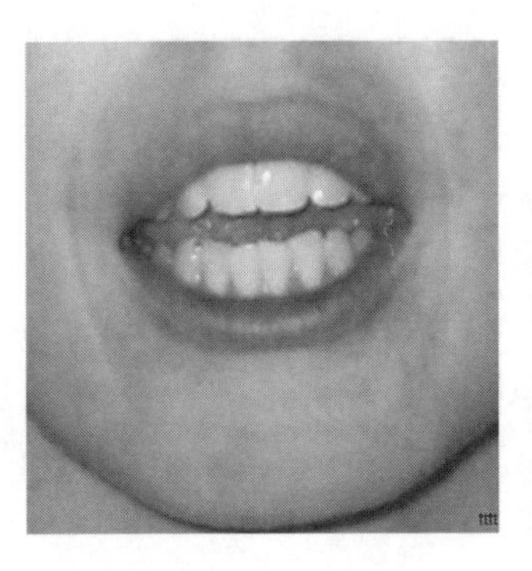

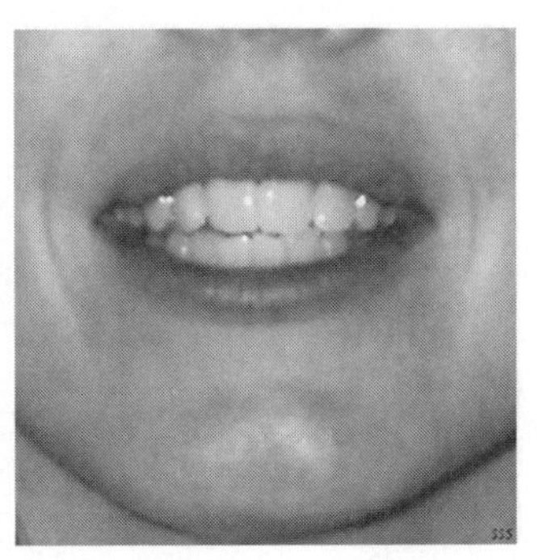

Teach this consonant blend after teaching the /t-/ and /s/. Momentarily dam air behind the tongue raised to the alveolar ridge. Then, say the /s/. Repeat this procedure until the /-ts/ occurs. This voiceless stop-fricative blend is indicated by a single Lissajous pattern, paper strip movement, or meter needle movement.

Prosodic Drill

otsotsots ots**ots**ots otsots**ots**

otsotsotsotsots ots**ots**otsots otsots**ots**ots

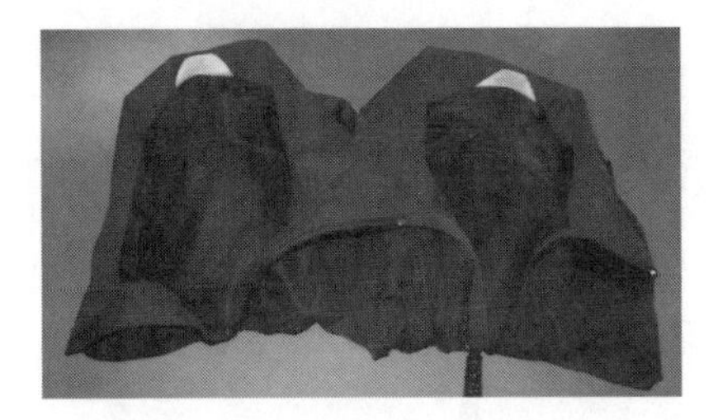

coats

Here are two ________.

beets pits nets bats shirts fights

toots boats cots shouts sights

Lesson 109 /-kt/

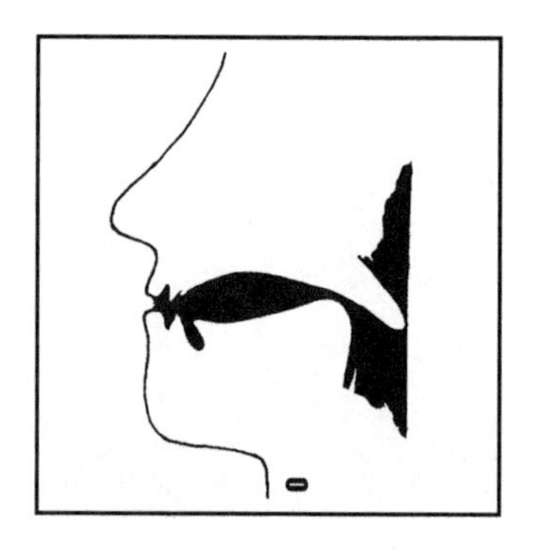
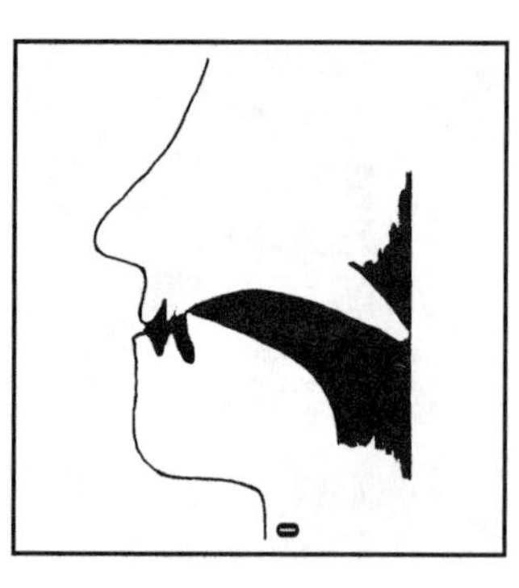
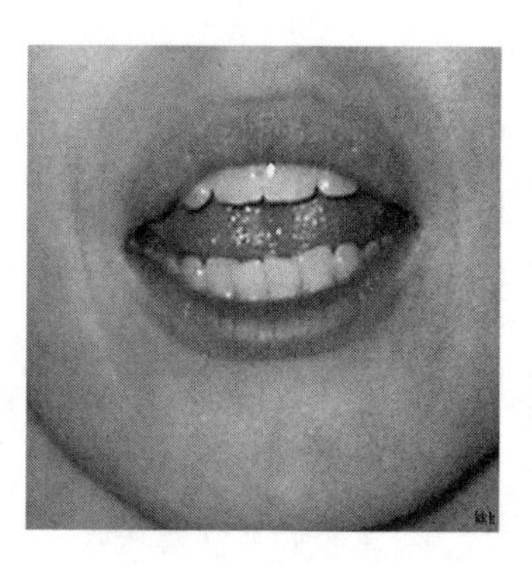
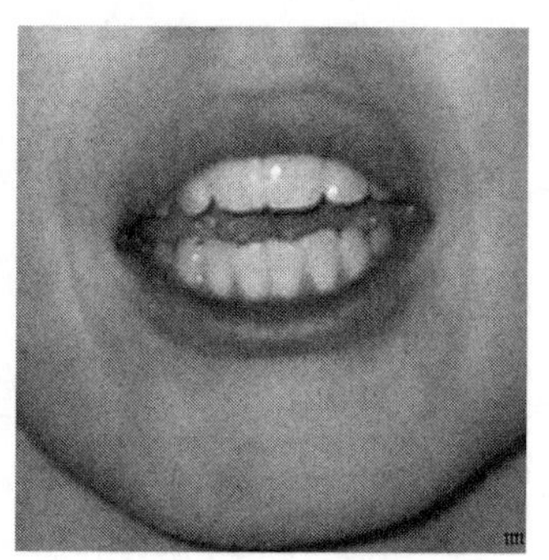

Teach this consonant blend after teaching the /k-/ and /-t/. Momentarily dam air behind the back of tongue raised to the velum. Then, say the /-t/. Repeat this procedure until the /-kt/ occurs. This voiceless stop-stop blend is indicated by a single Lissajous pattern, paper strip movement, or meter needle movement.

Prosodic Drill

æktæktækt æk**tækt**ækt æktækt**ækt**

æktæktæktækt ækt**ækt**æktækt æktæk**ækt**ækt

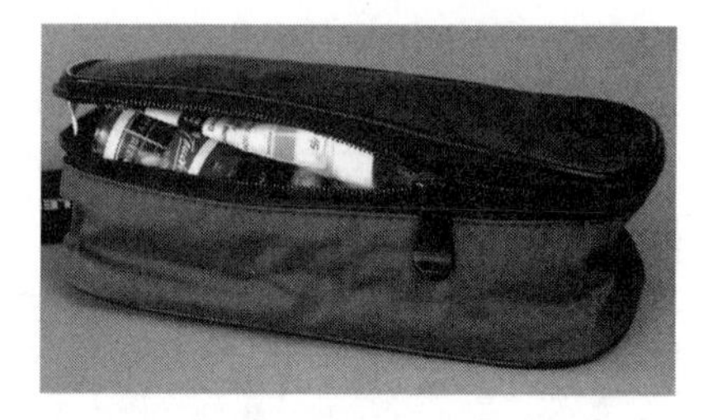

packed

The case is ________.

peeked kicked wrecked baked sacked ducked

lurked nuked poked locked hiked

Lesson 110 /-pt/

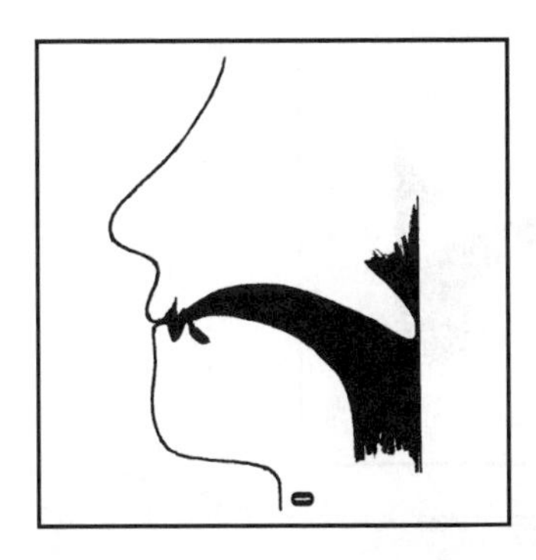
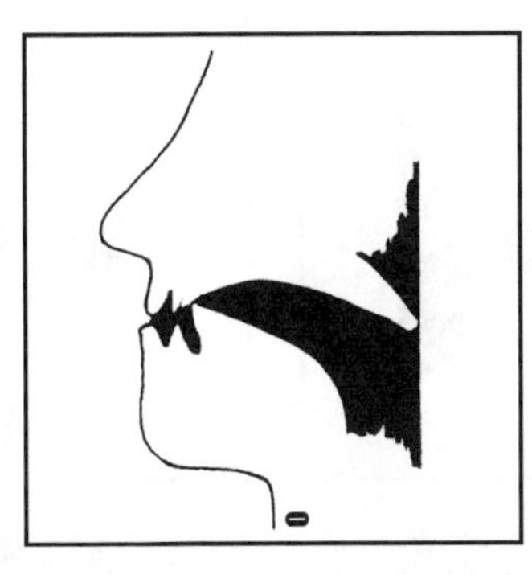
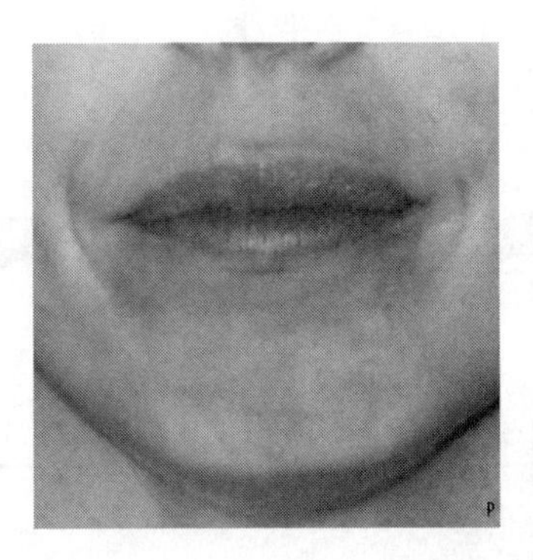
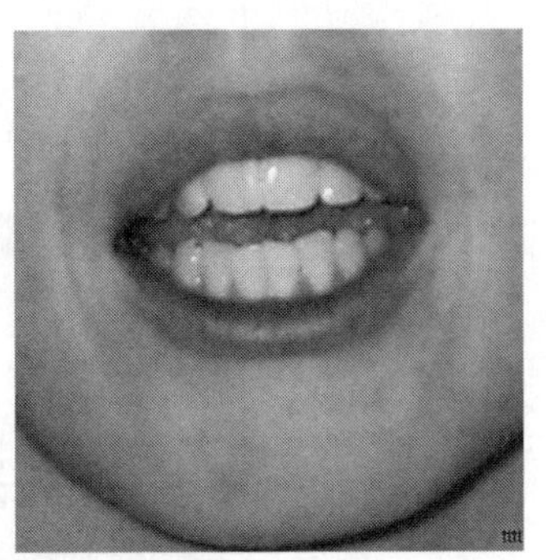

Teach this consonant blend after teaching the /p-/ and /-t/. Momentarily dam air behind shut lips. Then, say the /-t/. Repeat this procedure until the /-pt/ occurs. This voiceless stop-stop blend is indicated by a single Lissajous pattern, paper strip movement, or meter needle movement.

Prosodic Drill

epteptept ept**ept**ept eptept**ept**

eptepteptept ept**ept**eptept eptept**ept**ept

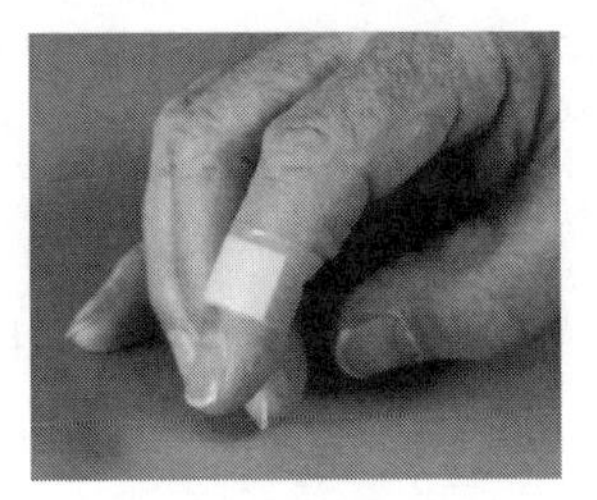

taped

The finger is ________.

leaped nipped kept mapped cupped burped

cooped doped mopped piped

Lesson 111 /-nts/

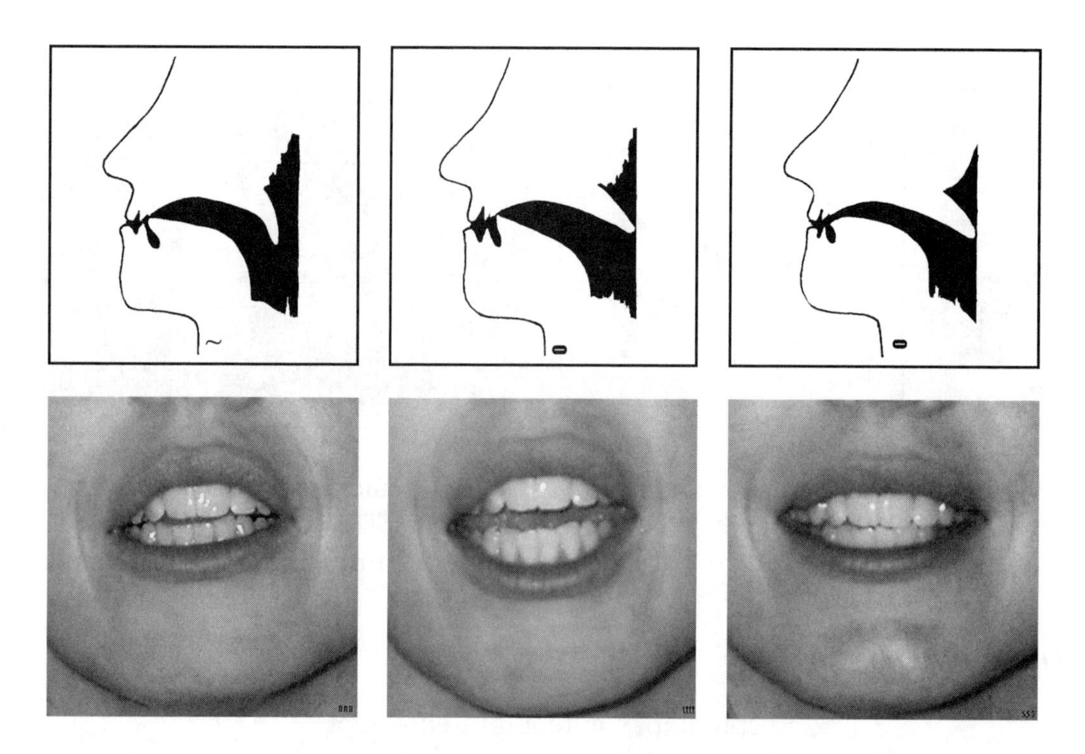

Teach this consonant blend after teaching the /n/, /t/, and /s/. Momentarily drop the velum and dam up air behind the tongue tip raised to the alveolar ridge. Immediately afterwards, say the /s/. Repeat this procedure until the /-nts/ occurs. This voiced nasal-stop-fricative blend is indicated by a single complex Lissajous pattern, paper strip movement, or meter needle movement.

Prosodic Drill

ɔɪntsɔɪntsɔɪnts   ɔɪnts**ɔɪnts**ɔɪnts   ɔɪntsɔɪnts**ɔɪnts**

ɔɪntsɔɪntsɔɪnts   ɔɪnts**ɔɪnts**ɔɪnts   ɔɪntsɔɪnts**ɔɪnts**ɔɪnts

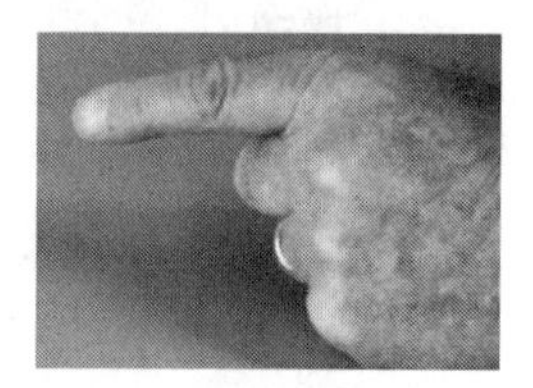

points

The finger ________.

dents   ants   bunts   currents

haunts   mounts   pints

Lesson 112 /-tnz/

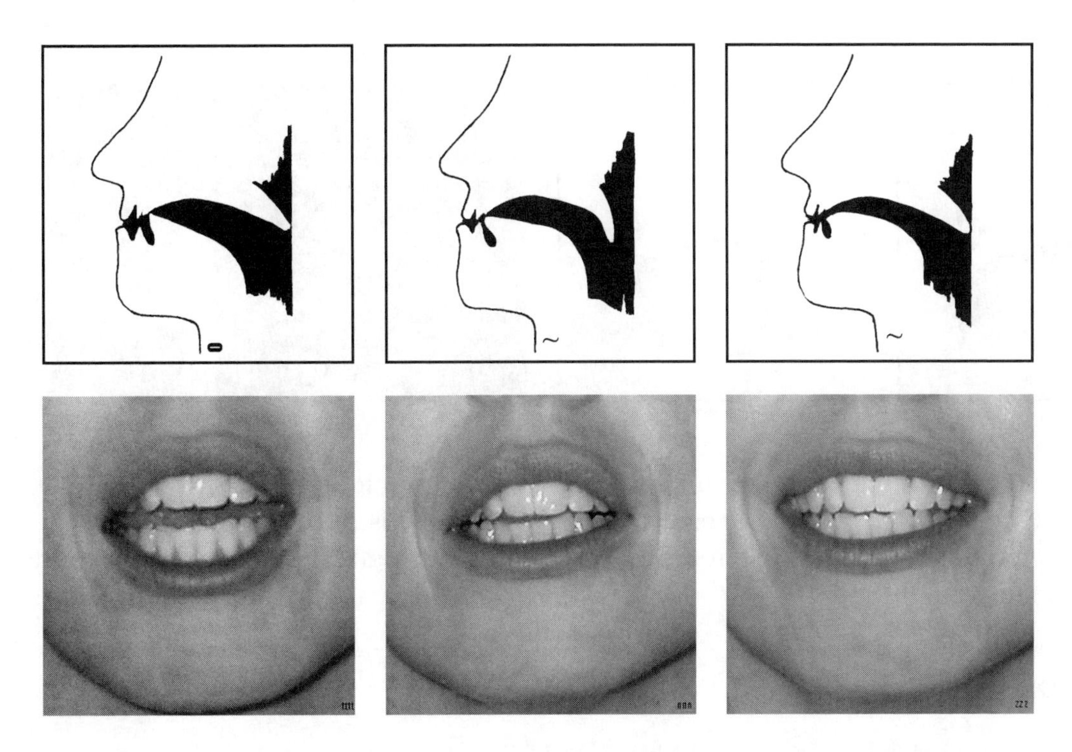

Teach this consonant blend after teaching the /t-/ sound and /-nz/ blend. Initially insert a /ə/ between the /t/ and /-nz/. Say /tənz/ repeatedly, faster and faster, until /-tnz/ occurs. The /-tnz/ blend is indicated by a single complex Lissajous pattern, paper strip movement, or meter needle movement.

Prosodic Drill

ɪtnzɪtnzɪtnz ɪtnz**ɪtnz**ɪtnz ɪntzɪtnz**ɪtnz**

ɪtnzɪtnzɪtnzɪtnz ɪtnz**ɪtnz**ɪtnzɪtnz ɪtnzɪtnz**ɪtnz**ɪtnz

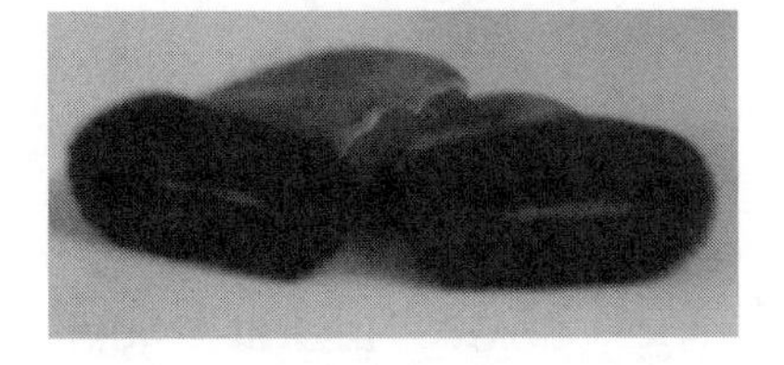

mittens

There are two ________.

kittens battens fattens buttons

cottons brightens lightens

Lesson 113 /-kl/

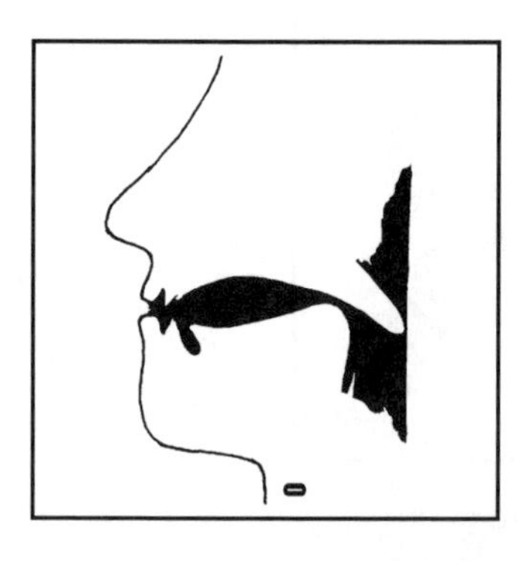
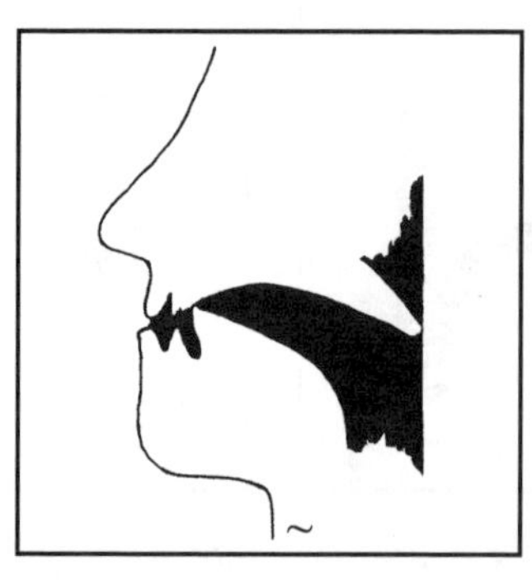
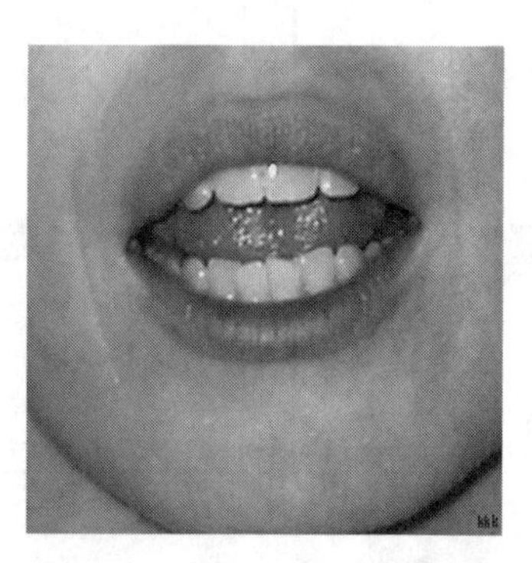
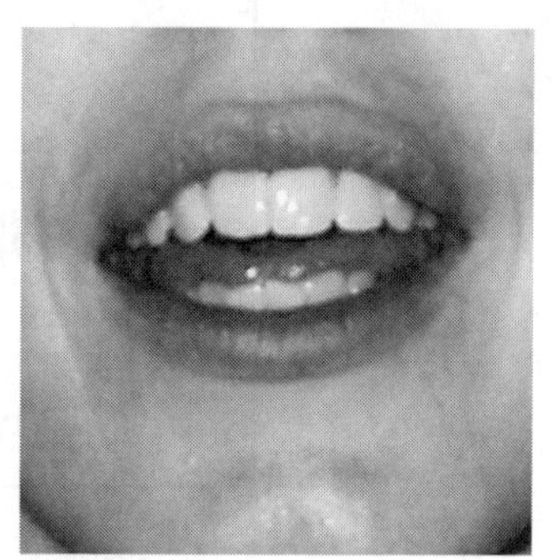

Teach this consonant blend after teaching the /-k/ and /-l/. Momentarily dam up air behind the back of the tongue raised to the velum. Then, say the /-l/. Repeat this procedure until the /-kl/ occurs. This stop-lateral glide blend is indicated by a single Lissajous pattern, paper strip movement, or meter needle movement.

Prosodic Drill

ɪklɪklɪkl ɪkl**ɪkl**ɪkl ɪklɪkl**ɪkl**

ɪklɪklɪklɪkl ɪkl**ɪkl**ɪklɪkl ɪklɪkl**ɪkl**ɪkl

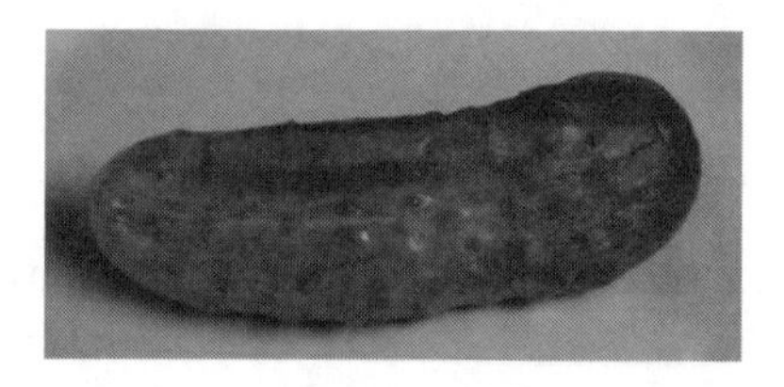

pickle

Eat the ________.

tickle fickle nickel sickle

heckle tackle cycle

Lesson 114 /-ks/

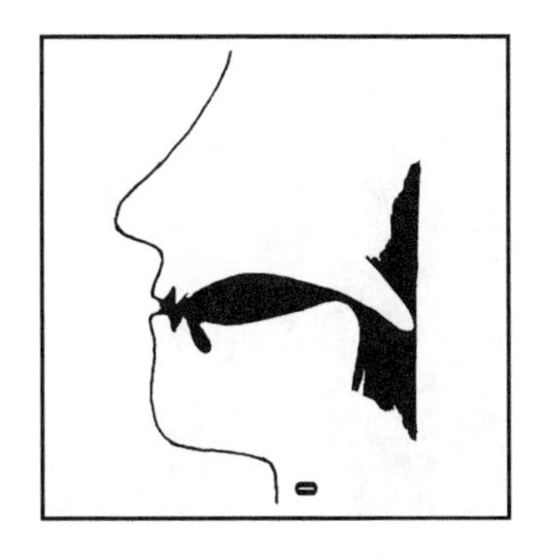
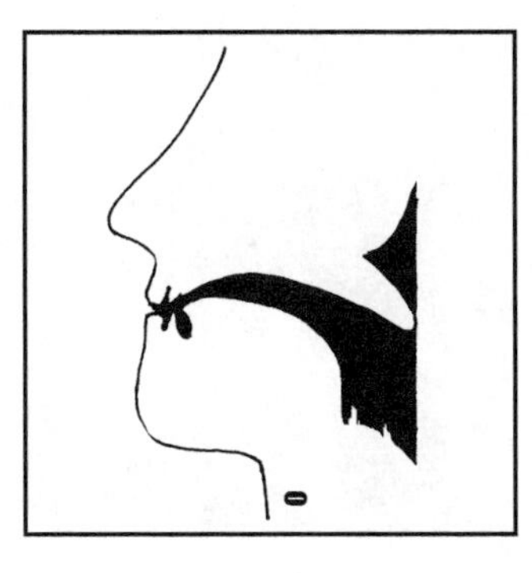
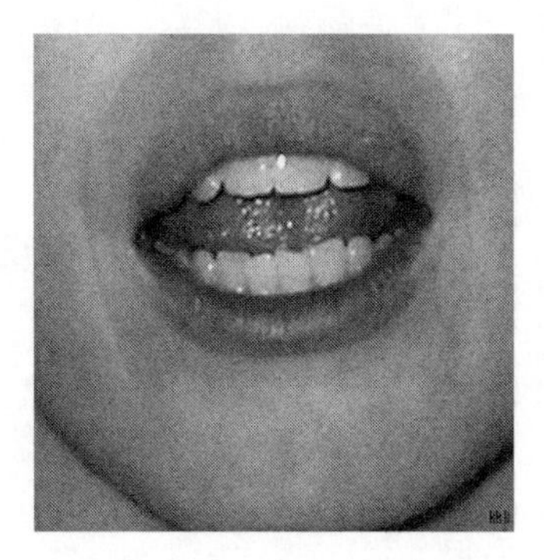
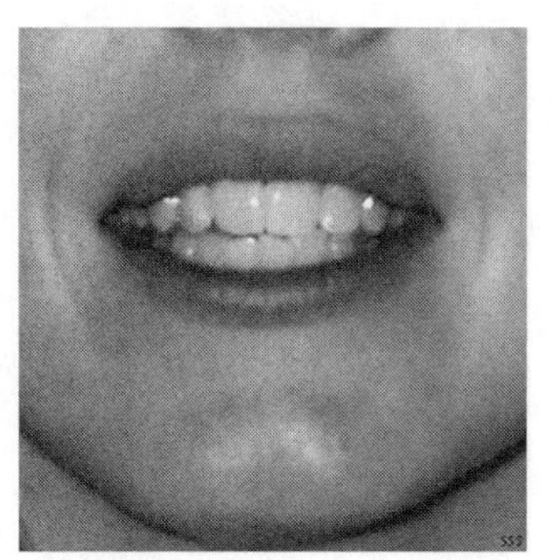

Teach this consonant blend after teaching the /-k/ and /s/. Momentarily dam air behind the back of the tongue raised to the velum. Then, say the /s/. Repeat this procedure until the /-ks/ occurs. This stop-fricative blend is indicated by a single Lissajous pattern, paper strip movement, or meter needle movement.

Prosodic Drill

aksaksaks aks**aks**aks aksaks**aks**

aksaksaksaks aks**aks**aksaks aksaks**aks**aks

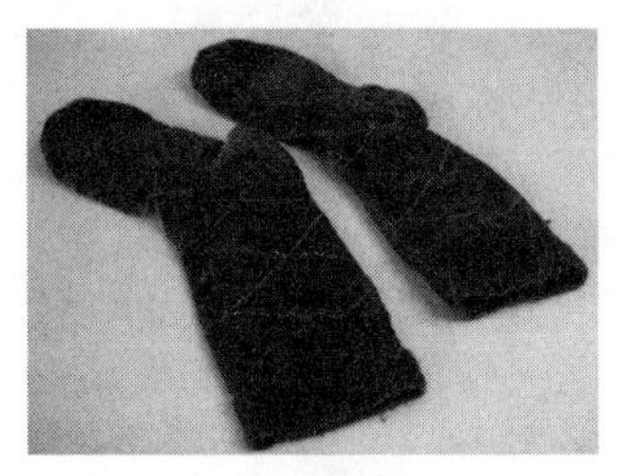

socks

Put on two ________.

peaks ticks takes pecks backs ducks perks

gooks pokes locks lurks bikes

Lesson 115 /-pl/

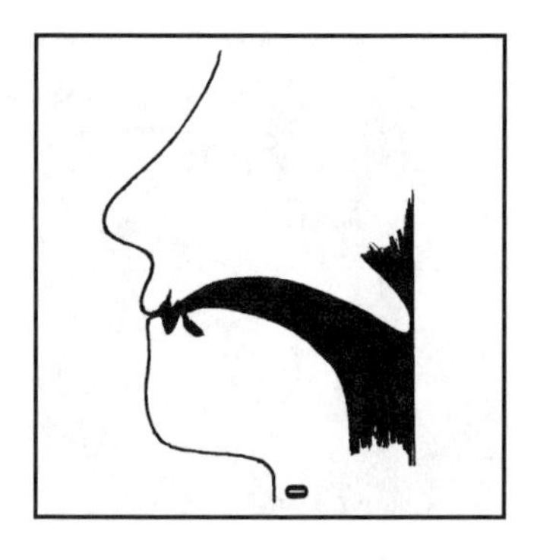
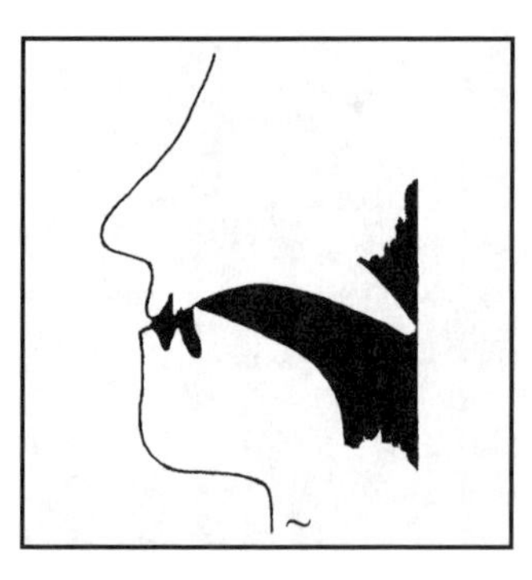
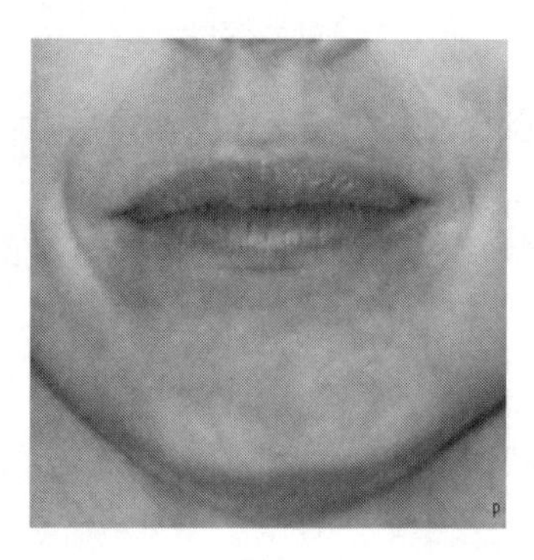
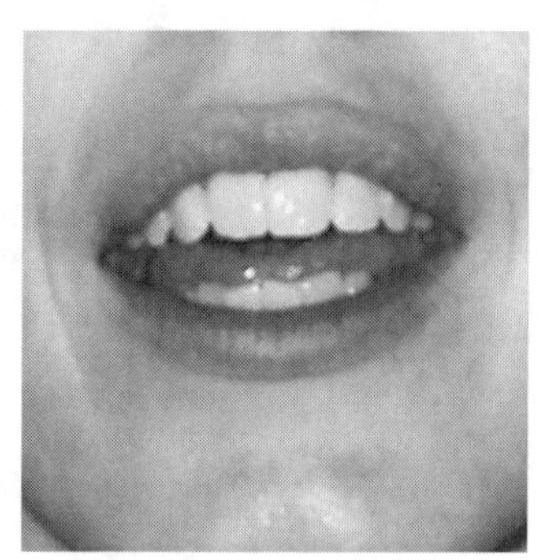

Teach this consonant blend after teaching the /-p/ and /-l/. Momentarily dam air behind closed lips. Then, say the /-l/. Repeat this procedure until the /-pl/ occurs. This stop-lateral glide blend is indicated by a single Lissajous pattern, paper strip movement, or meter needle movement.

Prosodic Drill

æplæplæpl æpl**æpl**æpl æplæpl**æpl**

æplæplæplæpl æpl**æpl**æplæpl æplæpl**æpl**æpl

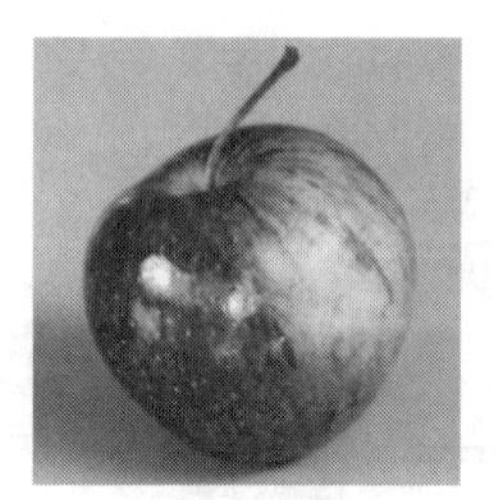

apple

Eat the ________.

people ripple maple chapel couple purple

opal disciple multiple

Lesson 116 /-fts/

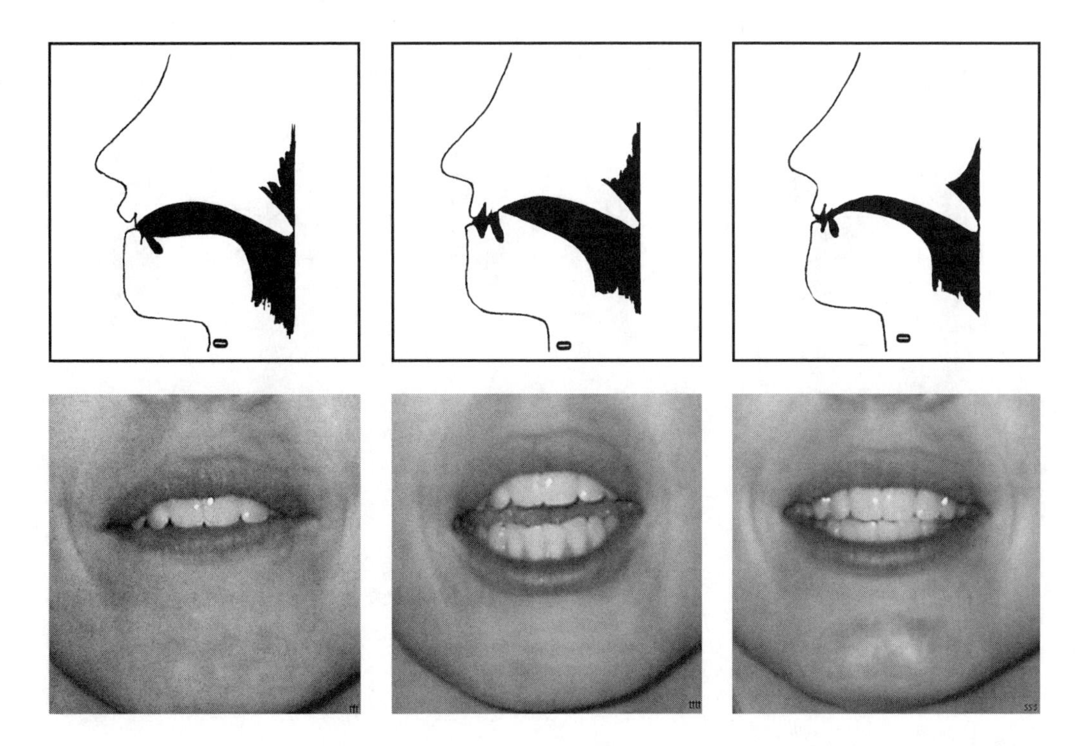

Teach this consonant blend after teaching the /f/, /t/, and /s/ sounds and the /-ft/ and /-ts/ blends. The /-fts/ is a fricative-stop-fricative blend. Say the /-ft/ and /s/ successively, faster and faster, until the /-fts/ occurs. It is indicated by a succession of Lissajous patterns, paper strip movements, and meter needle movements.

Prosodic Drill

ɪftsɪftsɪfts ɪfts**ɪfts**ɪfts ɪftsɪfts**ɪfts**

ɪftsɪftsɪftsɪfts ɪfts**ɪfts**ɪftsɪfts ɪftsɪfts**ɪfts**ɪfts

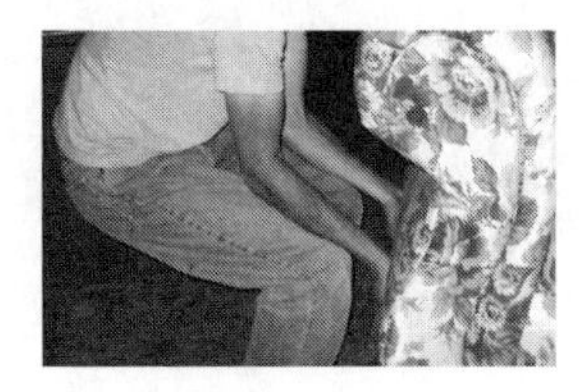

lifts

The man ________.

sifts rifts shifts drifts

rafts drafts lofts

Lesson 117 /-plz/

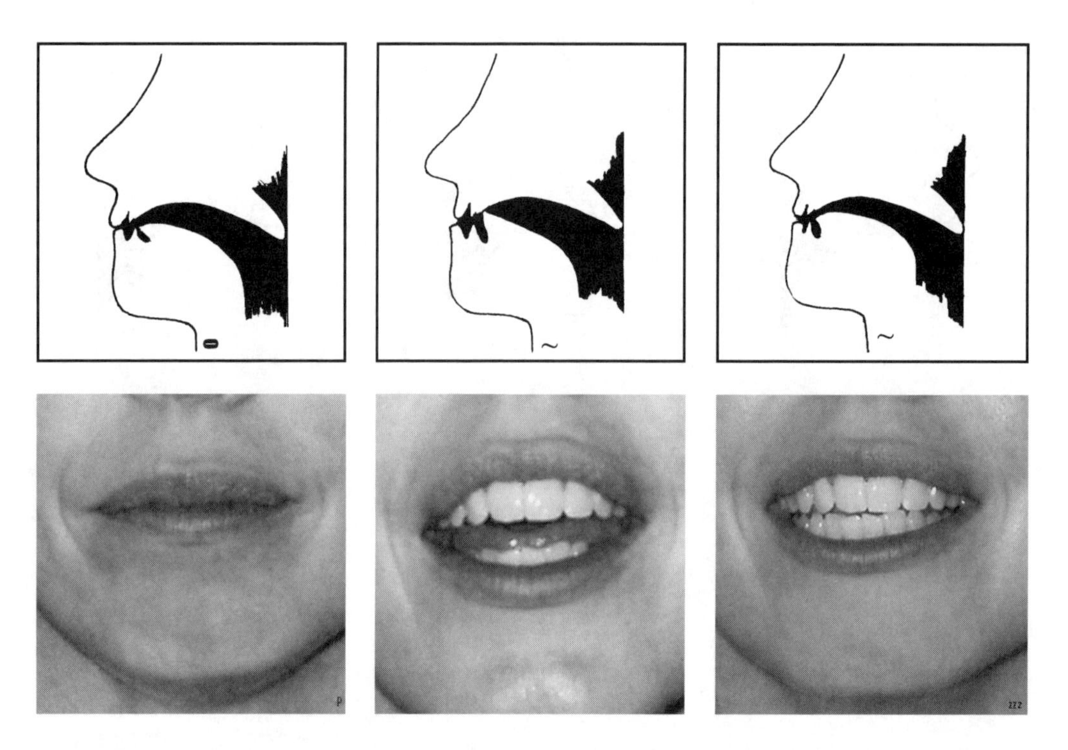

Teach this consonant blend after teaching the /-p/, /-l/, and /-z/ sounds and the /-pl/ blend. Say /-pl/ and /-z/ successively, faster and faster, until /-plz/ occurs. It is a stop-lateral glide-fricative blend. It is indicated by a single Lissajous pattern, paper strip movement, and meter needle movement.

Prosodic Drill

æplzæplzæplz æplz**æplz**æplz æplzæplz**æplz**

æplzæplzæplzæplz æplz**æplz**æplzæplz æplzæplz**æplz**æplz

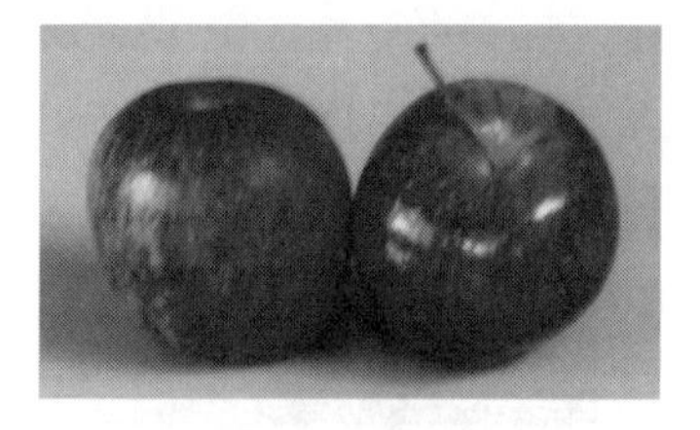

apples

There are two ________.

peoples nipples maples chapels couples purples

opals disciples multiples

Appendix

Incidental Learning of Speech

The emergence of speech in a young hearing child occurs naturally, through thousands of incidental situations he or she experiences. Osmond Crosby, father of a deaf child, described in his journal the emergence of speech in his deaf girl. "Dorothy Jane has finally started to communicate constantly, usually with Cued Speech (CS). We understand almost none of it until we replay it a few times. . . . " Her teacher also reported: "Lots of vocalizations all morning, easy to stimulate."

Suggestions of what parents can do to initiate speech and spoken language growth with their young deaf child through CS are given below.

1. Use many natural situations in the home, such as dressing, eating, and bathing, to cue and talk to the child.
2. Make use of each occasion when you have the child's attention to cue and say something of interest to him or her, including the names of family members and animals and objects of interest. Put each name in a sentence, e.g., *He is John. She is Mary.* etc., emphasizing them through gesture and facial expression.
3. Practice cueing words and sentences young hearing children use. Don't try to cue and talk fast. Your child will appreciate slow cues and speech. Concentrate on accuracy and coordinate the cues with your speaking. Use a mirror to monitor yourself.
4. Cue everything you naturally would say to a hearing child, even when your deaf child is not looking at you. That will give you the practice you need to become an accurate and fluent cuer without thinking about how to cue what you say.
5. Use props to contrive games, e.g., roll the ball and peek-a-boo, that hold the child's attention while you cue and say these simple sentences.
6. It will limit speech and language growth if you just cue and say words your child already knows.
7. Cue when you talk to other members of the family, especially your spouse.
8. Show consistent approval, enthusiasm, and affection for the child. Do not become frustrated.
9. Have faith in your progress and that of your child. Don't compare yourself or your child with others.
10. Keep a working list of words, phrases, and sentences that you have introduced to your child in a small notebook. This language should be used several times a day so it becomes a part of the child's permanent vocabulary. Even though a child will learn some words in a single exposure, repetition in meaningful situations is the key to speech and language growth.
11. In the same book, keep a comprehensive list of words, phrases, and sentences you are sure your child knows. This will give the child a sense of accomplishment, and document his or her impressions of what is happening and motivate the child to great achievement.
12. Check all entries that have become a part of the child's permanent speech and language so they do not have to reviewed any more.
13. Once the child knows the meaning of several hundred words, you can teach him additional vocabulary, sentence constructions, and concepts more rapidly.
14. Develop a scrapbook that includes magazine pictures of objects, photos of people, and

activities familiar to the child. Go through the scrapbook with the child and cue and talk about the pictures. Watch the child carefully to determine which pictures he or she wants to talk about on a given day. Repeat things of most interest. Say such things as: "I see a house. What do you see? I see something red. What is it?"

15. Develop another scrapbook that depicts experiences in the life of the child. An experience book helps a child develop sequencing skills, retention, and an importance of self. The child can show the experience book to others, relive the experiences, recall everything learned, and ask parents questions about what he or she does not understand.
16. Use a giant calendar to further develop vocabulary and language concepts and to refine the child's perception of time. Paste pictures on it to allow the child to associate past and future events with specific days of a week, dates of a month, and months of a year. Introduce the past, present, and future tenses of verbs in connection with days, dates, or time words and phrases like *yesterday*, *today*, *tomorrow*, *the day before yesterday*, etc.
17. Purchase or make a puppet with a mouth that opens and closes, so it can whisper to the parent, and suggest what the parent should "quote" to the child. It should have ears with one or more hearing aids. It should be given a name and introduced to the child. Anyone speaking to the puppet should cue, since it cannot hear well.

The time, effort, and creativeness that parents show will have short-term and long-term benefits for both child and family. Using CS will accelerate the progress of the child with hearing loss, including his or her emergence and refinement of speech (Cornett & Daisey, 1992).

The Vocal Scope

The Vocal Scope is a highly effective electro-visual speech training aid. It is an oscilloscope with microphone input. Its linear sinusoidal display, however, has been converted to a Lissajous or radial display. This makes the complexity of the speech signal displayed easier to identify than using a sinusoidal display or a spectrographic display.

The Lissajous display results by electronically splitting the incoming sound into two equal signals, one going to the vertical plates of the cathode ray tube and the other to the horizontal plates. Before reaching the plates, the signals go through an all-pass filter network which achieves a 90 degree phase shift between them. If incoming sound is a pure tone, a circle appears on the screen rather than the usual series of sine waves. If incoming sound is a complex sound, a combination of circles appears. The various Lissajous patterns for the different speech sounds are visual correlates of these sounds. A mouth-to-microphone distance of 2 inches or even less is recommended for consonants.

1. White noises for voiceless fricatives become juxtapositioned *circles*.
2. Bursts for voiceless stops become *splashes*.
3. Formants (frequency concentrations) for voiced consonants, nasals, vowels, and diphthongs become *loops*.
4. Buzzes for voiced fricatives become *whirls* or concentrations within loops.

Additional speech applications are summarized below.

1. *Voice control* is shown by the constancy of the Lissajous pattern for a sustained sound, e.g., the /o/.
2. The *pitch* of speech is shown by the configuration of the Lissajous pattern. Vary the pitch of /o/, for example, and note the configuration change.
3. The *loudness* of speech is seen by the size of the Lissajous pattern while keeping mouth-microphone distance constant. Practice producing various sizes of patterns. Speak or sing /o/ at first, and then other sounds and selections. Keep the patterns within the dimensions of the screen.
4. The *duration* of a sound is shown by how long the pattern or series of patterns can be held on the screen. Practice holding an /o/ pattern for 5 seconds, or producing as long a speech sample or vocal music selection as possible. Record duration of sound on a single breath in seconds using a watch.

Analog Sound Level Meter

An analog (not digital) sound level meter, of very low cost, can be used not only to measure overall sound intensities in a room but to assist in the teaching of speech sounds. A 9-volt alkaline battery makes the device portable. The meter is small and lightweight. It can be hand held or attached to a tripod. It can also be calibrated. Incoming sound is changed into electricity via the microphone located on top.

The meter will measure overall sound intensities from 50 dB to 126 dB. The particular dB range depends on which of seven dial range settings (120, 110, 100, 90, 80, 70, 60) are used. When the dial is turned all the way clockwise (60 will light on the dial), the meter needle for a 50 dB sound will read at −10, and for a 66 dB sound at +6.

The meter includes an A–C weighting switch. When the switch is set at A, the meter filters out low audio frequency room noise. When the switch is set at C, the meter is more sensitive; it does not filter out low audio frequency room noise. This is reflected in its having a more flat frequency response to incoming sound. The C switch setting should be used for speech training.

The meter also has a slow-fast response switch. For shaping speech sounds, it has to be set at *fast* to be sensitive to the rapid changes in duration and intensity that take place during articulation training.

Speech training should be given in a quiet environment. The background noise should not exceed 50 dBC. This will ensure that meter needle movements are responses of speech sounds said by the therapist or child, and not someone else.

During speech training, neither the therapist nor the child should focus on reading dB levels. Instead, focus on whether the needle moves, and to what extent it moves, for a given sound. Also, remember that speech sounds vary in intensity. The loudest speech sound, the /ɑ/, for example, may be 26 dB more intense than the faintest speech sound, the /θ/.

During speech training, rotate the range dial to 60. Hold the meter so its microphone is pointing toward you or the child. Tilt it down so you and the child can see the meter needle movement. The mouth-microphone distance may be about 4 inches. It should enable the meter to pick up your speech and that of the child. You will need to move it back and forth between yourself and the child.

The meter described above is available from your local Radio Shack store. It will come with a case and an instruction book.

References

Beck, P. (1999, February). *See hear: I cue.* Rochester, NY: National Cued Speech Association.

Berg, F. (1970). Language development. In F. Berg & S. Fletcher (Eds.), *The hard of hearing child* (pp. 111-124). New York: Grune & Stratton.

Berg, F. (1976). *Educational audiology: Hearing and speech management*. New York: Grune & Stratton.

Berg, F. (1987). *Facilitating classroom listening: A handbook for teachers of normal and hard of hearing students* (pp. 39-61). Austin, TX: Pro-Ed.

Berg, F. (2000). *Literacy and speech for the young deaf child.* Cleveland, OH: Cued Speech Discovery, National Cued Speech Association.

Berg, F. (2001). Educational management of children who are hearing impaired. In R. Hull (Ed.), *Aural rehabilitation serving children and adults* (pp. 169-184). San Diego, CA: Singular Thompson Learning.

Berg, F., & Berg, E. (1999). *Targeting speech articulation*. LDS Charities, USA/Ali Yavar Jung National Institute for the Hearing Handicapped.

Berlin, C. (1995). Encourages audiologists at the American Academy of Audiology convention to recommend Cued Speech. Cleveland, OH: National Cued Speech Association.

Borden, G., & Harris, K. (1984). *Speech science primer.* Baltimore: Williams & Wilkins.

Bowe, C. (1985). Memory issues in speech planning and production. In J. Lauter (Ed.), *Proceedings of the Conference on the Planning and Production of Speech in Normal and Hearing Impaired Individuals* (pp. 61-69). Washington, DC: ASHA Reports 15.

Cornett, O., & Daisey, M. (1992). *The Cued Speech resource book for parents of deaf children.* Raleigh, NC: National Cued Speech Association.

Geers, A., & Moog, J. (1994). Spoken language results: Vocabulary, syntax, and communication. The Sensory Aids Study at Central Institute for the Deaf. *The Volta Review, 96*, 131-148.

Hirsh, I. (1985). Conference summary. In J. Lauter (Ed.), *Proceedings of the Conference on the Planning and Production of Speech in Normal and Hearing Impaired Individuals* (pp. 79-80). Washington, DC: ASHA Reports 15.

Kent, R. (1985). Developing and disordered speech: Strategies for organization. In J. Lauter (Ed.), *Proceedings of the Conference on the Planning and Production of Speech in Normal and Hearing Impaired Individuals* (pp. 29-37). Washington, DC: ASHA Reports 15.

Lauter, J. (1985). Respiratory function in speech production by normally hearing and hearing-impaired talkers: A review. In J. Lauter (Ed.), *Proceedings of the Conference on the Planning and Production of Speech in Normal and Hearing Impaired Individuals* (pp. 58-60). Washington, DC: ASHA Reports 15.

Ling, D. (1976). *Speech and the hearing-impaired child.* Washington, DC: Alexander Graham Bell Association for the Deaf.

MacNeilage, P., Studdert-Kennedy, M., & Lindblom, B. (1985). Planning and production of speech: An overview. In J. Lauter (Ed.), *Proceedings of the Conference on the Planning and Production of Speech in Normal and Hearing Impaired Individuals* (pp. 15-21). Washington, DC: ASHA Reports 15.

Merrill, E. (1992). Forward. In O. Cornett & M. Daisey (Eds.), *The Cued Speech resource handbook for parents of deaf children* (pp. vii-viii). Raleigh, NC: National Cued Speech Association.

Picket, J. (1980). *The sounds of speech communication: A primer of acoustic phonetics and speech perception.* Baltimore: University Park Press.

Pronovost, W., Yenkin, L., Anderson, D., & Lerner, R. (1968). The voice visualizer. *American Annals of the Deaf, 113*(2), 230-238.

Speech Analysis and Feedback Products. (2006). Lincoln Park, NJ: KAYPENTAX.

Stelmach, G., & Hughes, B. (1985). Attention, motor control, and automaticity. In J. Lauter (Ed.), *Proceedings of the Conference on the Planning and Production of Speech in Normal and Hearing Impaired Individuals* (pp. 22-28). Washington, DC: ASHA Reports 15.

Stevens, K. (1985). Speech production and acoustic goals. In J. Lauter (Ed.), *Proceedings of the Conference on the Planning and Production of Speech in Normal and Hearing Impaired Individuals* (pp. 38–42). Washington, DC: ASHA Reports 15.

Templin, M. (1957). *Certain language skills in children*. (Institute of Child Welfare Monograph No. 26). Minneapolis: The University of Minnesota Press.

Templin, M., & Darley, . (1960). The Templin-Darley Tests of Articulation. Iowa City: State University of Iowa, Bureau of Educational Research.

Warren, D. (1976). Aerodynamics of speech production. In N. Lass (Ed.), *Contemporary issues in experimental phonetics* (pp. 105–137). New York: Academic Press.

World Cueing Alliance. (2006). National Cued Speech Association, *On Cue*, *20*(1), 12.

Glossary

Acoustic: sound, its physical nature

Articulation: the movement and positioning of the speech organs in sound production, especially that of consonants but also vowels and diphthongs

Audition: the act or sense of hearing

Auditory Oral Method: providing speech communication through residual hearing and speechreading in contrast to providing it only through residual hearing, referred to as the auditory-verbal method

Bilateral: two ears

Bone conduction: sound delivered to the cochleae (inner ears) of a person

Central nervous system: the part of the nervous system consisting of the brain and spinal cord

Cochlea: spiral-shaped organ of the inner ear

Cochlear implant: a device that electrically stimulates an auditory nerve with processed sound to partially compensate for a nonfunctioning cochlea

Consonant: a speech sound characterized by constricted voiced or voiceless breath flow through the vocal tract

Cognitive: having to do with cognition, knowing, perceiving, sensing, or being aware

Cued Speech: the system of hand cues invented by Orin Cornett that supplements speechreading clues to enable a child with a hearing loss to recognize speech sounds and learn spoken language

Digital: classifying into numerical categories, usually in sets of two, as opposed to analog, or continuously variable

Diphthong: a speech sound that combines two vowels

Expressive language: language that can be spoken by a child

Glottal: pertaining to the glottis, the space between the vocal folds

Intonation: pitch change within a syllable or from syllable to syllable in a word, phrase, or sentence

Kinesthetic: sensation of position, movement, or tension of parts of the body, perceived through nerve end organs in muscles, tendons, and joints

Larynx: a structure of muscle and cartilage at the upper end of the windpipe, containing the vocal folds and serving as the organ of voice

Lipreading: understanding speech by watching a speaker's lips and surrounding facial, gestural, and situational clues

Lissajous: a circular electro-visual speech display that varies in shape according to changes in the frequencies of sound

Mandible: lower jaw

Microphone: device that changes sound signals into electrical signals

Motor: involving muscle movement

Oral: sound that comes through the mouth during speech

Nasal: sound that comes through the nose during speech

Notation: prosodic marks or phonetic symbols

Palatometer: a device that registers the place and pattern of tongue contact against the palate, alveolar ridge, and inner margins of the teeth, and generates spatially accurate measures of the postures and actions identified

Phonetic: speech sounds or conforming to their pronunciation or articulation

Pitch: the perception of the frequency of a pure tone or lowest frequency of a complex sound such as a speech sound

Pharynx: the throat, the cavity of the vocal tract leading from the mouth and nose to the larynx

Phoneme: the smallest distinguishing unit of speech in a language

Prelingually deaf: loss of hearing before a child ordinarily develops basic language skill or before the child ordinarily starts school

Proprioceptive: kinesthetic and tactile sensation

Prosody: the system of stress and intonation included in a spoken language, including English

Pure tone: a sound with only one frequency or vibration rate

Receptive language: spoken language that can be understood by a child

Sensory: reception of information through the senses, such as the ears and eyes

Servo control: automatic control of a response due to feedback of information from the response

Sound level meter: instrument that measures intensity of sound waves in air, consisting of a microphone, an amplifier, a frequency weighting circuit, and a meter that reads in decibels

Spectrographic: a combined display of the frequencies and intensities of speech across time

Speechreading: (see Lipreading)

Stress: accent of syllable or emphasis of word

Tactile: sense of touch from contact of the structures of the mouth, from air constriction in the vocal tract, or from vibration of the vocal folds during speech

Velopharyngeal port: a passage in the back of the mouth which is closed for oral sounds and open for nasal sounds

Velum: the soft palate (roof) of the back of the mouth, anterior to the pharynx, that can be raised to shut the velopharyngeal port or lowered to open the velopharyngeal port

Vocal folds: ligaments and supportive tissues of the larynx that may be set into vibration to produce voiced speech sounds

Vocal Scope: an oscilloscope with a microphone that has been modified to display Lissajous rather than sinusoidal (sine wave) patterns

Vocal tract: the passageway from the larynx to the front of the mouth, and (for nasal sounds) to the front of the nose, which modifies the sound produced by the larynx or within which additional sound is generated during speech

Vowel: a speech sound characterized by unconstricted voice flow through the vocal tract

Index

A

B

C

E

G

H

L

P

R

S

T

V

W